"Centering is more than just giving care to people in a group setting. It's a powerful tool for engaging people in their care and living healthier lives. The evidence from many clinical trials confirms that it improves health outcomes, lowers costs, and leads to greater patient and provider satisfaction. This important book is crucial to spreading Centering as a fundamental approach for transforming health care delivery."

Diana J. Mason, RN, PhD, FAAN
Co-Director, Center for Health, Media & Policy
New York, New York

"CenteringPregnancy provides the opportunity for the clinician to be in true partnership with the pregnant woman through prenatal care in a group setting. This book provides the evidence base for nurses, midwives, and physicians to effectively change prenatal care in the United States. It is an important resource for both practice and academic settings."

Holly Powell Kennedy, PhD, CNM, FACNM, FAAN
Helen Varney Professor of Midwifery
Yale University School of Nursing
New Haven, Connecticut

"A book describing Centering group health care will be useful as a resource to provide background for learners in a variety of fields, including nursing, medical school, and postgraduate residency training. Understanding basic components behind this evidence-based concept of group care will be an important adjunct for future providers of health care in a wide variety of fields and settings."

Douglas W. Laube, MD
Past President of ACOG and Former Chair of Council on Residency Education in
Obstetrics and Gynecology

"This book provides an excellent review of the science, theory, practice, and evidence of Centering Healthcare all in one place. We need more of this kind of transformative innovation in health care delivery to improve the health of our nation."

Michael C. Lu, MD, MS, MPH
Associate Administrator for Maternal and Child Health
Health Resources and Services Administration
U.S. Department of Health and Human Services

"CenteringPregnancy has demonstrated the far-reaching positive consequences of bringing pregnant women together in interactive groups for their pregnancy care and ongoing support following birth. A sense of empowerment and the building of community through friendship networks can have a profound effect on reducing the potential stress and social isolation of new motherhood. In identifying the principles, practicalities, and evidence associated with CenteringPregnancy, this timely book opens doors of possibility across the world for clinicians who engage with pregnant women. It is a compelling resource for all those concerned with the development of cost-effective, woman-centered maternity services."

Nicky Leap, MSc
Adjunct Professor of Midwifery, University of Technology, Sydney, Australia

"March of Dimes has funded CenteringPregnancy programs in dozens of states for over a decade. It is a proven model that has fostered better outcomes for moms and babies, including demonstrating a significantly lower premature birth rate. We wholeheartedly support implementation of CenteringPregnancy and other models of group prenatal care."

Paul Jarris, MD, MBA
Senior Vice President, Maternal-Child Health and Deputy Medical Officer
March of Dimes Foundation

"The Centering Healthcare Institute is proud to have this comprehensive reference on the Centering model available for individuals and sites to explore, implement, and sustain Centering group care. We remain committed to this evidence-based model and its power to change lives and improve outcomes for both patients and clinicians."

Angie Truesdale
Chief Executive Officer, Centering Healthcare Institute

"The Centering Healthcare model, already a dynamic influence on efforts to improve quality and outcomes, including satisfaction, will be strengthened and energized by this important new book. Two experienced midwifery clinicians and academic leaders have prepared a volume that not only serves the reproductive health care provider community but society in general. The model is receiving broadening consideration and implementation and deserves the reference material, knowledge, and guidance this book provides."

George A. Little, MD, FAAP, FACOG
Active Emeritus Professor of Pediatrics and OB/GYN
Geisel School of Medicine at Dartmouth
Hanover, New Hampshire

The CenteringPregnancy® Model

Sharon Schindler Rising, MSN, CNM, FACNM, is a certified nurse-midwife who graduated from the Yale School of Nursing, taught on the faculty there, and then established the graduate nurse-midwifery program and the Childbearing Childrearing Center at the University of Minnesota. From 1993 to 1994, she developed and piloted the CenteringPregnancy® model of group health care in Waterbury, Connecticut and began doing instructional workshops nationally and internationally. She is the founder and president emeritus of the Centering Healthcare Institute, Inc. (CHI), a nonprofit organization dedicated to improving health by transforming care through Centering groups. She has been on the clinical nursing faculty at the Yale School of Nursing and is an adjunct professor at the University of Technology, Sydney, Australia. In 2006, she was named a distinguished alumna by Yale University School of Nursing, and in 2007 she was presented with the National/International Award for Outstanding Contribution to Maternal & Child Health by the National Perinatal Association. She was awarded the Purpose Prize by Civic Ventures in December 2008, and in 2010 she won the Trout Premier Cares Award, was named an Edge Runner by the American Academy of Nursing, and received the Hattie Hemschemeyer Award from the American College of Nurse-Midwives.

Charlotte Houde Quimby, MSN, CNM, FACNM, graduated from the Yale School of Nursing, taught on the faculty, and served as chair of the department of Maternal Newborn Nursing and chief nurse-midwife at Yale New Haven Hospital. In 1997, she received the Distinguished Alumna Award for Yale University School of Nursing. She developed the nurse-midwifery service at Dartmouth Hitchcock Medical Center and was a faculty member at Dartmouth Medical School, where she continues as an adjunct faculty of Community and Family Medicine. She has worked in nursing and midwifery programs internationally for the American College of Nurse-Midwives Global Division, providing training needs assessments, training, and project evaluation in Africa and Asia. She was a Visiting Senior Associate in 1993/1994 at Emory University's Lillian Carter Center for International Nursing. She served in the New Hampshire Legislature and received the New Hampshire Nurses Association Legislator's Award for Outstanding Contribution to Nursing Legislation. She was a consultant/faculty member for the Centering Healthcare Institute, Inc. (CHI) from 2004 to 2014.

The CenteringPregnancy® Model
The Power of Group Health Care

Sharon Schindler Rising, MSN, CNM, FACNM
Charlotte Houde Quimby, MSN, CNM, FACNM

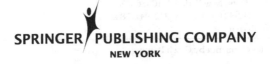
SPRINGER PUBLISHING COMPANY
NEW YORK

Springer Publishing Company, LLC
11 West 42nd Street
New York, NY 10036
www.springerpub.com

Acquisitions Editor: Elizabeth Nieginski
Composition: S4Carlisle

ISBN: 978-0-8261-3242-0
e-book ISBN: 978-0-8261-3243-7

16 17 18/5 4 3 2 1

The author and the publisher of this Work have made every effort to use sources believed to be reliable to provide information that is accurate and compatible with the standards generally accepted at the time of publication. Because medical science is continually advancing, our knowledge base continues to expand. Therefore, as new information becomes available, changes in procedures become necessary. We recommend that the reader always consult current research and specific institutional policies before performing any clinical procedure. The author and publisher shall not be liable for any special, consequential, or exemplary damages resulting, in whole or in part, from the readers' use of, or reliance on, the information contained in this book. The publisher has no responsibility for the persistence or accuracy of URLs for external or third-party Internet websites referred to in this publication and does not guarantee that any content on such websites is, or will remain, accurate or appropriate.

Library of Congress Cataloging-in-Publication Data

Names: Rising, Sharon Schindler, author. | Quimby, Charlotte Houde, author.
Title: The CenteringPregnancy model : the power of group health care / Sharon Schindler Rising, Charlotte Houde Quimby.
Description: New York : Springer Publishing Company, [2017] | CenteringPregnancy is a registered trademark. | Includes bibliographical references and index.
Identifiers: LCCN 2016040977| ISBN 9780826132420 | ISBN 9780826132437 (e-book)
Subjects: | MESH: Prenatal Care—methods | Patient-Centered Care—methods | Maternal Health Services—organization & administration | Self-Help Groups | Group Processes | Models, Organizational
Classification: LCC RG940 | NLM WQ 175 | DDC 362.1982—dc23 LC record available at https://lccn.loc .gov/2016040977

Printed in the United States of America by Gasch Printing.

This book is dedicated to the many clinicians, mothers, and families who have given and received care through the Centering Healthcare model . . .

. . . and to the clinicians, mothers, and families who informed our work over the years and made it possible for this model to give life.

It also is dedicated to our families: To Ron Rising, who has been at my side these many years and especially for his help through the conception, birth, and spread of the Centering care model and to the production of this book . . . his contribution and support continue to be enormous. To our children, Josh and Kristin, both physicians who practice in a "centering" way and who have provided a deep belief in the importance of this work. And to their spouses, Isabelle and Louis, who joined later in the process but shared their helpful insights and hope for health care reform.

To Tony Quimby for his abiding love and his belief in the importance of our work, and to my children, Bob, John, David, Judy, Beth, and Matthew Houde, their encouraging spouses, and all of our incredibly lovely grandchildren, who have cheered, inquired, supported, and helped in so many ways big and small . . . and to my dearest friends, who have been on the journey with me every step of the way.

We are hopeful that Centering Healthcare and other efforts to make relationship-centered care the standard will provide a better system of care for all of us and especially for our grandchildren.

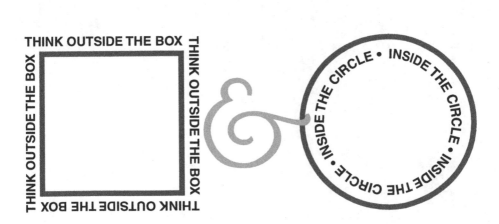

Contents

SECTION I: The CenteringPregnancy® Model

SECTION II: Centering Healthcare™: Transformative Change

SECTION III: The Centering Healthcare™ Model: Making Change Sustainable

Contributors

Sally H. Adams, PhD, RN Specialist, Division of Adolescent and Young Adult Medicine, Department of Pediatrics, University of California, San Francisco

Nancy Bardacke, CNM, MA Director, Mindfulness-Based Childbirth and Parenting (MBCP) Program, University of California, San Francisco (UCSF) Osher Center for Integrative Medicine; Assistant Clinical Professor, UCSF School of Nursing; Founder, Mindful Birthing and Parenting Foundation (MBPF)

Lisa Chung, DDS, MPH Associate Clinical Professor, Division of Oral Epidemiology & Dental Public Health, University of California, San Francisco, School of Dentistry

Larissa G. Duncan, PhD Elizabeth C. Davies Chair in Child & Family Well-Being; Associate Professor, Human Development & Family Studies; Associate Professor, Family Medicine & Community Health; Healthy Minds, Children, and Families Specialist, University of Wisconsin-Extension; Associate Director, Center for Child and Family Well-Being, School of Human Ecology, University of Wisconsin-Madison

Sheela Maru, MD, MPH Instructor in Obstetrics and Gynecology, Boston University School of Medicine; Women's Health Advisor, Possible and Health Care Systems Design Group; Research Fellow, Division of Women's Health, Brigham and Women's Hospital, Boston, Massachusetts

Kathleen F. Norr, PhD Women, Children & Family Health Sciences, University of Illinois at Chicago, College of Nursing

Crystal L. Patil, PhD Associate Professor, University of Illinois at Chicago, College of Nursing

Marlies Rijnders, PhD, RM TNO Child Health, Leiden, The Netherlands

Sandra A. Smith, PhD, MPH Director of Research, Center for Health Literacy Promotion, Seattle, Washington

Lisa Summers, FACNM, DrPH Former Director of Policy and Advocacy, Centering Healthcare Institute, Silver Spring, Maryland

Foreword

Despite spending more on perinatal health care than any other nation, the United States consistently ranks near the bottom among developed nations on most standard measures of perinatal outcomes. Furthermore, significant racial-ethnic and socioeconomic disparities persist. Doing more of the same will do little to move the needle. This book, *The CenteringPregnancy® Model: The Power of Group Health Care,* adds to the growing body of evidence compelling a reexamination of how perinatal health care is delivered in the United States.

For more than three decades, prenatal care has been a cornerstone of our national strategy to reduce infant mortality and improve birth outcomes. Federal and state efforts in the late 1980s and early 1990s to expand Medicaid coverage for pregnant women led to significant increases in prenatal care utilization, but not to significant improvements in birth outcomes. Two review papers published in 1995 began to question the effectiveness of prenatal care, citing problems with inconsistent results, insufficient adjustment for prematurity bias, and inadequate controls for the effects of critical confounding variables, as well as potential selection bias in earlier studies. In 2003, my colleagues and I published another review paper evaluating the evidence of effectiveness for prenatal care and concluded that "neither preterm birth nor IUGR [intrauterine growth restriction] can be effectively prevented by prenatal care in its present form. Preventing low birth weight will require reconceptualization of prenatal care as part of a longitudinally and contextually integrated strategy to promote optimal development of women's reproductive health not only during pregnancy, but over the life course" (Lu & Halfon, 2003). Our argument was drawn from the life course perspective, which conceptualizes birth outcomes as the product not only of the 9 months of pregnancy, but of the entire life course of the mother from her conception (or before) and onward, leading up to the pregnancy. Disparities in birth outcomes, therefore, are the consequences not only of differential exposures during pregnancy, but also of differential health trajectories across the life span. The life course perspective suggests a need for a paradigm shift in our national strategy to address infant mortality. It calls for an expanded approach to improve birth outcomes in America, one that emphasizes not only risk reduction during pregnancy, but also focuses on health promotion and optimization before and between pregnancies, and indeed across the life course. The approach needs to be *both* clinical and population-based, addressing *both* individual factors and social determinants of health.

Group health care exemplifies such an expanded approach. By receiving prenatal care in a group setting, women have more time with their providers to discuss not only clinical issues, but important concerns in their lives including social determinants. Instead of repeating the same information over and over to women, one at a time, providers in a group setting can cover many more topics that often are inadequately addressed in traditional, individualized prenatal care settings.

Some of these topics include nutrition, stress, and environmental exposures, the impact of which not only on pregnancy outcomes but also on developmental origins of health and disease is increasingly recognized. Providing care in this way allows women to get to know one another and their providers on a much deeper and meaningful level, which can lead to greater engagement, learning, and self-confidence. Members of the group form friendships and are connected in ways not possible in traditional care. As such, group prenatal care is a form of social support, which may buffer its members against the deleterious effects of psychosocial stress on birth outcomes. Recent expansion of the group health care model into parenting suggests an opportunity for greater longitudinal integration of the care continuum.

This book, a study of how a single innovation can transform health care, originated as an idea of its founder, Sharon Schindler Rising, to provide more effective prenatal care to her own patients. Centering has now spread to more than 400 sites across the United States. This book provides an excellent review of the science, theory, practice, and evidence of Centering health care all in one place. We need more of this kind of transformative innovation in health care delivery to improve the health of our nation.

Michael C. Lu, MD, MS, MPH
Associate Administrator for Maternal and Child Health
Health Resources and Services Administration
U.S. Department of Health and Human Services
Bethesda, Maryland

Reference

Lu, M., & Halfon, N. (2003). Racial and ethnic disparities in birth outcomes: A life-course perspective. *Maternal and Child Health Journal, 7*(1), 13–30.

Preface

We have chronicled the development of a model that is an alternative to what we consider to be the usual ambulatory medical care standard: one-on-one care in a closed exam room. The frustrations with our current health care system are legion. Too much of our Gross National Product is tied up in health care, but we continue to see disappointing results. The focus of this book is prenatal/postpartum/well-baby care. In our opinion this should be the major focus of health care today. Our most precious resource, our people, all begin as embryos, newborns, and young children. A family—yes, a village—is entrusted with nurturing this resource. Yet, the lack of social determinants of health in many of our communities has contributed to women often becoming pregnant with many personal health deficits—smoking, inadequate nutrition, poor management of medical and mental health issues—and they may also be dealing with the effects of racism, poverty, opioid addiction, and gun violence. Even women who have enjoyed privilege through much of their lives have real and perceived issues that keep them from being totally healthy and ready for parenthood. The longing for a support community is universal.

CenteringPregnancy® was piloted in 1993 to 1994 by Sharon Schindler Rising, a nurse-midwife who knew there must be a better way to provide care. She had spent 25 years working with women from all socioeconomic levels and found common concerns surfacing—concerns that needed more time to explore than was available in the short visits allowed by the system's expectations. It seemed natural to envision a different way to provide care, and so she just started—moving forward with careful attention, but also confident that women in her groups would show her the way.

Charlotte Houde Quimby has been a friend and colleague of Sharon's for more than 40 years. She, too, has taught students, cared for many women, and started an innovative midwifery care delivery service. She has led groups, marveled at the sharing that happens among women and couples, and longed for a better way to change our health care system. Pairing together to write this book made sense and has been a dynamic time for us both.

This book is a mixture of solid content on CenteringPregnancy and CenteringParenting®, circles, facilitation and implementation, and lots of stories. Some of the comments are short and come from reflections shared by group participants; some are longer profiles of people we have interviewed. One of these, Mindy's Musings, appears in several chapters as segments from a longer interview. We have boxed or italicized many of the comments to call attention to them and their origin, whether from patients served or from clinicians serving. To help represent to the readers what being in a group is like, we created a composite character, Ramona, and shared her pregnancy and transition into parenting. We also have brought to life Paul, a clinician who is a group facilitator.

The turtle has been important to Sharon for years. The turtle resides between the two worlds and has the important task of assuring safe passage of newborns into the world. It also "doesn't make progress until it sticks its neck out." We are using the turtle as an icon to identify stories that are contributed by group participants.

The book has three main sections. The first one is focused on the *Centering* model with Chapters 3 through 6 anchoring the CenteringPregnancy and CenteringParenting models. The second section has three chapters, one on implementation of the model and the other two on expansion of the model, including the need for interprofessional education. The third section explores policy, several research-funded studies, and an expansive chapter on international uptake of the model. Finally, we again look at health care with a focus on steps needed to continue to disrupt and transform. We hope this will give the reader vision and courage to move forward with possible change, clinical groups, research, or policy/advocacy work to further Centering Healthcare™.

We encourage all who want to find out more information about Centering Healthcare to visit the website of the Centering Healthcare Institute, Inc. The website outlines the process of exploring training and consultation options available and provides a contact e-mail and phone number to connect directly with a staff person: www.centeringhealthcare.org.

It has been our pleasure to work together and to touch base with the many who have shared their experiences and insights. We have focused on writing a book that contains many stories about real people and their involvement with the Centering model and its effects on the lives of patients, staff, and clinicians. We truly believe that this model has the potential to change health care and the health of communities. May the force be with all of us as we work for better care for those entrusting themselves to us and hope for more joy in our work as we continue to be present for ourselves, our communities, and our world.

Sharon Schindler Rising
Charlotte Houde Quimby

Acknowledgments

It has taken many years and the contributions of lots of people to get to this point in the implementation and dissemination of the Centering Healthcare™ model. Many people have generously given their time and expertise to provide support and current information on their experiences with CenteringPregnancy® and CenteringParenting®. We want to acknowledge them here and realize that the possibility of missing some is real, especially our numerous site group leaders and facilitators, who also have contributed much through the years.

We want to thank many people who have shared their thoughts about how Centering fits within the current and expanding health care system: Amanda St. Aubin, Amy Fine, Amy Picklesimer Crockett, Barbara Fildes, Cara Thompson, Carmen Strickland, Carol Brady, Carolyn Aoyoma, Debra Keith, Elysia Jordan, Fra Na Reddy, Gail Phillips, Gary Oftedahl, Jessica Densmore, Judy Butler, Karen Shae, Kimberly Couch, Kristen Sublett, Loral Patchen, Margie Rickell, Mark DeFrancesco, Merry-K Moos, Michelle Gallas, Michelle Munroe, Misae Vela Brohl, Richard Gilfillan, Suzanne England, Theresa Willie, and Toby Furash, among others.

Several people gave considerable time either to writing specific contributions to the text or agreeing to extensive interviews. They are Amy MacDonald, Art James, Carrie Klima, Gillian Fynn, Karen Baldwin, Jacqueline Grant, Jocelyn de Sena, Judy Levison, Katsie Cook, Kristin Vander Griend, Lisa Kugler, Margy Hutchison, Mari-Carmen Farmer, Matthew and Sarah Houde, Mindy Schorr, Paula Greer, Sarah Covington-Kolb, Sung Chae, and Sunshine Muse. We also had help from the Centering Healthcare Institute, Inc. (CHI) office, particularly from Tanya Munroe and John Craine.

We also acknowledge input from several students, including Carolyn Kieserman-Shmokler from the University of Wisconsin and Jessica Lyden, Julie Rivo, and Prisclle Schettini from Duke University.

Through the years there have been many people who have given special leadership, most notably through CHI. The founding board and early leaders who contributed substantially include Catherine Hamilton, Carrie Klima, Gina Novick, Lois Daniels, Colleen Senterfitt, Deborah Walker, Doug Laube, Karen McGee, Peter Bernstein, Kelli Viscounte, Ben Doolittle, and Vera Keane. Janet Ray was the anchor in the CHI office for several years and Becky Lindsay provided early graphic designs and content for grants.

We would be remiss for neglecting to name the group of CHI faculty and consultants who, in recent years, have worked with sites and taught others about facilitation skills and model implementation. These individuals are Amy MacDonald, Barbara Winningham, Beth Monahan, Carrie Klima, Charlotte Houde Quimby, Claire Westdahl, Cynthia Wade, Deena Mallareddy, Gail Phillips, Genie Rotundo, Gillian Fynn, Jane Ann Fontenot, Kathy Trotter, Laura Wise, Laurie Jurkiewicz, Lynn Scheidenhelm, Margaret Taylor, Margie Rickell, Margy Hutchison, Mary Alice Grady, Misae Vela Brohl, Peg Dublin, Sharon Matlock, and Toby Furash.

We owe special thanks to two friends who have helped with editing: Marjorie Smith and Kathy McAdams. We owe a big debt of gratitude to Ron Rising for his support through the years, but particularly for his help with pictures, illustrations, and other details necessary for this book.

And finally, we thank Elizabeth Nieginski and Rachel Landes from Springer Publishing Company for their help and encouragement.

Charlotte's Story

I came of age in nursing as a maternity nurse, working in Labor and Delivery in Maine in the 1960s when women received enormous doses of medication to dull the pain and reduce the memories of painful labor. The privilege of attending their births never waned. Being witness to the work, the pain, and the joy of watching them welcome their new infants validated for me that this was where I belonged. This was also a time of burgeoning upheaval in women's rights. Women were making decisions about childbearing and demanding to be awake during their labors and that their husbands be allowed to attend their births. As a young mother myself, I agreed: There had to be a better way. Midwifery became that way for me. At the Yale Graduate School of Nursing, I was blessed to have Sharon Schindler Rising as a mentor, and the millions of questions I had stored up began to have answers.

I stayed on at Yale to teach midwifery and work in a faculty practice. One night, on my way down the stairs to dinner, I met a young pregnant woman walking up the stairs, in obvious pain and out of breath. I learned that she had been contracting all day, had received no prenatal care, and was so frightened of elevators she was climbing the several flights to Labor and Delivery. She did not want her baby's first touch to be filled with her fear. When I shared this story with the midwives, one midwife said she had noticed that many of the young women we were caring for had received no prenatal care. She had begun keeping track of their addresses and realized they were coming from the same geographic area, a section of New Haven, Connecticut, known as Fair Haven, the home of our new young patient. We reached out to the community and found a nascent clinic, meeting one afternoon each week in the community elementary school, with volunteer nurses and doctors. No one was providing prenatal care yet. We contacted the clinic about providing care to pregnant women and had the joy of developing a prenatal clinic within the Fair Haven Health Clinic.

In the late 1970s, I joined a young physician in his new private obstetrical practice in New Haven. I loved and laughed with the women as they brought legal pads filled with questions to their appointments. We worked to get through their lists, seldom getting past question two or three. I wanted more time with them. I wanted to understand the context of their questions. I wanted to know what their partners were thinking.

I had begun to understand the power of groups in graduate school, and wondered what it would be like to bring couples together in groups to talk about their questions. What themes would emerge? What was really happening in their lives? We began to offer Transition to Parenting groups, six semistructured sessions for couples in mid-trimester, co-facilitated by a nurse colleague who had experience and insights about groups, to explore the experiences of couples as they moved through their pregnancies. Soon, women who were not our patients were calling the office to ask, "Is this the practice that has a group for pregnant couples to talk about what is happening?" We knew then that we were right: Women and their partners had concerns, questions, joys, and fears that they wanted and needed to talk about. We catalogued the themes over several years and it became clear the themes were heartfelt and universal: ambivalence about being pregnant; fears of not being capable, or of something being wrong with the baby; issues of the partners about money, work, and sharing their partner; dissonance between their desires and what they were hearing from the experiences of their parents or relatives; and planning for the baby, from naming to care after birth.

The sessions were rich in information that made me a better midwife and solidified my belief in offering groups for pregnant women. Couples frequently maintained the relationships with one another and with me for years after. My belief in offering pregnant women groups was solidified.

In 1983, as my own family began to move into their adult lives and I had adjusted to being a widow, I moved to New Hampshire to develop a new midwifery service at Dartmouth Hitchcock Medical Center (DHMC).

In 1990, I received a call from the American College of Nurse-Midwives asking me to do a site evaluation of a family-planning project in Senegal. I loved working with the midwives there, and my strong desire to do international work was rekindled. That trip led to 10 years of working with midwives in Africa, Vietnam, and Indonesia. My new husband and I spent a year in Uganda, where my work with a women's health collective led to many circle sessions under banyan trees, talking with the women, watching them sew goods to sell for their new business ventures, and hearing their questions while they talked about HIV/AIDS, contraception, raising teens who were beginning to be sexually active, and their fears of vaccinating their younger children.

During this same time frame, Sharon began to develop the model for group care that became CenteringPregnancy®. It made so much sense. I attended an early CenteringPregnancy workshop and I was completely hooked.

I worked as a site approval visitor for the Centering Healthcare Institute, Inc. (CHI), consulting with sites as they implemented this model. Over and over, sitting in the circle, I was moved and inspired by what I saw. I knew that as a midwife in traditional care, the women I cared for received good care. But as I participated in a group at each of the sites I visited, I realized again how much more the women gained by being in Centering groups, hearing one another's experiences, and learning new ways of thinking about pregnancy, birth, and parenting. I watched two midwives in an urban clinic cook traditional African food for their teenaged mothers-to-be; I saw male physicians in the South engage prospective teen dads in a way that made them want to be good fathers; I joined a group of Centering staff as they held hands and gathered in silence before beginning a group. I am very grateful to Sharon for her vision and for the privilege of sharing this journey.

A great deal of energy and attention is now being directed to changing and improving the health care system in this country. I believe the CenteringPregnancy model holds the promise needed to provide care that addresses better relationship-centered health, empowerment of women, and stronger communities. We hope it will make sense for you as we share our experiences and our learning about this wonderful model, Centering Healthcare™.

Charlotte Houde Quimby, MSN, CNM, FACNM

Starting Point Comments From Vera Keane, CNM, MA, FACNM

Strengthening of family values, preventing crime, and reducing violence are concerns that involve every American today; we are all looking for ways to achieve these goals. One untapped resource—perhaps the most important one of all in our search—is in the thoughts and hopes of women who are pregnant.

It has been well documented that pregnancy is a time of introspection and projection. During the months preceding her baby's birth, each woman undergoes a psychological as well as a physical metamorphosis. She reflects on her own growing-up years and her direct experiences in being "parented." Out of these perceptions, she builds an image of the kind of mother *she* wants to be. This process of decision making, with readiness to change, gives her a new chance to mature and use everything within herself and her environment to help her move into the maternal role. Obviously her mate, family, and friends can strengthen this process, as can those who are involved in her care.

However, our traditional system of prenatal visits focuses on physical progress and detection of "what might go wrong." Little advantage is taken of the repeated opportunities to help the woman along in her maturation. On the contrary, many of the procedures and counsels offered during prenatal visits may undermine her self-confidence, create distrust of her own body and her ability to cope, and may even foster within her feelings of being in the grip of powerful forces beyond her control.

Sharon Schindler Rising's system of care, on the other hand, by "centering pregnancy," puts emphasis on the *woman* who is pregnant, not just on the *pregnancy*. Each woman is an individual within a group that shares the bond of being pregnant at the same time. In this climate of mutuality, the group and its leader can help each member to understand what is happening, and to feel confident that she has the capacity to deal with events as they occur. The expectation that her pregnancy is progressing well is continually reinforced. As a result, each woman can recognize that while *all* is not within her control, *some* of it is!

The parent who starts out with faith-in-self and confidence in her own coping skills is going to handle the tasks of parenting differently than an uncertain, fearful person. The impact her behavior will have on the guidance and rearing of children can only be imagined. But, multiplied many times, it may be the lever that can turn society around! Sharon is showing us the way. In implementing this model we may, over time, change the world!

Vera Keane, MA, CNM, FACNM
Cheshire, Connecticut
July 1995. Published as part of the Foreword
to the first CenteringPregnancy handbook

Comments From Carmen Strickland, MD

Centering has quite literally changed my life. Let me share some of my treasured lessons:

Stay Centered

It is easy to lose focus in providing care. We can't be there for the patient if we are not present ourselves. I've learned to take the extra minutes to center myself before any clinical encounter. I've also tried to implement this concept in my personal life although it is definitely a work in progress.

Stay in Conversation

Also true both inside and outside of care, the circle allows and promotes conversation. As we get busier and more automated, we become disconnected from our patients, colleagues, and friends. We are forgetting how to listen. Centering has shown me how valuable minutes can be if we use them to be in conversation with each other.

Trust the Group

By extension, trust the patients. As a clinician, I'd like to think this occurs automatically. Centering has shown me time and again the ways in which we undervalue the patients' role in their own care, without even recognizing it. I have witnessed countless benefits that result from empowering the patients. By trusting our patients, we support them in community building and expand their capacity to reach their fullest potential.

It is my sincere hope that more of the health care system will come to know and appreciate the simple but powerful wisdom that Centering has to offer. Think of what might be possible!

Carmen is associate professor of Family Medicine, Wake Forest University. She is the chairperson of the Centering Healthcare Board of Directors.

The CenteringPregnancy® Model

1 The Origins of CenteringPregnancy®

The task of leading begins from within. It begins with a dream, a sense of what's possible, a commitment to a cause, a yearning to solve a problem, or a restless need to express one's creativity in service of the world.
—Intrator & Scribner (2007, p. 1)

Changing the paradigm of care delivery is difficult. Systems have entrenched rules and expectations that seldom reward innovation. Individuals, programs, and systems all resist change. While it is clear that a team approach to care has the greatest chance of being successful—and is of the most benefit to the women and families seeking care—creating the changes demanded by group care takes a commitment on the part of everyone involved, from desk clerks to top administrators.

Sharon Rising's Early Work

The idea of CenteringPregnancy originated during my graduate work at the Yale School of Nursing. There, I was challenged to hone my thinking in a symbolic logic course, encouraged to listen carefully to the pregnant and newly delivered women in my care, and be clear about "purpose" or why I was doing what I was doing. It was a rich environment for learning and for testing of my basic assumptions of nursing. Our small midwifery student group spent the summer delivering babies in Baltimore, Maryland. This provided me with my first opportunity to get into inner-city homes where very poor women were trying their best to care for their families. And it gave me an opportunity to begin thinking about how I, and our system, could be more effective in responding to the many needs present for these families.

On my return to New Haven, Connecticut in the fall of 1966, I spent several weeks in the clinic, talking with pregnant women while they waited for their appointments. I was curious about many aspects of their experience. How long would it take for women to develop trust in each other and share openly? Would their support for each other vary depending on gestation, parity, or cultural background? Would the group process I was using be effective even in this less-structured clinic setting? This was a golden opportunity for me to better understand the challenges the women faced, living in neighborhoods with safety issues, inflated prices for fresh fruits and vegetables, and schools with inadequate teaching supplies. It also introduced me to the richness of sharing that happens when women are together and feel safe in conversation with one other.

Minnesota

In the early 1970s, I joined the faculty at the University of Minnesota, School of Nursing to open a graduate program in maternal child health with an optional midwifery track. All the students who applied that first year for the maternity track wanted to become nurse-midwives. This provided me with the opportunity to implement an innovative site for care delivery, the Childbearing Childrearing Center (CCC). In an off-campus house, supported by hospital administration, obstetrics, pediatrics, and nursing, advanced practice nurses provided prenatal, postpartum, well-baby, and women's health care.

Although the health care visits were conducted individually, groups of seven to eight couples of similar gestation were formed during mid-pregnancy and continued meeting together through the first 4 months postpartum. The groups were facilitated first by a nurse-midwife and later, during the postpartum months, by a pediatric nurse practitioner. This became a time of preparation for the birth experience and parenting for the couples and provided an opportunity for them to build a community. My husband and I participated in one of those groups during our first pregnancy, personally experiencing the power of group support and appreciating the confidence those discussions gave us as we began our own parenting journey. We still are in touch with some of those couples some 40 years later. Three articles were published citing evaluation from this work at the CCC (Rising, 1975, 1981; Rising & Lindell, 1982).

The Problem: Coming Together

In 1980, our move from Minnesota to Connecticut brought us to a community that was not welcoming to a midwife who wanted to do full-scope midwifery, including the births. By 1993, I was providing prenatal care to women at three very different practice sites: a private office with obstetricians, a hospital clinic with obstetric residents, and a community health center where I was the only prenatal care provider. In the course of a week, I cared for over 100 different pregnant women from high school teenagers to 30-something professionals.

My interest in women and their challenges continued and included my observation that women raised common themes, regardless of their backgrounds. "If pregnancy is a normal event, why do I feel so terrible?" "What can I do to have the healthiest pregnancy possible?" "What are my options for birth?" Each needed similar assurance and practical information. And the women were isolated from each other despite the fact that they all shared a common experience: childbearing.

How did this affect my practice? Similar questions, similar answers, over and over from one woman to another took time and caused me to fall behind schedule. Also, women often returned for their next visit asking the same questions. Clearly, my responses weren't sufficient for the women, and this model of individual care wasn't working for me.

How did this affect the system? Schedules were full with delayed access to appointments for the women. The waiting room often overflowed as women waited to be seen. Then there was the wait for lab tests, discussion with the social worker, insurance questions for Women, Infants, and Children (WIC) or Healthy Start workers, and so on. Most women felt marginalized and confused by a health care system that was difficult to navigate, leading to irregular attendance. Many were new immigrants who were isolated from the support of their extended family. Clinicians weren't feeling much joy either as the administrators were asking for better patient flow and productivity. *We could do better, but it would require a drastic change in how care was provided.*

Addressing the Problem

Earlier experiences with groups made it natural for me to consider a model that brought women together for conversation and perhaps also included the components of care itself. But the question was: what kind of groups? Prenatal classes abounded, and participants often formed a type of support system for each other. However, fewer women were interested in formal childbirth classes, partly because their lives were busier and they were getting more of their education through media and books. Also, formal childbirth classes were not financially or practically feasible for all women.

I imagined a type of care that encouraged women to feel empowered to make their own health decisions that would provide a community for women to support each other and that facilitated sharing of the wisdom I knew women possessed. I also wanted to practice without repeating myself all day: genetics testing, nutrition, round ligament pain, and so forth. Thinking about the current prenatal experience available, namely, the short individual visits with little time to share on a deeper level, the fewer prenatal classes that women were attending and the didactic nature of most of those classes, and the obvious enjoyment of the women when they could talk with each other, I felt that care could be improved by bringing it into the group setting. Care should be more than "belly checks": care should also involve time for discussion and opportunity to make connections with other women/couples.

The Launch of a Group Prenatal Model

My initial task was to determine what it would take to provide prenatal care within a group space with a stable cohort of women of similar gestation? The system has many exam rooms designed for individual care. It would take some work on the actual logistics and also on the attitudes and expectations of both the staff and the patients to make a change in the way care had always been provided. Group care would need to be viewed as "enhanced," better than the short individual "sound-bite" visits. Initially, we could simply test it out to see if it could work. I started the first groups at the hospital clinic site that had a population of about 30 new prenatal women registering per month. Most women were healthy, young, of low income, and equally divided among Caucasian, African American, and Hispanic ethnic groups. The medical director, the clinic nurses, the women's health supervisor, and the social worker all responded enthusiastically to trying group care. So, 10 to 12 women of similar gestation, starting at about 16 weeks, were brought together for all 10 sessions of their prenatal care. This timing would ensure that the women were enrolled in the clinic, had received their initial exam and lab work, and had a viable fetus. The care was provided by a nurse practitioner or a nurse-midwife along with a nurse who followed the women throughout pregnancy, using the American College of Obstetricians and Gynecologists standard of spacing and number of visits. If women developed medical problems, they were referred to the medical staff for evaluation.

The women and the staff were excited, so we just started with about 12 in a group. "We are trying something new and we're inviting you to get care this way. We will want lots of feedback. Willing to give it a try?" was our invite to the women. We had no problem filling the groups. The first group was intentionally all primigravidas, the second was all multiparas, and the third was mixed . . . just to test what might work best. We all agreed that the mixed primigravida/multipara group had definite advantages, and so subsequent groups all were mixed parity. I drew on my 25 years of experience as a nurse-midwife to develop a notebook of materials to provide current information. These were prenatal-stage appropriate and were supported by clinical and theoretical understandings of pregnancy and maternal needs. Self-assessment sheets that each woman could use to get in touch with her thoughts and needs on a variety of topics related to pregnancy and childbearing were available for each session and were used to initiate facilitated discussions. As the clinician in these first groups, I had to learn to really listen to women. In that process, I found that I was learning much more than I was "teaching."

Women participated in self-care activities, assessing their own blood pressure and weight and then entering these data on the chart. The chart itself became demystified as terminology was explained and each woman was able to claim her own data. It was amazing to see how empowering this was for the women and how, when given a chance to speak, they were able to claim their own considerable knowledge.

A lack of appropriate space in which to conduct groups can be a formidable challenge since space is at a premium in most sites and the rivalry for space can create interdepartmental tensions. Conference rooms are also used for other activities, so the need to set up and take down the room for each use is not ideal. I was fortunate that there was a conference room available next to the birthing suite with storage space and no heavy table to move. Another major hurdle can be the recruitment of women into the groups, in part because the need to change registration mechanisms places an inadvertent burden on booking staff and clinic nurses. However, the clinic staff was enthusiastic about the program and helped with recruitment of the women. As the primary provider of prenatal care for the first groups, I was able to do much of the promotion. We found that we could easily involve half of our women in groups by starting one group a month, and in many months we were even able to start two. Women loved it!

The nurses working with the program also enjoyed spending more time with the women and sharing from their expertise. As one said, "This is what nursing should be!" Another commented, "In Centering, a connection is made between the women and the staff that is empowering to all." The initial pilot program included 13 groups, of which three were teen groups. At the final evaluation, 98% of the women said they enjoyed being with other women to receive their care (Rising, 1998). This figure is consistent with findings from across the country: 96% to 97% of all women, whether primigravidas or multiparas, say they prefer getting their care in this model. And midwives comment, "I was ready to get out of midwifery but this has totally reenergized me, by getting me back to why I became a midwife."

Once I began to experience the power of doing prenatal care in groups, there was no turning back. It was clear that the group members were much better at solving each woman's problems than I was alone. And relationship-centered care challenged our cultural assumptions, allowing us to learn together how to pursue good health and a healthy pregnancy. One midwife shared this story:

> Maria is an undocumented woman, from Mexico, who had been in California for a couple of years and was actually thinking of going back home when she got pregnant. She had thought to return because she just wasn't happy, was depressed—she described her life as being compartmentalized, with her going to work, going to school, and being home with her husband, with none of those parts of her life integrated. She showed up at our clinic, and the nurse who saw her for her first visit encouraged her to join a Centering group. She resisted, feeling that the last thing she wanted was to sit and talk to a group of women—that she was too depressed for this. The nurse was persistent and eventually convinced her to give it a try. She says she went to her first session and held back, and then over the course of the next couple of sessions came out of her shell, started participating, and became a leader in

the group. Looking back, she says that Centering "was a bridge for me between my culture and the United States culture. It is what got my feet on the ground in this country."

She had her baby and then returned to give back to Centering as a member of a group we called "graduadas," or "graduates"— Spanish-speaking women who had done Centering and who had shown leadership potential, who worked together doing community outreach, community education, and who also helped in our Centering groups. She now is on her way to nursing school, with a goal of becoming a midwife!

So what should this care model be called? I remember the day when I was driving my daughter to school and said, "CenteringPregnancy!" The three components of care—health assessment, education, and support—came together within the group space. In fact, they were "centered" within a circle that represented a safe holding space for each of the participants and that honored the many facets of care. Also, providing care within the circle in the group was a "centering" experience for me. I thought about the plumb line that keeps us anchored, holds our values, and provides a core for us to measure our thoughts and feelings. Group experience provided that anchoring for me.

Enthusiasm for the model grew from those first groups, and I soon began the model at other locations: a federally qualified health center and a private office with obstetricians. Spanish-speaking groups became important. All of these groups were successful, and the word spread. In 1995, I presented the first national description of CenteringPregnancy at the annual meeting of the American College of Nurse-Midwives with my friend, Marjorie Smith, PhD, CNM, who had done focus group research with group participants and clinic staff. The interest of the midwives was palpable and encouraged me to move forward with a training workshop in 1998. Joan Seabury, the nurse who was the co-facilitator in my groups, and Jane Tokunow, a midwifery student at Yale who did her thesis on the CenteringPregnancy model, helped lead this workshop. Twenty-five midwives, nurses, and one obstetrician came to the initial workshop, and their enthusiasm reinforced my conviction that the Centering model had the potential to change the lives of clinicians as well as pregnant women.

Other milestones followed the early workshops. In 2001, four midwife friends—Catherine Hamilton, Carrie Klima, Gina Novick, and Lois Daniels—joined me to form a 501c3 nonprofit organization. We named this the CenteringPregnancy and Parenting Association, which later was changed to the Centering Healthcare Institute, Inc. More than

20 midwives, nurses, physicians, and social workers became part of the faculty group, which conducted workshops and did consultation. Yearly faculty retreats built a strong sense of mission and belonging and kept our internal "flame" alive for this important work. These retreats provided time for exchange of ideas of what works, lessons learned, new approaches to particular issues, and true continuing education.

Centering had become a passion for me: I firmly believe that prenatal care, and most health care, does not belong in exam rooms. I didn't have a big vision when I started . . . I just knew this was something that I had to do. One obstetrician said, "Well, Centering certainly passes the commonsense test!" Yes, it made sense to provide care this way and the more I did it, the less willing I was to settle for care that wasn't meeting the needs of the patients, the providers, or the agency. But there was a need for more evidence of improved outcomes to make the case for support on a larger scale. A call in 2001 from Dr. Jeannette Ickovics, Yale Professor of Public Health, asking if I was interested in working with researchers on formal evaluation of the model led to a hearty "yes"!

The Evidence

The early evidence from the first two studies conducted by this Yale team showed a reduction in preterm birth (Ickovics et al., 2003; Ickovics et al., 2007). These were followed in 2012 by two other well-designed studies (Pickelsimer, Billings, Hale, Blackhurst, & Covington-Kolb, 2012; Tandon, Colon, Vega, Murphy, & Alonso, 2012). Preterm birth is the number one killer of newborns in the United States as well as a significant expense—it impairs the growth and development of babies and is a major drain on our health care dollars. From 2001 to 2006, the National Institutes of Health collaborated with Yale and Emory universities to conduct a 5-year randomized controlled trial of 1,047 young women randomly assigned to receive their prenatal care in Centering groups or by standard office visits. There was a 33% drop in the rate of preterm birth for women in Centering groups, and even more remarkably, there was a 41% reduction for African American women who received care in groups (Ickovics et al., 2007). Additionally, patient satisfaction was significantly higher in women who received care in Centering groups. The publication of these initial findings and continued published research from several sites helped fuel the huge upsurge in interest in Centering and led to early support from the national and state March of Dimes chapters, Strategic Grant Partners and, more recently, the Kellogg and Anthem Foundation. Now there are over 400 sites nationally and more than 200 published articles on the model.

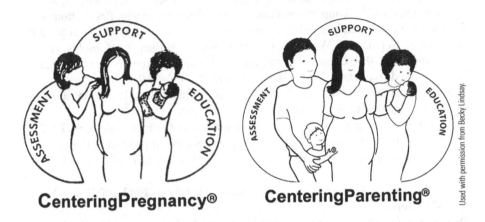

CenteringPregnancy®   **CenteringParenting®**

Research including randomized controlled trials supports the efficacy, effectiveness and transformative power of this 'disruptive design' of prenatal care that throws away the illness orientation and managing risk view of pregnancy in favor of a dynamic union of clients in a group setting, and facilitative providers. Few in health service delivery can claim to have created a new model of care; this alumna has.—Yale School of Nursing Distinguished Alumna Award, 2006

Centering is relationship-centered care that builds on the wisdom of each person in the group and that honors the deep cultural values present, leading to a dynamic environment of enrichment for all participants. This is a model that brings sustaining change to a system mired in inefficiency and ineffectiveness. "It is the one thing in my week that brings me joy," shared a physician. It started with my need to change how I provided care and developed into a vision that was embraced by other midwives, physicians and, most importantly, by the women in the groups . . . one by one, group by group.

It goes on one at a time, it starts when you care to act, it starts when you do it again after they said no, it starts when you say we and you know who you mean, and each day you mean one more.—Marge Piercy (2012, p. 305)

References

Ickovics, J., Kershaw, T., Westdahl, C., Magriples, U., Massey, Z., Reynolds, H., & Rising S. (2003). Group prenatal care and preterm birth weight: Results from a matched cohort study at public clinics. *Obstetrics & Gynecology, 102*(5), 1051–1057.

Ickovics, J., Kershaw, T., Westdahl, C., Magriples, U., Massey, Z., Reynolds, H., & Rising, S. (2007). Group prenatal care and perinatal outcomes: A randomized controlled trial. *Obstetrics & Gynecology, 110*(2), 330–339.

Intrator, S., & Scribner, M. (Eds.). (2007). *Leading from within: Poetry that sustains the courage to lead.* San Francisco, CA: Jossey-Bass.

Pickelsimer, A., Billings, D., Hale, N., Blackhurst, D., & Covington-Kolb, S. (2012). The effect of CenteringPregnancy group prenatal care on preterm birth in a low-income population. *American Journal of Obstetrics & Gynecology, 206*(415), e1–e7.

Piercy, M. (2011). *The hunger moon: New and selected poems 1980–2007.* New York, NY: Knopf.

Rising, S. S. (1975). Consumer-oriented nurse-midwifery service. *The Nursing Clinics of North America, 10*(2), 251–262.

Rising, S. S. (1981). Nurse-midwives in action at the childbearing childrearing center. In L. Jarvis (Ed.), *Community health nursing: Keeping the public healthy* (pp. 811–824). Philadelphia, PA: F. A. Davis.

Rising, S. S. (1998). CenteringPregnancy: An interdisciplinary model of empowerment. *Journal of Nurse-Midwifery, 43*(1), 46–54.

Rising, S. S., & Lindell, S. (1982). The childbearing childrearing center: A nursing model. *The Nursing Clinics of North America, 17*(1), 11–22.

Tandon, S. D., Colon, L., Vega, P., Murphy, J., & Alonso, A. (2012). Birth outcomes associated with receipt of group prenatal care among low-income Hispanic women. *Journal of Midwifery & Women's Health, 57*(5), 476–481.

2 Making the Case for Centering Group Health Care

Health care is not a product manufactured by the healthcare system, but rather a service, which is co-created by healthcare professionals in relationship with one another and with people seeking help to restore or maintain health for themselves and their families.—Batalden et al. (2015, p. 9)

Designing a new model of care that would respond to the needs of women and providers and still exist within the current reimbursement system was, and is, a challenge. There are few statements more powerful than, "but we've always done it this way." However, it was clear in the 1990s and is clear today that "the system is broken, and Band-Aids won't work."

This chapter explores the needs of childbearing women and their families in the context of current prenatal care, care that has frequently been referred to as the cornerstone of maternal and child health. In that context, the chapter reviews current traditional prenatal care practices and outcomes and delineates the basic assumptions, practices, and outcomes of the first group prenatal care model, CenteringPregnancy®.

Maternal and Infant Statistics in the United States

Increased costs, sophisticated professional education, and significantly augmented patient surveillance have become the new normal in obstetrics. The old adage about a big ship taking longer to turn mid-ocean certainly holds true when attempting to move decades-old practices into new models of care. Yet, the United States continues to witness alarming maternal and infant mortality. In the past 20 years, this country of abundance went from 7.2 maternal deaths per 100,000 in 1987 to a high of 17.8 per 100,000 in 2009 and again in 2011. Despite major efforts to decrease these alarming numbers (15.9 per 100,000 deaths in 2012), they continue to reveal social and racial inequities and disparities. Black women experience a 42.8% maternal death rate compared to a 12.5% rate for White women and a 17.3% rate for all other races (Krans & Davis, 2012).

In 2015, the UN General Assembly adopted a new agenda for Sustainable Development Goals for the period leading up to 2030. The new framework replaced the Millennium Development Goals (MDG), which expired in 2015. The Global Burden of Disease 2015 Collaborators compiled data to estimate the performance of 33 indicators for 188 countries from 1990 to 2015. The United States ranked 28th in this analysis; in part, because of poorer performance on maternal mortality ratios compared to other high-income countries and worse performance on non-MDG indicators, such as alcohol consumption and interpersonal violence (Global Burden of Disease Collaborators, 2016).

Women are more apt to die having a baby in the United States than in any other developed country. The United States places 33rd among 179 countries for maternal mortality. The complexity of causes has been articulated by the Centers for Disease Control and Prevention (CDC) with the discovery that many of these deaths could be prevented by a more aggressive attention to the chronic diseases experienced by many childbearing women (Centers for Disease Control and Prevention, 2016). Indeed, if the country were experiencing these numbers for any infectious disease, alarms would be at full throttle. Women of childbearing age intending to become pregnant *deserve to know* that a healthy lifestyle (good nutrition, avoiding obesity, abandoning all substance abuse, and seeking medical care for preexisting conditions) will serve them well as they begin their reproductive lives. It is estimated that every year in the United States, nearly 1 million women receive little or poor-quality maternity care, making their babies increasingly vulnerable. These babies are three times more likely to be born too small and five times more likely to die in the first year (March of Dimes, 2013). For Black infants, the chance of surviving to celebrate their first birthday is half that of their White counterparts, a gap that has not closed despite efforts to improve prenatal care (Lu, Kotelchuck, Hogan, Jones, & Halfon, 2012). Researchers, pediatricians, public health officials, and parents are increasingly aware of the persistent and pervasive causes of this tragedy, namely, the social determinants of health—poverty, economic stability, education, social and community cohesion, health and health care, and neighborhood environment—all of which play a major role (Social Determinants of Health, Healthy People 2020, 2016).

It is clear that much remains to be accomplished in solving the problems of preterm birth and infant mortality in the United States. According to the CDC National Vital Statistics Report of 2010 (MacDorman, Hoyert, & Matthews, 2013), in 2010 the United States ranked 26th in infant mortality, with an infant mortality rate of 6.1 infant deaths per 1,000 births. The mortality rate for preterm infants (born at 32–26 weeks gestation) was second highest among industrialized countries. Preterm births contributed to 39% of the U.S. infant mortality rate. While there has indeed been a reduction in preterm birth rates to 9.5% in 2014 thanks to an increased awareness of the dangers of preterm inductions and a subsequent decrease in nonmedically indicated deliveries, preterm birth rates were essentially unchanged for Black- and Hispanic-origin groups between 2013 and 2014 (Hamilton, Martin, Osterman, Curtin, & Mathews, 2013).

The March of Dimes estimates that the premature birth cost to our nation is $26 billion a year.[1] This fact does little to describe the emotional, fiscal, and potential lifelong costs of preterm birth, which wreak havoc on the beginning of a child's life and on their parents. Preterm births frequently set the stage for disastrously high and long-term medical and educational costs for the children as well as stress and potential marital discord for the parents. There is no accurate way to factor in the emotional toll to parents, siblings, and extended families (March of Dimes, 2013).

Concern about these issues in the 1980s moved the Public Health Service to form an interdisciplinary panel to review the evidence for the content of prenatal care. Two documents, *Caring for Our Future* and *New Perspectives on Prenatal Care*, were the result of this work (Merkatz & Thompson, 1990; Rosen, Merkatz, & Hill, 1991). The review surfaced a lack of evidence for many of the routine practices included in prenatal care and a lack of research to help inform changes. Recommendations for prenatal care include the promotion of healthy family development, the reduction of unintended pregnancy, and the promotion of community resources. Both publications underscored the need for more evidence to guide decisions regarding prenatal care.

In 2001, the Institute of Medicine published a seminal document, *Crossing the Quality Chasm* (Institute of Medicine, Committee on Quality Health Care in America, 2001). This report outlines steps to change the

---

[1]In November 2016, the March of Dimes reported that the preterm birth rate has worsened for the first time in 8 years, with widening differences in prematurity rates across different races and ethnicities (www .marchofdimes.org/mission/prematurity-reportcard).

environment to support needed redesign: applying evidence to health care delivery, using information technology, aligning payment policies with quality improvement, and preparing the workforce. It also identifies Aims for Improvement and Rules for Redesign, reconfirming the previous calls for better evidence and strategies for improved care.

Parallel to this national effort was the early development of the CenteringPregnancy group care model in 1994, which reflected a reduction in high tech surveillance with a focus on patient involvement in care. The model encourages empowerment and community building, as well as personal responsibility (Rising, 1998). The early data from studies dating from 2003 through 2007 underscored the ability of the model to reduce preterm birth, increase breastfeeding, and documented high patient satisfaction (Ickovics et al., 2003; Ickovics et al., 2007).

Basic Assumptions

These basic assumptions of the authors have guided their practice for over 100 combined years of working in maternal child health and underscore the material presented in this book:

- Pregnancy and the transition to parenting is a time of change, and most women (and their partners) are open to examining how this is affecting their lives and what strategies they can use to make it as smooth as possible.
- Most pregnant women are medically healthy and have medically uncomplicated pregnancies.
- As pregnant women focus more on the interrelationship of their body and that of the growing fetus, they are interested in altering potentially unhealthy behaviors such as smoking, recreational drug use, poor diet habits, and exercise regimes.
- Adult learning is complex as people use a variety of ways to gather, understand, and incorporate new knowledge. Social media and online social networking have opened new avenues for accessing information. Learning takes place in a variety of ways including professional one-to-one contact, informal sharing with friends and relatives, seeking out and exchanging books, Internet websites and other media, and sharing information with others who are experiencing similar life changes.
- The current system of care, which separates the risk assessment process from opportunity for substantive discussion, provides little help for true behavioral change.

- The system that for decades has supported individual visits has not shown substantial improvement in outcomes nor is it cost-effective or cost-efficient as noted by little change in the preterm birth rate and rising maternal mortality.
- Patient engagement in care is an essential component for empowerment. By maintaining a system that is focused on determination of risk, the provider continues to be in a position of control, making true partnership difficult and implying that the woman and her family do not bring knowledge or accumulated wisdom into the pregnancy.
- Participation in groups with others dealing with similar issues provides support and community for dealing with both the normal concerns and challenges of pregnancy.

These basic assumptions make it clear that traditional individual visits are not a model adequate to accomplish these beliefs. Prenatal care needs to be conceptualized as more than the belly check and other routines that are part of the definition of risk assessment. In fact, the routines that were common several years ago have been expanded to incorporate new technology such as multiple screening tests and serial ultrasounds, along with greatly enhanced genetics testing. A newly pregnant woman, who, at her first visit, receives a compact disk describing fetal deformities and rare genetic disorders, has embarked on a pregnancy course of anxiety and stress. Clinicians struggling with expectations for increased productivity have little opportunity to explore such information in depth with women. The introduction of electronic health records has further diminished the clinical interaction and removed the woman from her own information. These not only increased the cost of care and the complexity of visits, they have done little to engage the pregnant woman in meaningful conversation with her provider. Developing a system that honors the basic assumptions means the care definition needs to be expanded beyond the commonly accepted dimensions of prenatal care.

Over the years, new federal legislation has made it possible for the states to cover the cost of care for women living at or below the poverty level. Prenatal care utilization soared, but the content of the care changed very little. The increased number of visits did nothing to alter the rate of prematurity. The needs of this group of women were not being met.

The disparity in maternal child health is greatest in the outcomes for Black and White infants. Over the past two decades, public health efforts to address these disparities have focused primarily on increasing access to prenatal care. While the mortality rate for White infants declined as a result of so much prenatal care, this did not lead to closing the gap in birth outcomes. The rate for Black infants remained constant, or increased slightly. It is worth noting that the first randomized controlled trial of CenteringPregnancy published in 2007 documented a 33% reduction in preterm birth for women in group care and a 41% reduction for African American women who composed 80% of the sample (Ickovics et al., 2007).

More Than Prenatal Care

Researchers meanwhile continued to study the multiple risk factors and living conditions for women and infants, which impact on the outcomes of the persistent gap in populations. The Maternal and Child Health Bureau (MCHB), in a major concept paper, *Rethinking MCH: The Life Course Model as an Organizing Framework,* aimed to support and encourage the inclusion of Life Course Theory (LCT) in maternal and child health research, policies, and projects. This was an effort to reduce disparities and broaden the agenda for improving the lives of mothers and babies, not only the 9 months of pregnancy but also the entire life course of the mother before pregnancy (U.S. Department of Health and Human Services, 2010).

As Braverman notes, "A life-course approach considers how health later in life is shaped by earlier experiences." (2014, p. 368)

Maternal medical conditions, socioeconomic status, isolation, lack of social support, poor education, lack of jobs, and even previous health care encounters for Black women that have left many of them fearful or unwilling to return for more care have increasingly received attention. The complexities involved in any effort to improve these situations require multiagency, multiprovider strategies with the capability to encompass far more than prenatal care (Lu & Johnson, 2014). These complexities are expanded and highlighted in a study exploring the impact of discrimination and excessive weight gain during pregnancy for Black and Latina young women (Reid et al., 2016). Recognizing that excessive weight gain in pregnancy often determines later-life obesity among the women and their children, researchers also found that the influence of social discrimination further effected gaining more weight than recommended in pregnancy. Prenatal care is an optimal time for focusing on this issue (Reid et al., 2016).

Private and public organizations in maternal and child health continued the push for political and health care leaders to find ways to improve the outcomes of maternity care. Systems must be designed to not only provide prenatal care but also take into account the family's health and social service needs throughout adolescence, preconception care, pregnancy, childbearing, the postpartum period, and early childhood development. Medicaid currently pays for 50% of the births in this country. Most of these women are younger, less experienced, and less educated, often with language challenges, and could benefit from programs designed to meet multiple needs. Life course strategies were developed to support African American women and their families toward healthier lives and healthy birth outcomes.

An example of such a program, the Healthy Families Initiative, designed by a Partnership Program between Wisconsin School of Medicine and Public Health and a major endowment, developed four projects based on the following three goals: (a) improving infant health and survival, (b) improving the health status of African American women, and (c) eliminating racial disparities in birth outcomes. Specific community actions included such items as facilitating access to preconception, prenatal, interconception health care, increasing relationship-building skills, and strengthening partnerships to address barriers to quality health care. Among the lessons learned is how long it takes to build trust and a common understanding of the goal. Implementing this project meant creating specific messaging for the community, such as, "The birth of a child is not the product of 9 months of pregnancy, but the entire span of a woman's life leading up to the pregnancy," and "When dads are involved, moms and babies are healthier" (Frey, Farrell, Cotton, Lathen, & Marks, 2014). These messages were also reflected in findings of higher levels of antenatal anxiety, depression, and smoking among pregnant women who reported low partner support (Cheng et al., 2016).

Investigating What Works

The Strong Start for Mothers and Newborns initiative, an effort of the Centers for Medicare and Medicaid Services (CMS), the Health Resources and Services Administration (HRSA), and Administration on Children and Families (ACF), is a 5-year initiative, launched in 2012, to reduce preterm birth and improve health outcomes for mothers and babies (Krans & Davis, 2014).

One arm of the study is designed to reduce the rate of early elective deliveries. Another arm is testing three enhanced approaches to prenatal care: Maternity Home, Birth Center Births, and Group Prenatal Care/CenteringPregnancy for women enrolled in Medicaid or Children's Health Insurance Program (CHIP). Besides the intense focus on reduction of preterm birth, the study of these women with pregnancies at increased risk will document health outcomes for both mothers and babies through the first year of life and the anticipated reduction in cost of this care (Declercq, Sakala, Corry, Applebaum, & Herrlich, 2014).

Of the 27 awardees, 15 are implementing group prenatal care with a total of 54 sites involved. Year 2 evaluations reveal that women enrolled in Strong Start exhibit rates of depression that are substantially higher than generally reported rates of perinatal depression. Similar proportions of depression among women were observed within each of the Strong Start approaches. Strong Start interventions appear well-designed to support women with depression and other psychosocial stressors. The group aspect of CenteringPregnancy care is specifically intended to help women build relationships, support and learn from one another, and benefit from the knowledge that there are others experiencing many of the same risks, stress factors, and circumstances they are experiencing. All three approaches have implemented services that go far beyond the traditional, medically focused prenatal care (Alliman, Joles, & Summers, 2015; Centers for Medicare and Medicaid Services, 2016; Handler & Johnson, 2016).

A skyrocketing cesarean birth rate, from 21% in 1996 to 33% in 2011 and a slight decline to 32.2% in 2014—some 1.3 million babies born this way each year—further complicates the preterm and low birth weight dilemma (Hamilton, Martin, Osterman, Curtin, & Mathews, 2013). These are the highest rates ever reported in the United States, costly and unnecessary in far too many instances, exposing women to surgical infections, delayed recovery, increased costs, and future obstetrical difficulties. The rates for early preterm birth increased in that time frame by 36%, and for late preterm and term infants rose almost 50% (Centers for Disease Control and Prevention, 2016).

Consumer Reports conducted a study of 1,500 hospitals in the United States and found even women whose clinical course was unremarkable, with normal presentations of the fetus, had these high cesarean-section (c-section) rates. More concerning in their reports were the wide variations of rates in hospitals in the same city, with only a small number of hospitals achieving good marks for low rates (Rappleye, 2016).

In addition to Medicaid costs for maternity care, many women with insurance are expected to pay up to four times more, at sizeable additional costs (Rosenthal, 2013). The *New York Times* reported on an analysis done by Truven Health Analytics in 2013 about the tripling of charges for delivery since 1996. The services received for maternity care, while similar to those of other developed countries with much lower costs, are itemized individually and charged at higher rates. Women with normal pregnancies consequently receive far more testing and surveillance than warranted, increasing the costs exponentially. A second such study, conducted by a Yale University research team, looked at data from the 2011 Nationwide Inpatient Sample of 463 hospitals in the United States. The study found the range of cost to be $1,189 to $11,986. Even considering standard adjustments such as location (city/rural), volume of births, c-section rates, and so on, the team found the variation in costs could explain only a small portion of the cost increase (Xu et al., 2015).

What Women Want and Need

Researchers, providers, and the women themselves have well documented women's natural desires to learn all they can about how to care for themselves to grow and give birth to a healthy baby, what to expect in the first few weeks of life, and what they might expect at work and at home. They tell us in multiple ways that women are eager to learn, eager to connect with other women during their pregnancies, and eager to be the best mothers possible (Childbirth Connection; Transforming Maternity Care, 2013).

This is even more evident when we explore the behavioral patterns of young Millennnials—the generation of women born between 1982 and 1994, who are currently the largest cohort receiving maternal health care. Millennnials live in the social media world and on multiple connectable devices and platforms. They are in touch and on the move; they believe health care is a right, and they want providers who value connection and listen to their questions. They turn increasingly to web searches and social media for information and do not think of established health care as meeting their needs. They want "health care," not sickness care, and a system that honors their need for mind–body therapies, healthy foods, and one that allows individuals to make choices. "They want a system wherein preventive health and primary care is holistic, widely accessible and respected as a reflection of a community's core values" (Keckley, 2014). They are also choosing to have their babies at later ages. Birth rates have declined to a record low for women in their early 20s, but have risen for women in their late 20s and early 30s (Osterman & Martin, 2014).

Current prenatal care provides a considerable amount of technical information about genetics, various and multiple testing now required during the pregnancy, and the importance of technology surveillance in their births. Appointments are structured to be 15 minutes in the absence of high-risk issues. In addition, rotating providers who seldom have the time or the opportunity to develop a relationship that might yield important questions about a range of issues, from hidden anxieties and work-related discussions to exposure to harmful behaviors, are seeing patients on increasingly busy schedules. So much of the new information now being disseminated by science blogs can muddy the water even further: Do omega-3 fatty acids reduce aggression in children? What part of the newly emerging brain science should I take seriously or should I adopt? Do I put my children at risk if I vaccinate them, or if I don't?

An Evidence-Based Solution

CenteringPregnancy is a model that provides an opportunity for women to share strategies that are culturally appropriate and embrace new knowledge, which frequently leads to behavioral change, while interacting effectively with providers in what is often a woman's first health care experience. The model is perfectly designed to meet the multiple needs of women from varying socioeconomic, educational, and familial perspectives. The relationship of the women to each other provides a unique opportunity for women to support, encourage, and help each other.

Studies conducted to compare the psychosocial outcomes of CenteringPregnancy to individual care reflect a greater increase in the group participants' use of prenatal planning, preparation, and coping strategies (Heberlein et al., 2016; Ickovics et al., 2011). Women who were at increased psychosocial risk benefitted from participation in group prenatal care. Among women reporting inadequate social support in early pregnancy, group participants in this study demonstrated greater decrease in pregnancy distress and higher maternal functioning during the postpartum period. Other results from this study include the impact on education and preparation, which were deemed to be enhanced by the supportive group environment; group participants described more positive influences on stress reduction, confidence, knowledge, motivation, informed decision making and health care engagement. Group prenatal care provided an opportunity for the women to share experiences and knowledge, which even helped improve their food security, confidence, and skills (Picklesimer, Heberlein, & Covington-Kolb, 2015).

Reluctance

CenteringPregnancy care is ideally suited to the desires and needs of the childbearing population. Yet many young women receiving health care services for the first time may have never had the opportunity for one-on-one care, and so having a midwife or doctor relationship is a new experience. Their concerns about joining a group may include concerns about group inclusion and whether this model of care is "less than" what they or their families think they have a right to expect. The importance of educating staff and community about the benefits of CenteringPregnancy cannot be understated. Until women and men understand the multiple benefits of group care—quality care and education, and development of community and personal empowerment—enrollment remains a challenge. Yet, in a study to determine the willingness to participate in CenteringPregnancy, when given information about the model, 49.2% of respondents ($n = 477$) indicated they were "definitely" or "probably likely" to choose this model. Women placed a high value on learning about pregnancy, birth, and early mothering and being with other women who were pregnant, and about two thirds preferred to have their partners participate (McDonald et al., 2015). Such information may assist providers in engaging women to the model.

Cost Benefits

In a long-awaited article, group prenatal care has been documented to provide better outcomes with significant Medicaid savings in the state of South Carolina. CenteringPregnancy participation reduced the risk of preterm birth by 36%, with an estimated savings of $22,667 in immediate health expenditures. This same study documented the reduced incidence of delivering a low-birth-weight infant by 44% for a savings of $29,627. The state of South Carolina invested $1.7 million to implement the model in the state, and the estimated returns were nearly $2.3 million (Gareau et al., 2016).

Change Is Hard

Resistance to the implementation of CenteringPregnancy, while understandable in the face of bottom-line budgeting decisions and normal resistance to change, now flies in the face of evidence and in the years of experience of site consultants and data collectors who recognize that each site reports findings of important results: significantly reduced preterm births, 96% patient satisfaction on patient satisfaction questionnaires, increased breastfeeding, and increased numbers of women spacing their births. The vast majority of women receiving care in the CenteringPregnancy model in over 400 sites would not elect to do individual care in a future pregnancy and rated the relationship to each other as far more important in their learning that the relationship with a provider.

 As one woman wrote to her group, "Time to get pregnant again so we can have another group!"[2]

There is less opportunity with traditional care to develop friendships with other pregnant women trying to discern which information is the most important and to sort out for themselves what to believe, what to adopt as their own practices, and what does not meet their needs and they can reject. Nor does it help women become informed consumers with the ability to discern how they will make intelligent choices as their babies grow, as they are expected to make decisions about health care for their infants and young children, and further, how to make sense of all the information coming their way. If one ultrasound is good, would six be better? What if my partner and I disagree on an important piece of information? How do we come together to assess our own beliefs, our cultural heritage or our "gut feelings?" Gone are the days of their mothers' and grandmothers' "The doctors know best. Just do what they tell you."

The growth and development of mothers have undergone enormous change in the past 75 years, from when mothers were hospitalized for

---

[2]The turtle icon box used throughout the book references a comment from a group participant.

2 weeks to allow time for recovery and learning how to care for their infants to our current short-stay discharge policies, sending women home still reeling from the work of birth and the adrenaline rush of holding their newborns, and from rooming-in policies allowing families to participate in learning to care for their new baby and visit with new mothers to mothers working until their due dates and returning to work 4 to 6 weeks after the birth.

The group experience has led to the formation of friendships, a personal sense of having the knowledge needed, a new or renewed trust in oneself and one's abilities, and important strengthening of intimate relationships that are all central to the capacity to parent well. In the group setting, new knowledge has the capacity to expand compassion, such as the situation in an inner-city young mothers group when a woman at the end of pregnancy worried aloud to the group how she was going to bring her baby home, since the hospital staff had told her on her recent tour that babies would not be released without a car seat. "I don't have the money for that! How can I bring my baby home without one?" she asked the group. Another member of the group immediately replied, "I got two at my shower last week. I'll bring one in for you next week." Such a connection would have been unlikely in a waiting room of strangers.

New knowledge also has the capacity to change behaviors: smoking cessation and eating more foods you don't like and fewer of those that are not good nutrition is easier with group support. The sense of community, of personal responsibility, and of shared commitment to their babies is a powerful learning for men as well as women as they are beginning the journey into parenthood. Taking responsibility for yourself is contagious.

Clinician Benefits and System Challenges

In addition, the work satisfaction for providers involved in facilitating CenteringPregnancy groups is a proven deterrent to job burnout and frustration. Not having time to properly relate to pregnant women and their partners, needing to see more patients in less time, and needing to repeat the same normal pregnancy advice multiple times over the course of a day becomes tedious and frustrating. Enriching the work environment brings a new sense of satisfaction and pleasure. Group leaders voice their amazement at the "magic" that happens when the women engage each other. There is a powerful modeling of peer pressure and peer support, whether it is in a group's determination that babies should not be exposed to second-hand smoke, or making decisions about circumcision, discipline for the future, or whether or not to breastfeed, ideas that may not have been part of the lexicon but are now valuable constructs for new families.

"A Framework for Improving Health Equity" has been released by the Institute for Healthcare Improvement (IHI). It states, "A key concept in this framework is broadening the healthcare field's own sense of its mission and responsibility to reduce health inequities and disparities and appreciating that healthcare interventions are just one piece of the puzzle" (IHI, 2016, p. 82).

> *Dr. Art James, an obstetrician with special interest and expertise in health disparities and health equity, states that most health care is a downstream intervention trying to address many of the problems that occurred upstream. He sees Centering Healthcare™ as a midstream intervention that has the potential to deal with the upstream issues such as housing, segregation, unemployment, and unsafe neighborhoods. Involving interdisciplinary students and professionals in the workshops and in the implementation of group care has the potential to increase involvement in upstream issues. Many Centering sites already are active with Healthy Start, WIC (Women, Infants, and Children), and community programs focused on parenting, support for health challenges, and advocacy for improvement of community life.*

We have upstream/midstream/downstream discussions about what is and what could be. We scramble downstream, trying to deal with the health issues of heart disease and diabetes, much of which might have been prevented with mid/upstream initiatives. We struggle upstream to get communities to address issues of affordable housing, safe water, bike trails and playgrounds, adequate jobs, and drug and sex trafficking. Networks that connect social service agencies, business, and religious communities are also essential to improving health and health care. At times all of this seems insurmountable. The results of the CenteringPregnancy model on preterm births are strong and powerful. The savings in dollars, heartbreak, and pain are compelling reasons to implement this model. The additional values of strengthening young families, empowering parents to believe in their ability to parent wisely and well, and the growth of community bonds, while immeasurable in dollars and cents, have the capacity to change the future for children, families, cities, and states. A young couple who has learned to lean on each other, to seek help from others when needed, and to speak up when it is important has the capacity to speak up for quality childcare, better schools, and safer neighborhoods.

A clinician says, "I love the special relationship that forms between my patients and their support persons during groups while knowing all their physical, educational, and emotional needs are being met. Research shows women in Centering are less stressed, have a lower incidence of preterm delivery, and have more success with breastfeeding than those in regular care."

The CenteringPregnancy model is designed to include the means and supports to strengthen young families, empower new parents, protect the health and well-being of infants, and revitalize the clinical care for patients and providers. Realizations such as *when you get to know everybody you get to care about everybody* encourage active involvement in healthy community initiatives. The time is now to stand behind this transformative model. Our families, our clinicians, and society's health deserve our concerted efforts.

References

Alliman, J., Jolles, D., & Summers, L. (2015). The innovation imperative: Scaling freestanding birth centers, CenteringPregnancy, and midwifery-led maternity health homes. *Journal of Midwifery & Women's Health, 60*(3), 244–249.

Batalden, B., Batalden, P., Margolis, P., Seid, M., Armstrong, G., Opipari-Arrigan, L., & Hartung, H. (2015). Coproduction of healthcare service. *BMJ Quality & Safety*, 1–9. doi:10.1136/bmjqs-2015-004315

Braverman, P. (2014). What is health equity: And how does a life-course approach take us further toward it? *Maternal and Child Health Journal, 18*(2), 366–372. doi:10.1007/s10995-013-1226-9

Centers for Disease Control and Prevention. (2016). Pregnancy mortality surveillance system. Retrieved from www.cdc.gov/reproductivehealth/maternal infanthealth/pmss.html

Centers for Medicare and Medicaid Services. (2016, March 16). Strong start for mothers and newborns initiative: General information. Retrieved from https://innovation.cms.gov/initiatives/strong-start

Cheng, E., Rifas-Shiman, S., Perkins, M., Rich-Edwards, J., Gillman, M., Wright, R., & Taveras, E. (2016). The influence of antenatal partner support on pregnancy outcomes. *Journal of Women's Health, 25*(7), 672–679.

Childbirth Connection; Transforming Maternity Care. (2013). *Listening to mothers III: Pregnancy and birth: Report of the third national U.S. survey of women's childbearing experiences.* New York, NY: Author.

Declercq, E., Sakala, C., Corry, M., Applebaum, S., & Herrlich, A. (2014). Major survey findings of listening to mothers III: New mothers speak out: Report of national surveys of women's childbearing experiences conducted October–December 2012 and January–April 2013. *Journal of Perinatal Education, 23*(1), 17–24. doi:10.1891/1058-1243.23.1.17

Frey, C., Farrell, P., Cotton, Q., Lathen, L., & Marks, K. (2014). Wisconsin's life-course initiative for healthy families: Application of the maternal and child health life course perspective through a regional funding initiative. *Maternal and Child Health Journal, 18,* 413–422.

Gareau, S., Lopez-de Fede, A., Loudermilk, B., Cummings, T., Hardin, J., Pickklesimer, A., . . . Covington-Kold, S. (2016). Group prenatal care results in Medicaid savings with better outcomes: A propensity score analysis of centering pregnancy participation in South Carolina. *Maternal and Child Health Journal, 20*(7), 1384–1393. doi:10.1007/s10995-016-1935-y

Global Burden of Disease Collaborators. (2016). Measuring the health-related Sustainable Development Goals in 188 countries: A baseline analysis from the Global Burden of Disease Study 2015. *The Lancet, 388*(10053), 1813–1850. doi:10.1016/S0140-6736(16)31467-2

Hamilton, B., Martin, J., Osterman, M., Curtin, S., & Mathews, T. (2013). Births: Final data for 2013. *National Vital Statistics Reports, 62*(9). Retrieved from www .cdc.gov/nchs/data/nvsr/nvsr62/nvsr62_09.pdf

Handler, A., & Johnson, K. (2016). A call to revisit the prenatal period as a focus for action within the reproductive and perinatal care continuum. *Maternal Child and Health Journal.* doi:10.1007/s10995-016-2187-6

Heberlein, E., Picklesimer, A., Billings, D., Covington-Kolb, S., Ferber, N., & Frongillo, E. (2016). Qualitative comparison of women's perspectives on the functions and benefits of group and individual prenatal care. *Journal of Midwifery & Women's Health, 61*(2), 224–234. doi:10.1111/jmwh.12379

Ickovics, J., Kershaw, T., Westdahl, C., Magriples, U., Massey, Z., Reynolds, H., & Rising, S. S. (2007). Group prenatal care and perinatal outcomes: A randomized controlled trial. *Obstetrics & Gynecology, 11,* 330–339.

Ickovics, J., Kershaw, T., Westdahl, C., Rising, S., Klima, C., Reynolds, H., & Magriples, U. (2003). Group prenatal care and preterm birth weight: Results from a matched cohort study at public clinics. *Obstetrics & Gynecology, 102* (5, Pt. 1), 1051–1057.

Ickovics, J., Reed E., Magriples, U., Westdahl, C., Rising, S., & Kershaw, T. (2011). Effects of group prenatal care on psychosocial risk in pregnancy: Results from a randomised controlled trial. *Psychology and Health, 26*(2), 235–250.

Institute for Healthcare Improvement. (2016, May/June). A framework for improving health equity. *Healthcare Executive,* 82–85.

Institute of Medicine, Committee on Quality Health Care in America. (2001). *Crossing the quality chasm: A new health system for the 21st century.* Washington, DC: National Academy of Sciences.

Keckley, P. (2014, March 18). What do millennials want from the health care system? Retrieved from http://thehealthcareblog.com/blog/2014/03/18/what-do-millennials-want-from-the-healthcare-system

Krans, E., & Davis, M. (2012). Preventing low birthweight: 25 years, prenatal risk, and the failure to reinvent prenatal care. *American Journal of Obstetrics & Gynecology, 206*(5), 398–403.

Krans, E., & Davis, M. (2014). Strong start for mothers and newborns: Implications for prenatal care delivery. *Current Opinion in Obstetrics and Gynecology, 6,* 511–515. doi:10.1097/GCO.0000000000000118

Lu, M., & Johnson, K. (2014). Toward a national strategy on infant mortality. *American Journal of Public Health, 104*(S1), S13–S16. doi:0.2105/AJPH .2013.301855

Lu, M., Kotelchuck, M., Hogan, V., Jones, W. K., & Halfon, N. (2012). Closing the Black-White gap in birth outcomes: A life-course approach. *Ethnicity and Disease, 20*(1, Suppl. 2), S2-62–S2-76.

MacDorman, M., Hoyert, D., & Matthews, T. (2013). *Recent declines in infant mortality in the United States, 2005–2011.* NCHS data brief 120. Hyattsville, MD: National Center for Health Statistics.

March of Dimes. (2013). Long term health effects of premature birth. Retrieved from www.marchofdimes.org/complications/long-term-health-effects-of-premature -birth.aspx

McDonald, S., Sword, W., Eryuzlu, L., Neupane, B., Beyene, J., & Biringer, A. (2016). Why are half of women interested in participating in group prenatal care? *Maternal and Child Health Journal, 20*(1), 97–105. doi:10-1007/ s10995-015-1807-x

Merkatz, I., & Thompson, J. (1990). *New perspectives on prenatal care.* London, United Kingdom: Elsevier.

Osterman, M., & Martin, J. (2014). Primary cesarean delivery rates, by state: Results from the revised birth certificate, 2006–2012. *National Vital Statistics Reports, 63*(1). Retrieved from www.cdc.gov/nchs/data/nvsr/nvsr63/nvsr63_01 .pdf

Picklesimer, A., Heberlein, G., & Covington-Kolb, S. (2015). Group prenatal care: Has its time come? *Clinical Obstetrics and Gynecology, 58*(2), 380–391.

Rappleye, E. (2016, April). *Consumer Reports* rates hospitals on c-sections, finds 60% miss national mark. *Becker's HealthCare.* Retrieved from www.beckershospitalreview .com/quality/consumer-reports-rates-hospitals-on-c-sections-finds-60-miss-national-mark.html

Reid, A., Rosenthal, L., Earnshaw, V., Lewis, T., Lewis, J., Stasko, E., . . . Ickovics, J. (2016). Discrimination and excessive weight gain during pregnancy among Black and Latina young women. *Social Science & Medicine, 156,* 134–141.

Rising, S. S. (1998). CenteringPregnancy: An interdisciplinary model of empowerment. *Journal of Nurse-Midwifery, 43*(1), 46–54.

Rosen, M. G. (1989). *Caring for our future: The content of prenatal care. A report of the Public Health Service Expert Panel on the content of prenatal care.* Washington, DC: Public Health Service, Department of Health and Human Services.

Rosen, M. G., Merkatz, I., & Hill, J. (1991). Caring for our future: A report by the expert panel on the content of prenatal care. *Obstetrics & Gynecology, 77*(5), 782–787.

Rosenthal, E. (2013). American way of birth, costliest in the world. *New York Times*. Retrieved from http://www.nytimes.com/2013/07/01/health/american-way-of -birth-costliest-in-the-world.html?pagewanted=all&_r=0

Social Determinants of Health, Healthy People 2020. (2016). Retrieved from www .healthypeople.gov

U.S. Department of Health and Human Services. (2010). Rethinking MCH: The life course model as an organizing framework. Retrieved from http://mchb.hrsa.gov/ lifecourse/rethinkingmchlifecourse.pdf

Xu, X., Gariepy, A., Lundsberg, L., Sheth, S., Pettker, C., Krumholz, H., & Illuzzi J. (2015). Wide variation found in hospital facility costs for maternity stays involving low-risk childbirth. *Health Affairs*, 34(7), 1212–1219. doi:10.1377/ hlthaff.2014.1088

3 CenteringPregnancy® Group Care

Why do we limit ourselves so quickly to one idea or one structure or one perspective. Why would we stay locked in our belief that there is one right way to do something. We need more eyes to be wise. We have been invited to be part of the generative dance of life.—*Margaret Wheatley (2006, p. 73)*

This chapter explores the three CenteringPregnancy® group care components and the defining essential elements. In addition, it provides a visual representation of how group care actually works, discusses the space needed for CenteringPregnancy groups, and ends with a description of a CenteringPregnancy model designed for women with HIV.

What Is CenteringPregnancy?

And the day came when the risk to remain tight in a bud was more painful than the risk it took to blossom.—*Anais Nin*

Picture the current model of prenatal care. There are an expected number of visits, between 10 and 14, for the pregnant woman, starting in the first trimester and going through a postpartum visit. Initial intake may take more than one visit and include the following: nursing history, insurance assessment, laboratory tests, genetics testing, and enrollment in supplemental programs, maybe even a prenatal class. Then a return visit includes a physical exam and determination of risk status. Once in the system, the woman is scheduled for visits once a month for about 4 months and then every 2 weeks, or more frequently, depending on the medical monitoring needed.

A midwife arriving for a job interview sat in the prenatal clinic next to a woman who was waiting for her prenatal visit. The midwife, sitting in her heavy, winter coat noticed the clearly pregnant woman looking at her and then heard her say, "I see that you are here for your first prenatal visit. That's good because they will check you over to be sure that you are starting a healthy pregnancy. But then take it from me, don't come back until you are ready to deliver because nothing happens in the rest of the prenatal visits!"

These return visits become a routine consisting of collecting basic health data, a quick visit with the clinician, and any follow-up testing needed. Clinics struggle to have this time move efficiently, and clinicians find asking and answering the same questions over and over to be tiring, even boring. Patients experience crowded waiting rooms and

> "Imagine being escorted to a comfortable room, having refreshments, and spending that time in a pleasant, relaxed space with other pregnant women instead of sitting for hours in a crowded, noisy waiting area for a 5- or 10-minute visit with a harried care provider."

rushed individual visits. It's no fun for anyone. No wonder clinicians talk about burnout and patients skip visits.

Centering goes beyond standard definitions of prenatal care by promoting the concept that bringing women together in groups for care is quintessentially relationship-centered and honors the basic assumptions (see Chapter 2). The Pew-Fetzer task force report reinforces this concept by declaring that "the importance of the interaction among people is the foundation of any therapeutic or healing activity" (Health Professions Education and Relationship-Centered Care, 1994, p. 11). It further identifies relationship-centered care as "the vehicle for putting into action a paradigm of health that is focused on caring, healing, and community" (Health Professions Education and Relationship-Centered Care, 1994, p. 47).

There are many relationships within the care setting: (a) provider to patient, (b) provider to family, (c) provider to self, (d) care team to one other, and (e) patient to patient. In CenteringPregnancy the patient-to-patient relationship is at the core of the group cohesion and community building that supports and nurtures women through the childbearing experience.

I debated whether or not to put Sara in group. A recovering heroin addict, living in a residential treatment facility? How would the others react? I assured Sara she wouldn't need to share her story and invited her to join. People were startled when she blurted, during a discussion on nutrition, "They never give us fruit," but eyebrows really went high when she commented later, "We have lights out at 10." Before long, I heard "prison" being whispered around the circle, and I asked Sara if she'd be willing to tell her story. She explained everything—in vivid detail. As she finished, one of the women asked, "How do you get here?" "I take the train." "Let me and my husband drive you today." I don't worry any more whether a particular women will "fit" in a group—I know enough now to trust.

CenteringPregnancy is relationship-centered care that provides opportunities for a pregnant woman to interact meaningfully with her clinician, other women, her family, and her community (Klima, Norr, Vonderheid, & Handler, 2009; Massey, Rising, & Ickovics, 2006; Novick, 2004; Rising, 1998; Rising & Jolivet, 2009; Rising, Kennedy, & Klima, 2004; Rotundo, 2011/2012; Tanner-Smith, Steinka-Fry, & Lipsey, 2012). This care engages each woman and provides extended opportunity for her growth and development as a mother. Physiologic care monitoring is done in conjunction with the same clinician along with the opportunity for women to engage directly with their charts. The publication, "No Decision About Me Without Me," came out of the CenteringPregnancy's work in the United Kingdom that encourages responsible decision making by both the woman and her clinician. This wisdom is reflected in Centering care (Gaudion & Menka, 2010).

 "The providers didn't just give you medicine and not tell you what was wrong. Even if they tried to do that you had a chart there that told you what was wrong."

Relationship-centered prenatal care, the foundation for CenteringPregnancy, provides standard health care and, equally important, provides for interactive learning and community building. This design ensures that care includes all the usual assessments and occasional interventions as needed to help ensure the best possible outcomes for the mother and the baby. The exchange of information and conversation occurs in a format that is fun and that encourages open dialogue among all the members. To further support this effort, there is time within the group for participants to get to know one other. This structure leads to a building of community that may continue long after the pregnancy has ended. All three of these components of care—health care, interactive learning, and community building—happen within the group setting with a stable cohort of women who stay together through the 10 sessions of prenatal care.

Three Components of CenteringPregnancy

CenteringPregnancy has three major components: health care, interactive learning, and community building. Essential elements help to define each of these components. Fidelity to the model's structure is critical to its success (Novick et al., 2013). The elements below are specific to CenteringPregnancy prenatal care but equally applicable to any health population. They are also used to describe CenteringParenting® in Chapter 5.

Health Care

Health Assessment Happens in the Group Space

Within the group space is a private area for brief discussion between the woman and her provider; the actual belly check is done on a low table or mat. Music playing in the room enhances the privacy of this encounter. During this time, the clinician and woman review her health data and discuss any problems of a personal nature. General questions are brought to the group since many women are likely to have the same concern. This is what is viewed as the billable component of prenatal care since each woman has her own private assessment with the clinician.

One woman reported decreased fetal movement so we went down the hall to do a non-stress test. I asked two moms to bring her some sandwiches and juice. When I finished belly checks, I went to check on them. The test was reactive, and the three women were talking and relaxed. I said, "I'm glad the food made the baby perk up; you have passed the test." She replied, "Oh, I haven't eaten yet, we've just been talking!"

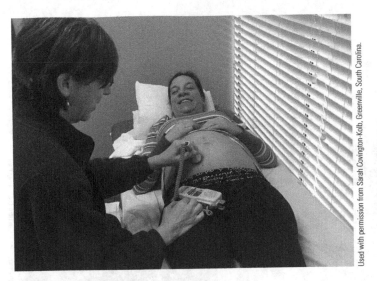

Assessment of mother and fetus.

Women Are Involved in Self-Care Activities

Each woman collects her own health data including weight, blood pressure, and gestational age. These data are recorded by her in her chart, electronic or paper, and also on her own progress record found in her CenteringPregnancy notebook. Each woman also has access to pertinent chart information, including results from lab and ultrasound testing. Before the formal "circle-up," she completes the self-assessment sheet for the session and revisits personal goals.

 "I learned to take my blood pressure. I thought only doctors could do that."—A teen mother

There Is Ongoing Evaluation

The site has set benchmarks for improvement and has a system to collect and record health outcomes. Regular view of their data assures the site that outcomes are improving through use of the group model. Data are also sent to the Centering Healthcare Institute's (CHI) CenteringCounts™ data system (or other central data bank) at regular intervals. This helps maintain site approval status with CHI and contributes to the aggregate data set maintained by this national organization. A minimum data set includes such items as number of group sessions attended, delivery method, baby gestation and birth weight, breastfeeding initiation, and return for postpartum visit.

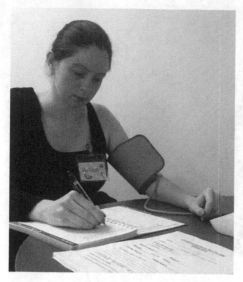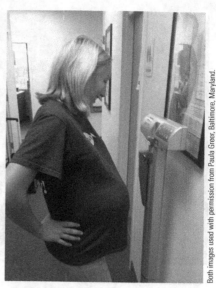

Both images used with permission from Paula Greer, Baltimore, Maryland.

Blood pressure assessment and charting, and self-assessment of weight.

Interactive Learning

Groups Are Facilitated to Be Interactive

Once the health assessment has been completed, participants join together in an open circle for discussion. The clinician and co-facilitator sit apart from each other in the circle. A circle opening such as, "Share one fun thing that happened to you this last week," helps start the discussion. Facilitators refer questions back to the group and encourage women to share from their own experience. Interactive activities help to discourage didactic presentations. Facilitators draw on the wisdom of the women in the group, sharing from

> "Group was a lot more enjoyable than sitting in a waiting room. We had personal, private time with the midwife and then shared our experiences, questions and concerns in group. I enjoyed being able to discuss discomforts and not being the only one experiencing them. I loved how personal our experiences became with one another. I learned so much. I will miss my group."

their own expertise as appropriate. Training sessions for all staff and providers who touch the group are essential to model skills needed for active listening. Facilitators also need to develop comfort with interactive strategies that encourage meaningful sharing among group members.

Groups Are Conducted in a Circle

To facilitate sharing and the ability to perform activities that may involve movement, the group meets in an open circle with no large table in the middle. Seating should be comfortable, either in chairs or on pillows on the floor. The space should be private, ideally with natural light. All people in the room should be seated within the circle so no one is thought to be an "observer." Extra chairs are removed so the circle has just enough seats. A circle "center" is encouraged to help focus attention. This could be a vase of flowers, a small table with a cloth and suitable centerpiece, or women could bring something special to them and place it in the center.

"I liked getting to know other women and sharing different opinions, the help and advice we exchanged was beautiful. I liked this format of prenatal care."

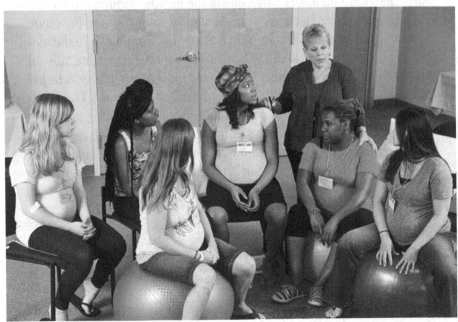

Informal sharing with the clinician.

Used with permission, Paula Greer, Baltimore, Maryland.

Each Session Has a Plan, But Emphasis May Vary

Both facilitators complete a Facilitator Process Evaluation at the close of each session. This helps the facilitators to prepare for the next session with such content as where the facilitators should sit to maximize group sharing, content areas that need further discussion, activities that might promote better group cohesion and sharing, and particular concerns about any group members. Before each session begins, the facilitators review their notes from the previous session. Needed supplies for the group are gathered. All participants have written materials in their own language. Pictures are used in some groups to help facilitate discussion. Improvement of health literacy is seen as one of the goals of CenteringPregnancy.

Particular sessions may need some formal discussion of content (e.g., genetics screening and flu vaccinations). Although the women take leadership in the discussion, there are several content threads that run through the 10 sessions. These threads include nutrition, breastfeeding, safe sex, stress management, exercise, preterm labor, and gestational diabetes. The facilitators hold the safety of accuracy and knowledge for the content of each group.

There were several couples in the Centering group who had met for several sessions. The clinician was "on the mat" doing a health assessment for one of the group members when one of the members entered the room and promptly started to cry. The co-facilitator (a nurse) and the group members gathered around her. When the young woman got to the mat for her assessment she said, "When I came into the room and saw all those guys with their partners it really hit me that my fellow is in jail and won't be there to be with me when the baby is born." The topics for the day were put on hold so we could spend time talking about the importance of support and ways that the group could reach out to this woman. It again emphasized to me the importance of not being alone and the power that the group can bring to undergird its members.

Group Size Is Optimal for Interaction

Group guidelines in appropriate languages are posted in the room, and written materials are available with translations as needed. Confidentiality is discussed and forms are signed and stored at the site. When a new member joins the group, confidentiality is again reviewed. Personal information shared with the group, stays with the group. Each woman is encouraged to share within the group, but there is never pressure for a woman to disclose beyond her comfort level.

Group facilitators do not wear lab coats or carry cell phones or pagers. While they are responsible for the ultimate safety of group members' knowledge, their behavior supports the concept that the women themselves are experts on what they need, have wisdom to share, and bring different perspectives to the group.

The optimal size for a Centering group is about 10 women. This number meets most productivity expectations and also provides time for each woman to share. Groups have been smaller than six and larger than 12 and have still been successful. Small groups generally aren't cost-effective and may be more likely to lead to didactic presentations if the women are hesitant to contribute. Large groups will take more time for individual assessment and also decrease the opportunity for each person to share. If partners or support people are present, they add to the complexity of the group.

> At the first session of a mixed group of women and their partners, a teen Hispanic dad said that he just couldn't talk in a group. By the fourth session one of the other dads pointed to him and asked him to be quiet so he could hear directly from his pregnant partner. This was a real "coming out" for him.

Community Building

Group Members, Including Facilitators and Support People, Are Consistent

The group cohort is stable throughout the many sessions. This isn't a therapy group with tight boundaries, but the group sharing, the information exchange, and the building of community happen best with the same group in attendance. Most sites find that the cohort firms up at about the third session, but a woman who arrives late to care often can still be added if there is room in the group and the members agree. Studies find that women who received most of their care in groups reported the highest level of satisfaction and the best outcomes (Cunningham et al., 2016; Ickovics et al., 2016).

> Many of our Centering groups have baby showers. Moms set the price and (like a secret Santa) buy a gift for the name they pull out of a hat. The English-speaking group prices usually are $5 to $10 while the Spanish group moms are much more lavish (could be $20 or more). The group leaders always have some extra items on hand in case someone forgets to bring a gift.

There is an opportunity in most groups for partners or support people to be part of the group. The woman's support person should be the same from session to session. Children are not to be present during the formal "circle-up" since this is a special time of sharing for the women and children cannot be counted on for confidentiality. Group leaders are very conscious of the Health Insurance Portability and Accountability Act (HIPAA) regulations that include confidentiality standards. Many sites make special provisions for childcare during Centering sessions.

At the second session of my first Centering group a woman arrived, thumping up the stairs, carrying a heavy backpack. Her blood pressure was elevated and remained so at the end of group. I asked her to wait while I finished up so I could escort her to the labor triage area to be checked. "I'm going now," she declared, getting ready to leave. "Do you know where it is?" I asked. "No, but I can find my way and I'm going to go now," she harrumphed, shouldering her pack. One of the other women came up to her. "You're in a group now. You don't have to go alone. I'm going with you." That was when I knew that group care was the way to go!

The continuity of care, provided by the same clinician and co-facilitator through the entire series of 10 sessions, helps to ensure that health care

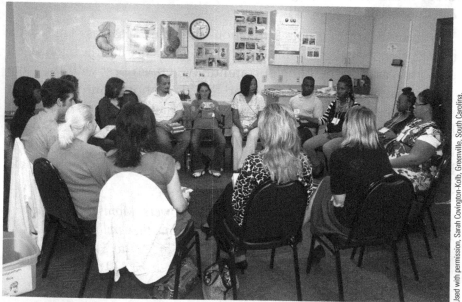

A group in session.

standards are met and that content threads are woven throughout the sessions. The setting also has backup in the event of an unexpected absence of one of the facilitators. Professional students who are part of the group are committed to attend all the sessions and also have appropriate supervision.

There Is Time for Socializing

The third component of the model, community building, calls for women to have opportunity for informal discussion and connection. Having fruit or other healthy snacks available and encouraging informal exchanges before and after the circle-up time, contribute to this, as does requiring nametags for all participants at each session. At one of the later groups, women could be invited to share their contact information to allow for continued interaction after delivery. In some sites, women set up a blog or other contact system for staying in touch. Since there is a stable cohort of women who meet together for the entire pregnancy, women get to know each other, reach out to those who need special attention, and form friendship bonds that often continue long after the pregnancy ends.

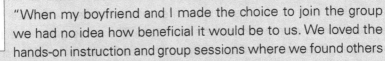

"When my boyfriend and I made the choice to join the group we had no idea how beneficial it would be to us. We loved the hands-on instruction and group sessions where we found others were going through exactly what we were. But the main thing the group gave us was our newfound friends. My fellow Centering mommies and I have a Facebook chat that dates back to when our babies were born. If you were to look through the messages you will see that we literally talk 24 hours a day, 7 days a week. We talk about life, babies, development, and even poop! Our babies are 5 months old and last night we all met for dinner. My boyfriend and I are so grateful to have those ladies and their husbands in our lives and we owe it all to CenteringPregnancy."

RAMONA

A Visual of the Group: How Does It Work?

Let's imagine how care in CenteringPregnancy will look for Ramona. Ramona is in early pregnancy and receiving care at a community health center near her neighborhood. She has had her prenatal intake that included her medical history, essential lab work, genetics testing options, and a physical exam. Her insurance status was reviewed and she was encouraged to sign up for Women, Infants, and Children (WIC).

The clinician and the nurse both encouraged her to join the CenteringPregnancy group that would be starting in 2 weeks for women with pregnancies of 12 to 16 weeks gestation. The staff said that she would be with 10 to 12 other women of similar due dates and would meet with these women for all 10 of her usual visits throughout pregnancy. The group takes 2 hours and starts and ends on time with no waiting in the waiting room. She is shown the group space and told to go directly there without stopping at the desk when she comes for her next visit in 2 weeks. Ramona thinks that not having to wait in the waiting room will be a welcome change. Most visits she waits for at least 30 minutes before being seen and then another 15 to 20 minutes in an exam room before her provider comes in and does a quick check.

Ramona now has arrived for her first CenteringPregnancy visit and she goes directly to the group room. A nurse (medical assistant), Louise, and a clinician, Jane, who will be her care provider throughout pregnancy, meet her there (midwife, physician, nurse). The room is attractively furnished with music playing and a table in the corner with food and water. She goes to a check-in table and joins two to three other women who also have just arrived and who are making their nametags. The nurse gives each mother a CenteringPregnancy notebook and shows each where to record the health data. She then shows them how to weigh themselves on the digital scale and how to take their blood pressure using a digital cuff. The women even help each other to get the cuff on easily. She is oriented to the body mass index (BMI) chart and helped to plot her current weight and height and set her own weight goal for pregnancy. The nurse helps each woman to use the gestational wheel to figure out her pregnancy weeks. Ramona is happy to understand the difference between weeks and months of pregnancy. Each woman then records all of her own data in her pregnancy notebook and also may record it directly in her paper or electronic chart. Ramona asked some questions about what her numbers mean and feels that already she has learned important things about her pregnancy.

The nurse, Louise, shares with them the other parts of the intake flow. They have a self-assessment sheet for each session in their notebook that will take a few minutes to complete. This activity provides Ramona with an opportunity to think about timely pregnancy issues. The sheets are personal for her, a tool to use with her partner and family, should she choose, and to share within the group . . . but there is no pressure to do so. The topics include such areas as common discomforts, breastfeeding, family dynamics, comfort measures for labor, emotional adjustment, and baby care.

Each woman has her own private, short assessment including a "belly check" and fetal heart tones with the clinician. This is the time for both of them to share particular concerns, many of which will be discussed in the group since they are common issues. Ramona notes that even though this assessment area is in the group space, because it is off in the corner and the mat is low, it feels absolutely private to her. Jane, the midwife, talks with her about her health data and personal concerns and says that she will be her care provider throughout her pregnancy. Ramona says that she will like having the same midwife every time.

There is a circle of chairs in the middle of the room and the nurse encourages Ramona to find a seat, look through her materials, and complete the self-assessment sheet for the day. Other women are also getting settled in the circle. Ramona hopes that she will feel comfortable in the group and that she will become friends with at least some of the women. She looks at the snack table, noticing that there is water, some fruit, and cheese/crackers. She asks the nurse if they can have a snack and the nurse invites all of them to have water and some food. This just reinforces Ramona's thoughts that this visit is very different from regular care and is starting out to be fun.

When all the mothers have checked in and been seen by the midwife, both the facilitators join the circle. They don't wear lab coats and they don't sit next to each other. Now there are nine other moms in the circle each wondering what will happen next. The midwife, Jane, welcomes them to the circle and asks them to find another person to talk with. In a minute, each mom will introduce her partner to the group. Since everyone has a name tag it is pretty easy to remember names and Ramona enjoys her partner, Ida, and easily introduces her to the group. Jane then goes over the general flow of the sessions and gives the women their 10 appointments that will take them to their due dates. The group meets at the same time and on the same day so this will make it easy for them to plan work schedules and childcare. The discussion around confidentiality is an important one and includes reasons why children should not be present during this talk time. There are group guidelines with reminders to shut off cell phones, to come on time, and to be respectful of each person's contributions. Part of this discussion usually includes the potential for bringing dads, partners, and friends to the group, especially to ascertain whether the women would be comfortable with having men in the group. Ramona thinks about her husband, Dave, and hopes that he will come with her to at least some of the sessions.

Jane and Louise work together to facilitate the discussion and start by talking about the importance of setting goals for this pregnancy. The women open the goals sheet in their pregnancy notebook and set two or three goals for the pregnancy. Ramona thinks that daily exercise and regular time for relaxation are important for her. She also makes a note that she wants to make time each day for Dave. The self-assessment sheet for the first session, "My Pregnancy: What's Most Important," focuses on topics that are most important to the group members. All the women identify "eating healthy for pregnancy and breastfeeding" as major interest areas so that leads into a discussion of nutrition. As part of this discussion the group is encouraged to share what they know about diabetes and why healthy eating might help prevent gestational diabetes.

Ramona enjoys playing a quick game that focuses on healthy food choices and important decisions around smoking, soft drinks, alcohol, over-the-counter drugs, and other possible toxic ingredients. As each mom pulls pictures out of a basket, all of the women talk about why a choice might be affirmative or negative. Ramona agrees with the other moms that she still has some important things to learn about having a healthy diet and staying away from items that might be bad for her and the baby.

Before she knows it the time is up and the nurse and clinician invite the group to stand, hold hands, and repeat these words: "I am a strong woman; I will eat well to stay healthy; I will do it!" The members continue to talk with each other as they leave, and several grab another snack to take along.

After the group leaves, Louise and Jane finish up charting and talk about the flow of the group. How did it go? What would have made it go better? What should be planned for the next session? Both of them comment on their own feelings about starting another group. Although there was work in the setup of the room, seeing the mothers get to know each other was a major benefit. Jane also comments that it felt good not to be rushed but to have time to really listen to the concerns of the women.

Space for Centering Groups

Space for Centering should feel like "a nest," a place to go to that feels safe, warm, comfortable, and private.

Imagine an ideal space. How big? It's square, at least 25 by 25 feet and located near an entrance or the parking area for accessibility. The room has a pleasant color scheme with murals or appropriate pictures. Since the room is used only for groups, it doesn't need constant setup/

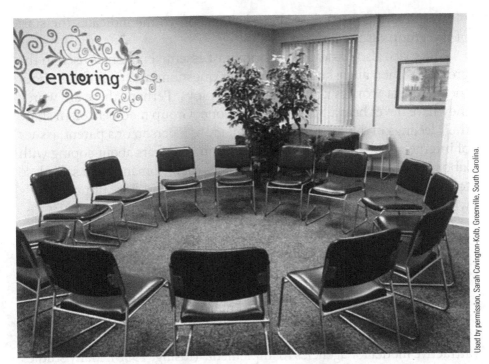

Centering group space. Note physical assessment area behind the "tree" in the back of the room.

takedown, therefore supporting efficiency of the model. There are windows with translucent curtains or other appropriate covering if privacy is an issue, and there is no window on the door.

There is a check-in area with a room for at least two women to sit and measure their blood pressure, a digital scale with an arm for weight check, and room on the table for any other materials such as gestational wheels, and so forth. The assessment area is in another part of the room. Here there is a low massage table or an inflatable mattress, a spot for the clinician to sit, and two large plants to provide privacy. The clinician sits or kneels at the level of the patient. There is music playing in the room to provide both atmosphere and white noise.

The majority of the room is composed of an open circle to hold up to 24 chairs or pillows. The middle of the circle is bounded by a round rug that frames a centerpiece that may change from session to session and could be flowers, a candle, a visual that pertains to the main focus of the day, for example, a plate of healthy food/snacks, a pedometer (some sites give one out), a large birthing ball, or perhaps a baby blanket. The two facilitators take seats across from each other and may decide ahead of time next to whom they should sit. A soft chime indicates the start of the group discussion.

The space also has room for storage of essential materials used in the group. Women are asked to freely offer questions and comments about their deepest worries as well as personal joys. Perhaps these are words they have never before shared with anyone. Group members often share their feelings of depression or inadequacy as a person or a parent, issues of interpersonal violence, cultural isolation, and fears about coping with labor or breastfeeding. The group provides each woman with a safe place to listen, develop strategies for herself, and test out her cultural beliefs without fear of being misunderstood. Peter Block notes:

> *Community is built when we sit in circles, when there are windows and the walls have signs of life, when every voice can be equally heard and amplified, when we all are on one level.* (2009, p. 151)

In the initial pilot of Centering, it was clear that women were very satisfied to get care in CenteringPregnancy groups. "The combination of satisfaction, good outcomes, and effective delivery of care makes this an attractive model for agencies to implement" (Rising, 1998). Many studies of the model have continued to document high satisfaction of women and clinicians with the model (Baldwin & Phillips 2011; Earnshaw et al., 2016; Grady & Bloom 2004; Ickovics et al., 2007; Klima, Norr, Vonderheid, & Handler, 2009; McDonald, Sword, Eryuzlu, & Biringer, 2014; McNeil et al., 2013; Teate, Leap, & Homer, 2012).

Mindy's Musings

We did the exercise where everyone writes down one thing from their family of origin that they thought was great and one thing from their family of origin that they did not think was great; everybody scrunches the paper, throws them on the floor, and popcorn style people pick them up and read them. Group consensus decides if it is going into the waste paper or this lovely other wicker basket. So most pretty cut and dried, there isn't a whole lot of conversation about it. Then someone uncurled this piece of paper that said, "My mother was more my best friend than my mother" that the group did not find so cut and dried. There was a lot of conversation about it, the group decided to toss it into the trashcan. There was another thing that talked about competition, to not bring so much competition among the siblings and to make their child so competitive. There was a woman who defended this as a great thing. The fact that there was a competitive spirit brought to her family made her feel like she was compelled to be the best she could be. And then one of the men said, "I so did not want to do this when my wife signed up for it, and I am so glad I did." He said his father brought competition to his children in everything as he grew up. He feels that he can never do anything well enough. He has talked with his wife about this and he is very worried that it's a legacy he is not going to know how to break. Now, what place in traditional care could a man say that? There is no room for men to process their concerns about parenting in traditional care. *If we don't think these discussions impact family well-being, we are mistaken.*—Mindy Schorr, MSN, CNM

Special Challenges

Pregnancy has always been a time of challenge, joy, and change. But few other eras have presented the challenges we see today faced by parents in the first part of the 21st century: new and strange illnesses such as HIV and Zika, underemployment, discrimination, food and housing insecurity all piling on top of the usual concerns facing young families (Gordon et al., 2016). New approaches are needed to be confident, supported 21st-century parents, not focused on fear but on possibility. CenteringPregnancy provides the opportunity for parents to explore their deep concerns and receive validation as well as concrete solutions that will help them navigate these new waters. The following reflection describes one such group model focused on the particular health issue of HIV and pregnancy.

Reflections From a Clinician: CenteringPregnancy and HIV

Judy Levison, MD, MPH

Dr. Judy Levison recalls being at a CenteringPregnancy workshop when it was like a "light bulb went on . . . and I got it! If women attend all the Centering sessions, they will get what they need to know. We realized we had at least one HIV-related topic we could introduce into each of the 10 sessions."

Groups were started in the fall of 2013. During the second year, the program got a nutrition grant from the Harris County Hospital District Foundation to purchase ingredients for healthy snacks such as peanut butter and banana sandwiches; black bean, corn and red pepper salad; and vegetables in a yogurt-based dip. With this grant, the program could provide a snack with its recipe at each visit, the women could take ingredients home with them, and they got a cookbook at graduation. One woman said, "I never would have bought red peppers before." Judy prepares the snack ahead of time and laughs, "How many people can say their obstetrician cooks for them!" Starting in 2016, the local food bank is partnering with them by providing 30 to 40 pounds of fresh produce combined with shelf-stable items such as peanut butter, canned chicken, lentils, and whole grain pasta.

One of the important outcomes of the group is to make sure that the women are actively involved with their primary care clinician when the pregnancy ends. An asset will be the establishment of CenteringParenting, which will keep the groups together for another 1 to 2 years. Judy says, "In traditional care our HIV positive women define themselves as having HIV, but in Centering groups women define themselves as being pregnant and, by the way, having HIV. I couldn't think of a better outcome."

Judy Levison, MD, MPH, is a professor in the Department of Obstetrics and Gynecology at Baylor College of Medicine in Houston, Texas.

Here are two stories that help with further understanding the power of the model. The first is told by a midwife who facilitated this group. The second is told by the mother herself.

From a Group Facilitator: Monica's Centering Experience

Monica and her husband moved to our state from Honduras, found jobs and a place to live, became pregnant, and joined one of our CenteringPregnancy groups.

They planned to send money home and finally bring their other two children to the States, but Monica lost her job and her husband left her. During a discussion on support, Monica explained that she was living with strangers and our group was her only support.

Unbeknownst to the midwife, the women in group decided to have a surprise shower for Monica at our next session. They arrived at that session with a lovely stroller, other small gifts, and some cash, only to learn that Monica was in the hospital with pregnancy complications. After group, they packed up their shower supplies and carpooled to her hospital room.

Following the birth of her healthy, full-term baby, Monica became roommates with one of the other single moms in the group, who also found employment for her at her workplace. The group saved Monica.

Emily's Centering Experience

"I was surprised to find that sharing such an intimate experience as pregnancy with a small group of people was more comforting and holistic than I had anticipated. It took more than one session to feel comfortable and at ease with the group dynamic, but we gelled and it worked and I can't imagine not having had that experience now. We laughed and cried together, we shared pieces of parenting and labor experiences, we gave each other positive encouragement and well wishes to find what worked for us as individuals, and it was incredible. It felt good to feel like I had a group of people in my corner. I wasn't just a name on a file, and I wasn't waiting by myself in an exam room, I was with real people who shared pieces of themselves with me for almost an entire year."

These stories demonstrate a strong alternative to the traditional care model that has driven our health system as long as any of us can remember. It presents an answer to many of the issues raised in Chapter 2. Mother/baby health outcomes are far from what we should be seeing despite the investment of enormous dollars. CenteringPregnancy data affirms that this model of group prenatal care will do just that—better outcomes for lower cost. "What's the question? Centering may be the answer!"

References

Baldwin, K., & Phillips, G. (2011). Voices along the journey: Midwives' perceptions of implementing the CenteringPregnancy model of prenatal care. *Journal of Perinatal Education, 20*(4), 210–217.

Block, P. (2009). *Community: The structure of belonging*. San Francisco, CA: Berrett-Koehler.

Cunningham, S., Grilo, S., Lewis, J., Novick, G., Rising, S., Tobin, J., & Ickovics, J. (2016). Group prenatal care attendance: Determinants and relationship with care satisfaction. *Maternal and Child Health Journal.* doi:10.1007/s10995-016-2163-3

Earnshaw, V., Rosenthal, L., Cunningham, S., Kershaw, T., Lewis, J., Rising, S.,... Ickovics, J. (2016). Exploring group composition among young, urban women of color in prenatal care: Implications for satisfaction, engagement, and group attendance. *Women's Health Issues, 26*(1), 110–115.

Gaudion, A., & Menka, Y. (2010). No decision about me without me: Centering-Pregnancy, *Practicing Midwife, 13*(10), 15–18.

Gordon, D., Campbell, C., Washington, K., Albritton, T., Divney, A., Magriples, U., & Kershaw, T. (2016). The influence of general discrimination and social context on young urban expecting couples' mental health. *Journal of Child and Family Studies, 25,* 1284–1294. doi:10.1007/s10826-015-0313-5

Grady, M., & Bloom, K. (2004). Pregnancy outcomes of adolescents enrolled in a CenteringPregnancy program. *Journal of Midwifery & Women's Health, 49*(5), 412–420.

Health Professions Education and Relationship-Centered Care. (1994). *Pew-Fetzer Task Force on Advancing Psychosocial Health Education.* San Francisco: University of California.

Ickovics, J., Earnshaw, V., Lewis, J., Kershaw, T., Magriples, U., Stasko, E.,... Tobin, J. (2016). Cluster randomized controlled trial of group prenatal care: Perinatal outcomes among adolescents in New York City health centers. *American Journal of Public Health, 106*(2), 359–365.

Ickovics, J., Kershaw, T., Westdahl, C., Magriples, U., Massey, Z., Reynolds, H., & Rising, S. (2007). Group prenatal care and perinatal outcomes: A randomized controlled trial. *Obstetrics & Gynecology, 110*(2, Pt. 1), 330–339.

Klima, C., Norr, K., Vonderheid, S., & Handler, A. (2009). Introduction of CenteringPregnancy in a public health clinic. *Journal of Midwifery & Women's Health, 54*(1), 27–34.

Massey, Z., Rising, S., & Ickovics J. (2006). CenteringPregnancy group prenatal care: Promoting relationship-centered care. *Journal of Obstetric, Gynecologic, and Neonatal Nursing, 35*(2), 286–294.

McDonald, S., Sword, W., Eryuzlu, L., & Biringer, A. (2014). A qualitative descriptive study of the group prenatal care experience: Perceptions of women with low-risk pregnancies and their midwives. *BMC Pregnancy and Childbirth, 14,* 334.

McNeil, D., Vekyed, M., Dolan, M., Siever, J., Horn, S., & Tough, S. (2013). A qualitative study of the experience of CenteringPregnancy group prenatal care for physicians. *BMC Pregnancy and Childbirth, 13*(1), S6.

Novick, G. (2004). CenteringPregnancy and the current state of prenatal care. *Journal of Midwifery & Women's Health, 49*(5), 405–411.

Novick, G., Reid, A., Lewis, J., Kershaw, T., Rising, S., & Ickovics, J. (2013). Group prenatal care: Model fidelity and outcomes. *American Journal of Obstetrics & Gynecology, 209,* 112e1–112e6.

Rising, S. S. (1998). CenteringPregnancy: An interdisciplinary model of empowerment. *Journal of Nurse-Midwifery, 43*(1), 46–54.

Rising, S. S., & Jolivet, R. (2009). Circles of community: The CenteringPregnancy group prenatal care model. In R. Davis-Floyd, L. Barclay, B. A. Daviss, & J. Tritten (Eds.), *Birth models that work* (pp. 365–384). Berkeley: University of California Press.

Rising, S. S., Kennedy, H., & Klima, C. (2004). Redesigning prenatal care through CenteringPregnancy. *Journal of Midwifery & Women's Health, 49*(5), 398–404.

Rotundo, G. (2011/2012). CenteringPregnancy: The benefits of group prenatal care. *Nursing for Women's Health, 15*(6), 508–518.

Tanner-Smith, E., Steinka-Fry, K., & Lipsey, M. (2012). *A multi-site evaluation of the CenteringPregnancy programs in Tennessee.* Nashville, TN: Vanderbilt University. Retrieved from https://my.vanderbilt.edu/emilytannersmith/files/2012/02/Contract19199-GR1030830-Final-Report.pdf

Teate, A., Leap, N., & Homer, C. (2013). Midwives: Experiences of becoming CenteringPregnancy facilitators: A pilot study in Sydney, Australia. *Women and Birth, 26*(1), e31–e36. Retrieved from http://dx.doi.org/10.1016/j.wombi.2012.08.002

Tresolini, C. P., & the Pew-Fetzer Task Force. (2000). Health professions education and relationship-centered care. San Francisco, CA: Pew Health Professions Commission.

Wheatley, M. (2006). *Leadership and the new science.* San Francisco, CA: Berrett-Koehler.

4 Why Circles Work

*A circle is essentially a gathering of equals . . . an energetic social
container capable of helping a group draw on wellsprings of insight,
information, and story that inspire collective wisdom and action.*
—*Baldwin and Linnea (2010, p. xvi)*

This chapter illustrates how a Circle/Centering model may impact and
even improve the quality of life for new parents. Circles of the past,
as well as group theory, inform ways in which groups work to create
community and comfort. The chapter ends with a series of stories focusing on how parents and groups dealt with unexpected outcomes of
the pregnancy in ways that resulted in aid and comfort.

Giving birth stands alone as a transformational experience. For each
woman and her family, birth overflows with emotions that are personal, many
so intimate that only some may be shared. Even the news of an upcoming
birth can bring joy—coupled with ambivalence, hope, anticipation, and even
fear. At the same time, this experience unites partners, families, and friends
who can share in the miracle of welcoming a new child into their circle.

Women are affiliative by nature, and this becomes particularly true of
pregnant women who want to share their pregnancies with others in the
same situation. Pregnant women have questions and are eager to know
how other women think, feel, and react to the process of giving birth;
they want to know what foods to eat, how much to exercise, how long
to work, and what method of birth control to use in the future. There
may be new conversations with mothers, grandmothers, siblings, and
friends, which may be interesting or confusing. Old wives' tales and
superstitions persist despite reams of new information on social media.

Most first-time mothers and their partners realize that giving birth means that they will begin making decisions for another human being. Dilemmas ranging from choosing genetic testing to where to give birth may overwhelm new parents, while the choosing of names can be fun. Important choices seem never to end for parents-to-be, who must choose methods of feeding, as well as understand and process the implications of various feeding methods. Myriad cultural and familial expectations for child rearing are processed and discussed. Each of these choices is a decision made on behalf of the newly born, taking parents into daunting new territory.

RAMONA

Ramona thought about her group experience during the month between her first and second sessions. Her time in the Centering circle was her first real group experience outside of getting together with friends and she wondered whether she would get to know any of these women really well. She was a bit anxious about sharing in the circle that first session, and she was careful not to say anything that might embarrass her or anyone else. One of the women, Lisa, lived in her neighborhood and Ramona thought she would try to sit by her at the next session.

Parents Need Centering Circles

For expectant and new parents, experiences surrounding birth can lead to powerful personal and interpersonal changes. Mothers and partners benefit from processing these events—and their own thoughts and feelings—in the company of other new parents.

Both the primary partner and the birth mother feel the strains of new roles and multiple task alignments. Some fathers and partners in group circles have debated the wisdom of staying home with babies, while some others questioned the safety of staying on the job as policemen or fire fighters because suddenly life seems more vulnerable. Giving up her sports car became a major focal point for one partner, anticipating the need for a baby car seat. Most partners feel, and articulate, an increase in anxiety that comes with the loss of a known lifestyle and with its replacement: an unknown future and a tangible fear of losing the new mother's attention.

When pregnant couples gather in Centering circles, they may find much in common. One researcher observed the impact of being in a circle: "Listening, witnessing, role-modeling, reacting, deepening, laughing, crying, grieving, drawing upon experience, and sharing the wisdom of experience. . . . Women in circles support one another and discover themselves, through talk" (Bolen, 1999, p. 14). These are the observations of Dr. Jean Bolen, a psychiatrist with decades of work with women's circles. Bolen suggests that when interaction leads to change for members in the group, a "tipping point" may be reached for people in the group. The "Hundredth Monkey" allegory suggests that at the tipping point, a critical number of people change how they think and behave, so that eventually the changes become normalized.

Circles in Our Past

Circles, as structured groups where participants discuss common concerns, have long been recognized as an effective and productive method for sharing ideas, forming allegiances, improving quality of life, and strengthening communities. Anthropologists and archaeologists have traced ancient interactions through records of circle-based villages. Cave walls show circles of connectedness and family. Also, remains of Native American camps and villages often are structured in concentric circles around a central totem or ceremonial fire. Ancient fire circles drew people together for heat, food, and companionship. In these circles they were educated and socialized by people about whom they cared. Joseph M. Marshall III was raised on the Rosebud Indian Reservation in South Dakota. He has written: "The greatest principle the circle symbolizes for me is the equality that applies to all forms of life. In other words, no one form of life is greater or lesser than any other form. . . . And we all share a common journey . . . the Circle of Life" (2001, p. 225).

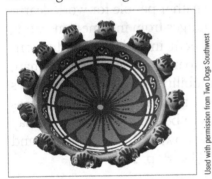

Bowl from Zuni representing women in a talking circle.

Used with permission from Two Dogs Southwest Gallery, Chandler, Arizona.

Theorists and psychologists see and explain the world—including political, social, and spiritual dimensions—as concentric spiritual circles. Circles have long indicated that the members share some special communication and that all members share rights to contribute and to be listened to, with needs respected.

Circles in Daily Life

Today's circle groups, though rarely labeled as such, are familiar parts of daily life in the 21st century. On any given day, community members share pleasures by learning in book groups, studying new fields in adult education programs, and building team skills in schools, colleges, and corporate think tanks. Many group circles support personal behavior change and coping skills, with networks of circles growing to involve millions of people in successful nationwide programs such as Alcoholics Anonymous, Al-Anon, and Weight Watchers. Religious groups also can be powerful forces for dealing with issues of concern to the community.

Circles have a well-earned reputation for supporting personal empowerment. By respecting one another in conversation and learning from others' experiences and knowledge, members of a circle share goals, solve problems, and take on serious commitment to the purposes of the group (Thompson, 2011). No one individual in the group stands out or stands alone.

Around the world, circles are used to gather people for work, learning, pleasure, and problem solving that ranges from income-generating lending circles for community development in India to production-improvement circles in Fortune 500 companies (Lawler & Mohrman, 1985). Seniors and people with limited mobility often credit their circles with being sustaining forces in their lives. Christina Baldwin emphasizes that "The circle as social practice asks us to be willing to arrive, to pay attention, to speak as clearly as we know how, and to help action and accomplishment arise out of the group" (1998, p. 221).

▪ Centering Healthcare With Indigenous Communities

Indigenous ancestors understood that the powers of the universe work in circles. Using the power of the circle, CenteringPregnancy® is an innovative example of a social and cultural context within which public health messaging and health literacy can be increased. It's extremely difficult to change people's behavior. CenteringPregnancy offers an innovative social and cultural environment in which people can make decisions about personal health behaviors with peer support along with medical assessment, improving access to health literacy.—Katsi Cook, Mohawk midwife

Work with several tribal sites across the country has occurred through Indian Health Service (IHS) and also through direct contract with some of the sites. Even though circle work is part of Indian culture, the implementing of a new care model that happens in circles still is unfamiliar. Katsi Cook, elder Mohawk midwife and researcher, shares the following thematic analysis of a series of 18 focus groups conducted in six tribes of the Northeast resulting in a set of recommendations that support a systems shift in how prenatal care is delivered in tribal communities:

- Nurture initiatives that empower women, especially within the context of reproductive health and childbearing.
- Encourage and build on community social support, increase community interaction and cohesion, and diminish social isolation.
- Increase the capacity for tribal members to develop community-led and culture-based initiatives.
- Increase the knowledge of community members and public health staff in communications concepts regarding age-appropriate human sexuality.
- Provide trustworthy cultural resources to help guide the integration of conscientious cultural knowledge.

Several clinicians working at tribal sites contributed their experiences with CenteringPregnancy to a discussion of implementation of the model at their locations.

CenteringPregnancy provides a powerful social and cultural construct within which tribal families can achieve public health goals using the strengths of our kinship networks.—IHS clinician

While all felt that CenteringPregnancy was a good fit for care provision, they mentioned common implementation issues, such as frequent staff turnover, that present challenges. Sites mentioned that already their data are showing better breastfeeding, with one site having 99% initiation, a decrease in cesarean births, and fewer patients with anemia. Another mentioned that women are coming to the health center earlier and continuing to get prenatal care at the center, which is increasing their numbers.

The democratization of public health knowledge and building trusty bridges to Indigenous ways of knowing and being are critical to establishing culturally safe and structurally sound systems of wellbeing and health in Indigenous communities.—Katsi Cook, Mohawk midwife

Tribal elders are often involved with the model, with some being co-facilitators. In one site, the clinic nurses commented that they had never heard native women laugh the way that they do in the Centering groups. The women develop close relationships with each other, "this is really neat . . . they are going to be friends for life." One site has many mothers who continue on with CenteringParenting®. Some of the patients now are interested in becoming nurses and midwives. Many of the groups have dads and grandmothers involved. Grandmothers, in particular, are happy to have this model available for their daughters. Tribal customs are still shared, and in some sites the women make cradle boards and talk about special traditions that include the placenta and cord.

The model also has helped the staff get out of silos and talk with each other about how they can support the women and make the groups better. As one clinician noted, "The different entities that are working together have to depend on each other. That's exciting. It's clear that people really care."

An IHS midwife shares, a 42-year-old woman experiencing her seventh pregnancy came in for care. She was a long-term drug user who never delivered past 32 weeks and had all babies removed from her care. The staff said, "She's not right for Centering," but the woman came anyway. She was outspoken in the group but also shared her story. She stayed clean for the whole pregnancy, came to all visits, delivered at term, kept her baby and then continued on in CenteringParenting. We saw her blossom. Now she is getting visitation rights for her other children. An amazing story.—IHS clinician

Circle Theory in a Nutshell

In a circle, silence is accepted and all members are assumed to have equal ownership and authority. Circle structures upset the balance of power often experienced by patients in a traditional model of medical care—where the patient is undressed and seated, while the provider stands alongside in a white coat. In a Centering circle, members have expertise about their own lives. They may consider ways in which they want to emulate or change the behaviors of their parents.

"Talking with other women makes you think about all the issues you hadn't thought about yet or were too embarrassed to mention."

During circle conversations, participants dig deep. They bring forth memories, some of which are sweet and tender—bedtime stories, after school snacks, family movie nights, and so forth. Other contributions may be harsh or painful—from being ignored or being rebuked without a chance to explain, from spankings to impossibly high expectations. The group members hold these thoughts, and as they listen to each other, they begin to imagine a gentler way, more loving and tender, toward this baby they are carrying. The clinician and co-facilitator are members of the group, "holding" the comments and occasionally sharing from their own experiences. Their guidance provides a boundary of safety for all participants.

The women began an animated discussion about eating starch. "What kind of starch do you eat?" A woman put her box on the table. "I used to eat starch and now I eat clay," responded another. "Where do you get your clay?" "Well, I used to eat starch but now I eat dirt." This exchange challenged the clinician to avoid a knee-jerk response and instead listen carefully and then prompt a discussion focused on the nutritional and cultural challenges posed by pica.

Lifting Up Women in Need

Young and poor women who may have limited education are often not in the habit of speaking their mind, being respected for their experience and knowledge, or of speaking their truth to medical providers. The Centering Circle provides a powerful opportunity to experience a model of care that can be life changing. Here in this circle, they can "try on" new behaviors, such as experiment with saying aloud what they like or dislike and what they need and want during their pregnancy.

In the group, each woman is ensured the opportunity to question and clarify what she reads or hears from the media and from others in her family and social circle. Facilitators learn to be sensitive to differences in the group.

Circles change the power dynamic from one of all-knowing experts to something new: a shared exploration of what works, for whom, and how. Circles offer women room for exploration of options not common in their life experience. Participation in such circles expands the potential for growth on both personal and community levels. These safe circles provide opportunities to clarify thinking and practice asking for what is needed. Women in circles see models of behavior they haven't experienced at home, school, or work.

Centering groups can explore solutions to problems, try new strategies, discuss outcomes, and support peers in taking new and difficult steps such as talking to a partner about what feels abusive or hurtful, or telling the women in her life she *does* plan to breastfeed, or trying new techniques to stop smoking. These exercises become powerful determinants for future action. Simply attempting to motivate someone to eat "better" does little to overcome the inertia that prevents change, but sharing culturally appropriate recipes with suggestions and ideas

"When I hear other women in the group say something I have heard my wife say a hundred times but I didn't take seriously, I get a wake-up call."

of where to shop and how to cook is an action step that does change behavior.

Partners too share by frequently bringing an important question or issue into the discussion. Watching other men struggle with positioning exercises, or being unsure of how they feel about circumcision, can be very helpful.

Mindy's Musings

I love the satisfaction of the women. But to be perfectly honest, *it is the satisfaction of the men that gets to me.* And we have had female partners too. In individual care, a good partner shows up at visits but doesn't speak much. He is just totally there and supportive of his wife. There is no place in individual care for a man to say, "I am really scared about this." or "I cannot imagine how this is going to happen." or "My family thinks this. . . . Your family thinks this. . . . What do you think? How do you think?"

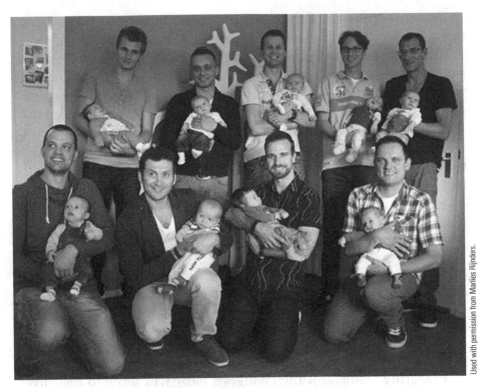

Used with permission from Marlies Rijnders.

Dads and their babies in a Netherlands Centering Group.

There is no room for a man's process about becoming a father in prenatal care. Not in prenatal care, not at the birth . . . we reinforce that men are supposed to be selfless and needless and not in touch. And *Centering gives men an opportunity to actually be in touch with this momentous time in their own life. What might be coming up for them?*—Mindy Schorr, MSN, CNM

The Power of Story

Stories matter more than we understand. Stories are prayers of terrific power, we are collections of stories, we are vast houses in which stories come and go. If we don't listen for them, and share them, then we have nothing . . . stories are how we live, and stories are compasses and lodestars. (Doyle, 2013, p. 35)

Many pregnant women are "cognitive copers" who want answers to all the questions real and imagined. The lives of American women in the second decade of the 21st century are models of multitasking, managing work, family, study, and then 3- to 5-minute prenatal visits. For the provider of care, the pressure to see women in shortened time slots is intense, as is the need to repeat information and document all interventions. Engaging women to commit to a CenteringPregnancy group can be most challenging. Taking the time for a 2-hour session may seem like an extravagant amount of time for a health visit for working women. "Can't we make these visits shorter? I don't have this kind of time." And yet, the comments of women who join the group frequently include: "Are we done already? I wish we could have more talk time." It's not unusual to see women leave arm in arm, perhaps with a plan to have lunch or a snack together.

 "We came at the same time and left at the same time and something happened the whole time we were there."

Preparing women for the changes a baby will bring to their lives requires hearing shared experiences as well as time to think and discuss issues realistically with others who are facing the same challenges. All too often, the recommendations to rest when the baby sleeps and decrease expectations after nights of interrupted sleep fall on deaf ears as new mothers visualize an early return to work, a contented baby, and a clean house, or perhaps wonder how they will change beliefs of family members who remember "how it used to be." A major example from such discussions is that infants no longer should sleep on their stomachs, but rather now sleep on their backs and in their own beds.

While narratives can frequently be used to reenforce stereotypes, they are also powerful sources of personal affirmations reminding us of our better selves, our ability to change and grow, and our enormous resourcefulness and strength. For example, women who face family members who do not believe in breastfeeding hear each other share stories of pleasure and success, combined with the benefits to the baby of breastfeeding, find within themselves a new strength to pursue and persevere in their desire to do the same. Such experiences also help build a sense of adequacy (Ochs, Taylor, Rudolph, & Smith, 1992).

Partners Reflect on Centering

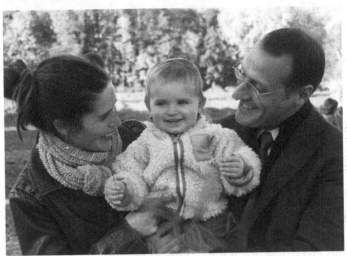

Used with permission from Matthew Houde.

Matthew and Sarah are a young, professional couple who live in New Hampshire and participated in a CenteringPregnancy group.

S: The beginning was always informal, and it gave us a little time to warm up. The chance to put ideas on a board about things that you wanted to have addressed during the session was like a little warm-up where we got something done and got fed. What stood out for me about group was being able to develop a relationship over the course of a pregnancy, which is huge to have somebody there with you for the duration. I liked the space a lot. I loved that there were snacks. I loved that you had some control over getting your own data. It made me feel more in control or more a part of what was actually being measured.

M: I think in a group setting, all of these different parents bring different ideas and questions; often in a quick hospital visit you don't have the ability for discussion or things don't always come up. In group, you have all these people who are reading different things and thinking about different things and they're able to articulate questions and get other questions that may not have been in your consciousness but they bring them to the forefront. That was awesome. . . . The biggest challenge during this pregnancy for me was the discovery of my wife's hypertension. It raised the specter of worrying about two people as opposed to one.

I think the unknowns of pregnancy in general were sort of a bit unsettling. . . . Then we got into a Centering group, and it made a great deal of difference. At the beginning of each group the women would take their own blood pressure and weigh themselves, the midwife would listen for the fetal heart beat and ask how we were doing. And then we'd come together and discuss whatever was on the agenda for that day . . . . I didn't have the same aversion to medical institutions that Sarah did, and it was important to me that she find a grounding that she was comfortable with . . . and Centering unquestionably provided that. We were at a major medical center teaching hospital, and as a result we saw a different midwife each time we went into the hospital.

S: I think it's like finding a therapist. You need to find, or you hope to find, somebody you relate well with.

M: In our group, everyone was partnered and that was terrific. It really mattered to be able to share my thinking with other men. The men got together outside of group, too, just to share our thoughts about what was coming. You don't know what to expect until you do this. I'd love to have had a session where there were several new parents just to talk about the challenges they faced.

S: I think having an infant can be very isolating, and it would have been won-derful to have Centering continue with a group of parents who are going through the same thing. I would have jumped at that opportunity.

M: We would do Centering again in a heartbeat.

Why Circles?

How can a circle of care achieve the intimacy, knowledge, and personal characteristics of high-quality medical care and supervision that often seem possible only in a one-on-one relationship with a health care provider? Groups exist and are formed to help people achieve goals that would be either unattainable by individuals alone or far more difficult to accomplish solo. The reflection and discussion brought by others to the group help members grow in knowledge and strength that will help them meet the common challenges they face. In facilitated groups in Centering, reflection and discussion revolve around mutual needs and expectations of the pregnant women, partners, and facilitators.

All groups experience similar phases in their development over the course of their existence. Members typically experience feelings of uncertainty, mistrust, anxiety, and stress during the initial stage of group development. Group members tend to avoid conflict and direct confrontation and may look for ways to provide support for each other. Individual group members must each find a place to fit in with one another. At the same time, individual members are also deciding on their identities within the group and the amount of interaction, or involvement and communication, they wish to have with the other group members. Group members frequently deal only with safe, familiar, and noncontroversial topics and attempt to conceal their feelings and personal concerns during the initial phase of group development.

Group learning is best accomplished in a cohesive group that has shared goals that are articulated by the members with guidance from the facilitators. The women are also encouraged to set personal goals that focus on challenges they see as personally important, such as improving their nutrition, getting more exercise, and focusing on stress reduction. Group activities have been designed to support women as they work on these goals over the 10 sessions. The group facilitators and group members formulate a contract together that clarifies such norms as prompt starting and ending of group, the importance of confidentiality, mutual respect, shutting off cell phones and pagers, and sharing talking time.

Confidentiality underscores the group contract and helps to build the trust and comfort of group members. It allows people to speak more

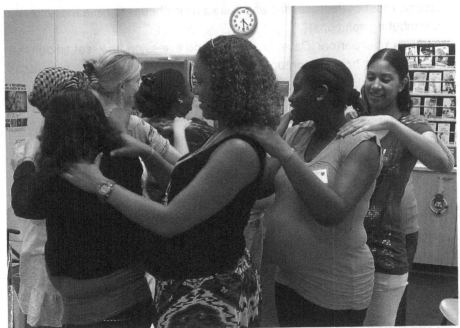

Netherlands Centering Circle.

Used with permission from Marlies Rijnders.

freely about personal and intimate issues, assures them they will not be discussed outside the group, and provides a safe arena for trying new ideas and changing their minds as they assimilate new information. As Baldwin notes in her seminal work on Peerspirit Circles, the circle allows women to "listen, sort, and speak without having to be right." Someone else's opinion doesn't make her opinion right or wrong. It's just different (1998, p. 221).

RAMONA

As her pregnancy progressed, Ramona continued to reflect on the group, its members, and the interaction with the facilitators. Lisa had become a friend, and they regularly met at the local community center between the group sessions to talk and participate in an exercise program offered by the center. Their partners attended the sessions as often as possible and were also providing support to each other around their anxieties of parenting. Ramona also realized that she was comfortable sharing more personal thoughts and concerns with the group. The open dialogue within the group and comments of the other members helped her to relax about her own concerns. She remembered one woman saying, "We each have issues, most of them similar, and it is so much better to have many heads contributing solutions!"

When her partner, Dave, couldn't attend a session, they set aside time to talk about how the group went, especially any new content or ideas that were helpful to her. Together, they looked through the Centering-Pregnancy notebook, and occasionally she shared her thoughts related to the self-assessment sheet for the session. Ramona was happy that their communication was improving and both of them were feeling more excitement about their coming baby.

As group development evolves, the members find that their comfort with the process, and with each other, allows them to make progress in their learning. In a CenteringPregnancy group, the learning follows a natural plan as women bring up important issues that also coincide with the stages of pregnancy. This stage is often the most enjoyable for group members since they feel a part of the group and know what is expected of group members. There are few barriers to communication, and the behavior of the members is purposeful and constructive.

The end of a Centering group usually brings a multitude of emotions. Women and their partners are grateful for the friendships they have made and the support they have received. They are also very aware that the birth is near.

It is important to the successful closure of a Centering group that a celebration of the group's efforts and accomplishments occurs after the babies have all been born. Members can then leave the group feeling satisfied with their experiences after sharing their birth stories and new learnings with their fellow group members. It is quite common for the women to continue meeting, creating play dates for their toddlers, and referring to the members of their cohort as a support group. This is a critical phase and should include a summary and evaluation of the events that have occurred over the life span of the group. Evaluation of both the group process and the extent to which the group is fulfilling its original goals is crucial.

RAMONA

In preparing for the eighth session of the group, Ramona thought about how her own anxiety regarding the birth and handling a new baby was increasing. She was noticing, too, that other women—they now were well into the last trimester—were more physically uncomfortable and looking for advice from the women in the group who weren't having their first baby. From the beginning, they had been doing some focused meditation, and now that work felt even more important. They were reviewing some of the content around breastfeeding and comfort measures in labor, and this session, she knew, was going to focus on mental health issues including better understanding of depression.

Ramona also thought more about the other group members and how much she cared about them. "We really have become friends." They had exchanged phone numbers and e-mail addresses early in the pregnancy and were having regular between-session contact with each other. In one of the last sessions, they made bracelets and agreed to wear them until all had delivered. Although she still got together with Lisa, often there were several other women who joined them for a walk, or a snack over coffee. They also were planning for a picnic that would include all the members, partners, and other children. Ramona realized that having this group with which to share was just as important as all the new things she was learning.

Problems Happen

In a Centering group—as in pregnancy and all of family life—serious events have the potential to destabilize any group. Perhaps a woman shares her concern that her partner now is unemployed. Or one of the women has learned that her baby has congenital anomalies and probably won't survive. No matter the challenge, group members have kept the circle together with powerful support: a mother who goes off to have a fetal heart test and finds members of her group bringing food and drink and company; a group forming a prayer circle around one of their members who has just found out there is no heart beat; or another member diagnosed with gestational diabetes who benefits from diet tips from the collective experience of the group members. There is no end to the way a community that is organized and recognized as having shared values can bring problem solving, empathy, and compassion to its members. Sue Monk Kidd captures the power of this sharing:

> Sometimes another woman's story becomes a mirror that shows me a self I haven't seen before. When I listen to her tell it, her experience quickens and clarifies my own. Her questions rouse mine. Her conflicts illumine my conflicts. Her resolutions call forth my hope. Her strengths summon my strengths. All of this can happen even when our stories and our lives are very different.—(1996, pp. 172–173)

Stories Around Loss and Recovery

 A woman who was part of a group of eight couples commented, "We think of each of these babies as being our babies and we want each of our babies to be healthy."

Worries that frighten facilitators as they think about group work may sound something like this: "What if someone in the group experiences a loss?" or "What if there isn't a fetal heart beat?" or "What if a partner disappears or has to serve time in jail?" or "What if the parents are told their baby has a significant anomaly?" There are many powerful stories of dealing with loss in Centering groups; several are presented here without additional comment. At least part of the message is that although bad things do happen and are outside of our control, there is a community of support to lean on in the Centering group.

Some could see the need to share bad outcomes in the group as a negative of the model, but after experiencing this firsthand I see the group as a positive experience for the woman in spite of a negative outcome. She has support people with whom to share. CenteringPregnancy speaks to the value of peer support.

▪ Story 1

"I saw a woman for her first prenatal exam and realized that she was here from East India with absolutely no family. Her husband has been denied an immigration card. I encouraged her to join a CenteringPregnancy group which she did. Clearly it provided her with community. One of the women whose grandmother always came with her, asked about her labor support. When she found out that she had no one her grandmother offered to be with her. One day before her due date she had a fetal demise. The grandmother volunteer still was with her during that labor and the family took her in with them for a week postpartum. The woman, herself, came back to the group and shared with them her experience. A very special community had developed for her."

▪ Story 2

"A woman experienced an early loss of her baby. She asked me not to tell the group because she didn't want them to worry. After I shared that I was sure the group would miss her and worry about her, she worked with me on what to share. In the group, the women wondered why it is so hard for us to trust each other with difficult experiences. . . a whole deep discussion followed. At the ninth session the woman who had experienced a loss came back to the group. During the previous weeks she had knit baby booties for each woman in the group and went around the circle stopping in front of each woman wishing her and her baby safe passage. So touching for the group and healing for the woman too."

▪ Story 3

"One of our groups had a couple with a stillbirth at term. The first person the dad called was another dad in his group. In another group that also had a stillbirth at term the dad came back to the group to tell the story. Later at the postpartum reunion his wife wrote a letter to the group sharing her grief and thanking them for their support. The group decided to plant a tree in honor of the baby who was lost."

▪ Story 4

"We had two women lose their babies in a group. One an unexplained intrauterine demise at 32 weeks; the other died 10 days after birth from complications of cystic fibrosis. I was concerned about how the seven other women in the group would deal with the news. I circulated an e-mail, which the parents of both babies had helped compose. I then followed up the e-mail with an individual discussion with each woman. They all had concern for the parents. Two women attended the memorial of the baby with cystic fibrosis days before they gave birth. This baby's memorial was also attended by the couple who had the stillbirth.

"At the postpartum group session for that same group, the members collected money to send the bereaved parents for a weekend away. I was astounded at this powerful acknowledgment of the grieving parents' experience and at the affirmation of their babies' beautiful but short lives. This experience has made me realize that when we don't talk about adverse outcomes as possible 'normal' parts of life and we don't share the experiences when they happen, we do two things: First, we marginalize the parents whose experience of birth and/or early parenting has been different—less than optimal. Second, we also create greater stress for ourselves as caregivers, as the silence supports the idea/myth that maybe we could have done something to prevent the outcome, when in truth neither mother nor caregiver in the majority of these situations did anything to make it happen."

The stories of loss remind us of the power of the circle to hold, support, and heal each of us and particularly those who are grieving. The message of "you are not alone" is one that each of us longs to hear at times of special need. The group facilitator's "hold" the circle rim during these times, ensuring that everyone in the circle is safe and that needs are met.

"Being in a circle is a learning and growing experience that draws upon the wisdom and experience, commitment, and courage of each one in it" (Bolen, 1999, p. 15). "In fact we survive only as we learn how to participate in a web of relationships" (Wheatley, 2006, p. 20).

References

Baldwin, C. (1998). *Calling the circle: The first and future culture*. New York, NY: Bantam Books.

Baldwin, C., & Linnea, A. (2010). *The circle way: A leader in every chair*. San Francisco, CA: Berrett-Koehler.

Bolen, J. (1999). *The millioneth circle: How to change ourselves and the world*. Berkeley, CA: Conari Press.

Doyle, B. (2013). *The thorny grace of it*. Chicago, IL: Loyola Press.

Kidd, S. (1996). *The dance of the dissident daughter: A woman's journey from Christian tradition to the sacred feminine*. San Francisco, CA: Harper.

Lawler, E., & Mohrman, S. (1985). Quality circles after the fad. *Harvard Business Review, 63*(1), 65–71.

Marshall, J. (2001). *The Lakota way*. New York, NY: Penguin Compass.

Ochs, E., Taylor, C., Rudolph, D., & Smith, R. (1992). Storytelling as a theory building activity. *Discourse Processes, 15*(1), 37–72.

Thompson, T. (2011). Circles of change. *Stanford Social Innovation Review*, 42–47.

Wheatley, M. (2006). *Leadership and the new science: Discovering order in a chaotic world*. San Francisco, CA: Berrett-Koehler.

5 CenteringParenting®: From Pregnancy Through Postpartum and Beyond

Babies are tough. They don't come with instructions, and it's really nice to have a community of parents going through the same things.
—*Dr. Kara Bruning, Pediatrician*

This chapter describes the dynamic CenteringParenting® model focusing on the mother–baby dyad. The model provides care in a group space to both individuals utilizing the three components: health care, interactive learning, and community building. Parents interact with each other, their clinician, their babies, and share joys and concerns around parenting, health needs, and family dynamics.

Either the CenteringPregnancy® group cohort stays together during the postpartum year and beyond, building on the skills, learnings, and friendships developed throughout pregnancy or the model stands alone for a completely new group of parents. The model is designed to have at least six sessions starting at approximately 2 weeks postpartum through the first year, with another three in the second year. Visits are set to correspond with directives from Bright Futures, including the schedule for baby immunizations (Hagan, Shaw, & Duncan, 2008). Note that immunization schedules are updated yearly and posted on the American Academy of Pediatrics website.

The Postpartum Period

Think about all the excitement but also the fears, worries, and anxieties that new parents have when dealing with the reality of holding a new

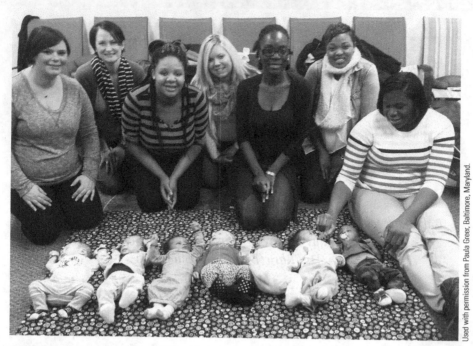

Mother–baby Centering group.

Used with permission from Paula Greer, Baltimore, Maryland.

baby in their arms. As one new mother said a few minutes after birth, "Look Tim, we have a baby. Now what do we do?!" Perhaps the biggest adjustment a family makes is incorporating a new baby into the mix and at a time when they are just coming down from the adrenaline rush of birth. As Susan Brink notes, this "fourth trimester is an outside-the-uterus period of intense development that is an extension of the work begun during the first 9 months" (2013, p. 2).

Would the transition time be easier if a group of other mothers and support people were just a phone call away? Or perhaps one newly delivered mom is hospitalized next door to one of the women in her Centering group. One midwife commented, "I had two patients in the hospital; one had delivered and the other was in labor. I visited the postpartum mom first. She had been texting with a woman in her group who was in labor and she knew more than I did about her progress! The next day when I made postpartum rounds I found both moms in the same room and a couple others from group visiting them!"

RAMONA

Ramona comes to CenteringParenting, happy that her group is continuing to stay together for at least a year. Her daughter, Marianne, is 2 weeks old, and Ramona thinks that parenting is even more challenging than giving birth. This is time to share experiences and get new ideas from moms who she knows will be so comforting. Since this is care for her baby too, there will be a clinician skilled in baby care in the group and her midwife will be present at least for the first session. She is glad that Dave was free and could come with her. He has some anxiety holding the baby and seems a bit resentful of the time that it takes for her to breastfeed.

Ramona talks with the nurse about the check-in process for herself and Marianne. The baby stays in the carrier while Ramona checks her own weight and blood pressure, picks up the CenteringParenting notebook and watches Dave make name tags for all three of them. She notices that the room is set up with a baby scale/measuring board where she will be taught to gather Marianne's data. The clinician is off in the corner sitting on the floor examining a baby and talking with the mother. It feels just like the CenteringPregnancy group except that it is noisier. There are seven moms/babies in the room along with all the baby stuff of carriages, car seats, and diaper bags. Lots of room needed!

She has her own assessment with the clinician who does a quick baby exam, asks about immunizations, and checks in about Ramona's health and personal goals. She is pleased that Dave is included in the conversation. The co-facilitator for the group is a social worker who asks each mom to do a short depression screen; then there is time to look at the notebook for the self-assessment sheet for the day.

The discussion time happens on the floor. There are comfortable pillow seats arranged in a circle with a nice rug in the center for the babies. Ramona finds a place to sit and puts Marianne on the colorful mat on the floor in front of her; she talks with the other women, her friends from CenteringPregnancy, as they wait for the formal circle-up to begin. She notices that Dave is still talking with a couple of other dads in attendance. It is wonderful to exchange comments, questions, and get strategies for dealing with all of the issues of this postpartum transition. The formal discussion feels so appropriate.

At the end of the session, the babies each have their immunization; Ramona is glad for the support of others. She makes sure that she has correct contact information for the other moms so they can connect between groups and maybe even meet for an outing with the babies.

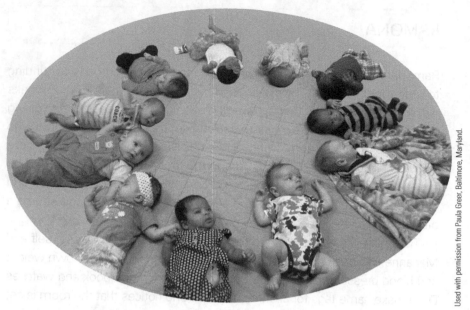

A multi-cultural circle of babies.

Dyad Care

As in pregnancy, during this early postpartum period the health of the mother and the baby are closely tied. If the mother is depressed, the baby suffers. If the mother struggles with breastfeeding and feelings of inadequacy, the baby will struggle too. If the baby is small, or has a physical challenge, or is extra fussy the mother (and dad/support people too) will expend more energy that already is in short supply.

Without looking at the total picture, the clinician caring for the baby has only a partial data set upon which to act. Moreover, postpartum care is lacking for most women, and so their depression screening, follow-up for gestational diabetes, support for breastfeeding, challenge to set personal goals especially around weight and stress management seldom happens. Even though our system isn't designed to care for two patients at once it makes sense to keep the mother and baby together during the first year of life and beyond.

Where can mothers go to get advice and support from other women and skilled professionals? Postpartum care most often has been the 6-week check, a HEDIS measure, meant to ensure that the woman has recovered from childbirth. Additional visits might be scheduled around birth control needs. The baby's evaluation has been more scripted with six to seven visits expected during the first year of life. The focus of these visits is on immunizations and assessment of growth and development parameters. Is it enough?

A study published in 2015 from a team at Johns Hopkins that analyzed over 26,000 Medicaid claims shows that one-quarter of these postpartum patients made an emergency room visit within 6 months of delivery. Women with pregnancy complications had a 14% increase in visits, even more profound if they were 25 years or younger. The article supports more attention to postpartum care and also suggests that mother–baby care visits might improve care and reduce these expensive emergency department visits.—(Harris et al., 2015)

Leaders in the field of women's health have continued to work on the content of pre- and interconceptional care. A consensus recommendation for preconception wellness was published in 2016 from a national clinical workgroup (Frayne et al., 2016). The nine wellness measures are:

- Pregnancy intention
- Access to care
- Preconception multivitamin with folic acid use
- Tobacco avoidance
- Absence of uncontrolled depression
- Healthy weight
- Absence of sexually transmitted infections
- Optimal glycemic control in women with pregestational diabetes
- Teratogenic medication avoidance

These measures, along with appropriate follow-up from pregnancy complications are equally appropriate for the interconception period. "The words/concepts overlap as every woman is 'preconception' prior to any next pregnancy, whether planned or not, and she is always interconceptional (period between pregnancies) as long as there is a chance she might become pregnant again in the future," stated Merry-K Moos, a pioneer for preconception health promotion and reproductive life planning.

I went to the first CenteringParenting group with women who had been in CenteringPregnancy together and found that the women already identified two women who didn't have a contraceptive plan and they fixed that. I didn't have to say a word! And in the second session, they

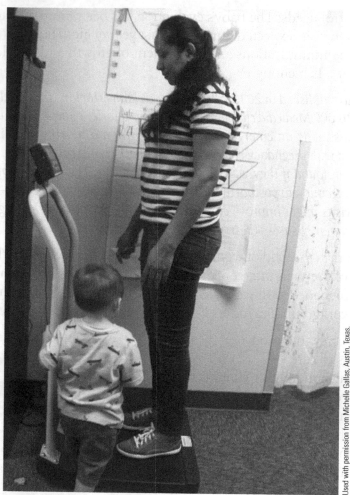

Used with permission from Michelle Gallas, Austin, Texas.

A woman assessing her own weight.

identified a woman who was depressed and reached out to her to provide support. Was lovely to see and gave me a heads-up of issues that needed to be addressed.—A family physician

To further promote the needs of mothers, babies, and families, the dyad CenteringParenting model outlines three components—health, safety, and development—and then specifies general focus items for each of the components (Table 5.1). A combination of clinicians focused on the baby, family life, and women's health will provide a rich environment for assessment, interactive learning, and community building within the group.

TABLE 5.1   Maternal–Baby Dyad Components

Component	Mother	Baby
Health	Postpartum care	Growth parameters
	Mental health	Immunizations
	Breastfeeding	Nutrition
	Oral health	Oral health
	Family planning	
Safety	Safe sex	Car seats
	Substance abuse issues	Childproofing
	Relationship issues	Emergency first response
	Smoking	Safe sleep
		Childcare
Development	Mothering role	Milestones
	Attachment	Behavior
	Life balance	Cognition
	Stress management	Motor skills

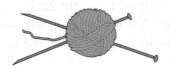

Although this content list can look daunting, there are several content threads that run through the model. Like in CenteringPregnancy, these threads are picked up when an opening surfaces in the facilitated discussion. There are several content threads that run through the model. In the *Health Component* the threads are (a) nutrition and the setting of weight goals, (b) exercise, (c) breastfeeding, (d) family planning, (e) mental health, and (f) baby nutrition; in the *Safety Component*, (a) relationship issues (b) safe sleep, and (c) substance abuse including smoking cessation; and in the *Development Component*, (a) life balance and (b) baby milestones. The clinician also focuses on any specific health issues of the dyad, such as follow-up for gestational diabetes, vaginal infections, abnormal lab tests, substance abuse, and physical and developmental issues for the baby. Assessment of appropriate growth and development for the baby is integral to the model, along with observation of the mother–baby–family relationships.

A site group facilitator shares, "We started CenteringParenting yesterday and it was a smashing success. Eight women came with their babies and then the other facilitator arrived with many flowers and balloons that set a festive tone. The group was very multicultural: Chinese, Indonesian, Haitian, Brazilian, and four African American women. Several of the women were quite disclosing of their situations and people seemed to have a lot of fun, including the three of us who were doing the facilitating. Although there were cultural differences regarding weaning and toilet training, the women were very nonjudgmental."

Mother/Baby Focal Areas

It may seem intimidating to a pediatrician or other well-baby provider also to focus on the mother's needs during the visits. Clinicians credentialed for both mother and baby care will find it relatively easy to have both of those charts available. Those not dually credentialed will rely on a women's health provider to follow up on issues that arise and are outside of their scope of practice or comfort. However, all facilitators can pay attention to the goals set by each woman. Questions such as: "How are you doing meeting your weight goals?" "Is your family planning method working for you?" "How is it going with your partner?" should be comfortable for all to ask and will continue the focus on woman's health.

Physical Health Issues

Some women will have had medical issues during pregnancy and childbirth that need follow-up. These could include diabetes testing, testing for sexually transmitted disease, and blood pressure monitoring (Kershaw, Magriples, Westdahl, Rising, & Ickovics, 2009; Schellinger et al., 2016). The baby may have congenital or birth issues that need continued monitoring.

Nutrition and Exercise

If mothers are encouraged to set weight goals and monitor them during this postpartum period, they may be more apt to lose extra weight gained during pregnancy. A recent evaluation of weight-gain trajectories in pregnancy and postpartum showed that women randomized to group care gained less weight and lost more postpartum than women in

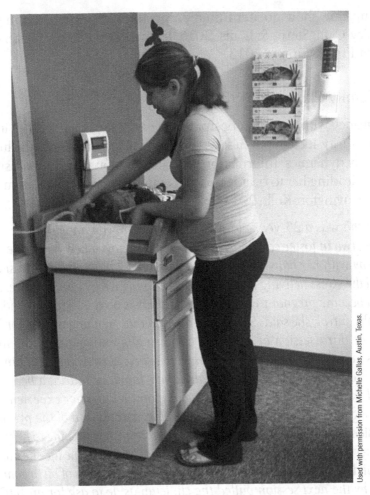

A mother assessing her baby's weight and length.

individual care. This outcome was especially significant for women with prenatal depression and distress (Magriples et al., 2015; Tanner-Smith, Steinka-Fry, & Gesell, 2014).

Infant Feeding

The American Academy of Pediatrics recommends exclusive breastfeeding for 6 months and breastfeeding for at least a year. Numerous studies have documented the benefits of breastfeeding for both the mother and baby. Research studies comparing breastfeeding outcomes for women in group care show greater initiation postpartum for women in groups (Brumley, Cain, Stern, & Louis, 2016; Ickovics et al., 2016; Tanner-Smith, Steinka-Fry, & Lipsey, 2013).

Family Planning

A pregnancy within the first postpartum year is associated with an increase in prematurity. It often puts a stress on the family resources, also influencing the family dynamics. Information on contraception may be confusing to a woman, leading her to decide not to use anything (Hale, Picklesimer, Billings, & Covington-Kolb, 2014; Ickovics et al., 2016; Trotman et al., 2015).

Tonisha was a 25-year-old African American woman with three children, two in foster care with her mother, and now a new baby. She was happy with her baby but struggled with type 2 diabetes, sleeplessness, and the stress of living in a neighborhood plagued by gun violence. She had become pregnant with each of her babies on a different method of birth control, she said. She was convinced that "nothing works" for her. At the third session of Tonisha's CenteringParenting group, the topic was family planning and women were asked to envision what kind of life they wanted for themselves and their families. Maria, a beautiful and charismatic 20-year-old biracial mom, related her experience of getting an IUD [intrauterine device] placed at the end of the previous session, and how being on long-term birth control was going to help her achieve the goals of finishing school and moving out of the life she had as a child. Tonisha repeated her negative view of all forms of birth control, but by the next session pulled the clinician aside to ask for an IUD.

Depression

Guidelines are more specific now about the importance of screening women for depression during the prenatal and postpartum periods ("Editorial: Screening for Perinatal Depression," 2016; Ickovics et al., 2016; Siu 2016).

"In addition to the Edinburgh depression screening tool, which we already know we administer more frequently and consistently than in individual clinic care, we discuss postpartum depression in group, demystifying it. Most groups are facilitated by an LCSW [licensed clinincal social worker], so the ongoing familiarity with the therapist as a person, destigmatizes accepting services." When the data was reviewed, it was clear that women in Centering got screened more often than the women in traditional care and got referred for follow-up clinical assessment (G. Fynn, personal communication, 2009).

As we were discussing postpartum depression and the importance of support after the baby is born, one girl said that nobody would be able to help her or give her a break from the baby. Immediately, three other women in the group gave her their phone numbers and said "call me." They figured out how they could trade off babies for 30 minutes at a time. "I can hold two babies for half an hour while you go for a walk as long as you let me pee before you leave!"

Interpersonal Violence

Women gain trust in the group and are willing to disclose issues of abuse that they haven't shared individually with their clinicians. Depression often is related to interpersonal risk factors (Westdahl et al., 2007).

A mother was feeling upset that she had lost patience with her baby and shouted at him. The other moms normalized it, talking about times they had messed up and had to say sorry. They all strategized about how to walk away, even if it meant leaving the baby crying in its crib, so that you can collect yourself. The mother said she felt much better and thanked the others for being able to share their mistakes.

Immunization

Group is an excellent time to remind women about the flu and other appropriate vaccines for them. There has been much debate in the popular literature about the possible influence of immunizations on the baby's health, including an increased chance of becoming autistic. Some parents refuse vaccines because of religious reasons. In a small Yale randomized controlled trial on CenteringParenting, results showed more anticipatory guidance, better attendance, and babies immunized on time (Fenick et al., 2011).

A mother was reluctant to get her baby immunized, but because she came to trust the staff in the group over time, she eventually agreed to some vaccines, as long as they were administered by the staff with whom she had built relationships.

▇ Group Support

Women make long-lasting relationships in group and may have gatherings for years after the baby is born. Chapter 4 addresses the kind of support the group can give to families with unexpected outcomes. The group sessions also provide an early opportunity for babies to socialize. This story talks about the power of group for both this mother and father.

Vanessa joined the CenteringParenting group shortly after she arrived from Mexico. She had three other children, but this new baby had club feet, which worried her especially since he was so different from her other children. She also had a Pap smear report from an exam in Mexico and gave it to the pediatrician leading the group who promptly gave it to a women's health provider. The report was abnormal, and efforts were made to get her some immediate care. At the 1-year birthday party for the group, Vanessa shared how important the group was to her especially in helping her to see that her young son was actually developing normally. Shortly thereafter, she began to have health problems related to the abnormal Pap smear, and her husband came to the group with her son. Vanessa died 6 months later, but her husband continued to come to the group throughout that second year, receiving support from the women and carrying on the focus of family health so important to Vanessa.

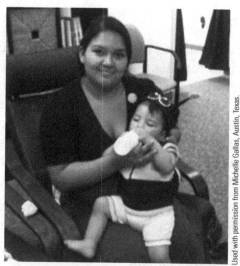

Used with permission from Michelle Gallas, Austin, Texas.

Vanessa with her baby.

So Does It Work?

CenteringParenting is definitely one of the best things that have happened to me! Initially, when I first "inherited" the facilitator role, I was incredibly nervous and apprehensive; my immediate thought was "What am I going to do with a room full of crying children for 2 hours?" Soon, after my first group I realized how important continued support in the postpartum and parenting period is. We invest so much time in preparing women to have healthy pregnancies and term babies but tend to forget the challenges they face when they become mothers. I love that this is a space where mothers can just be mothers. It's a place they can come share their joys, worries, experiences, questions, and fears; all without judgment and most importantly be heard.—A co-facilitator

The data on CenteringParenting is strengthening as more sites continue their groups into the postpartum period and share their outcomes with the data system, CenteringCounts, at the Centering Healthcare Institute (CHI). An evaluation was done by CHI in 2012 of 15 geographically diverse sites that had implemented CenteringParenting. The goals were to explore the successes and challenges experienced by the sites and the needs of the staff involved with the model. Several themes were identified:

- The importance of support of participants for each other. "We share a lot of information and a woman can ask anything in this space without feeling judged." The clinician added that these women are learning to be moms and need lots of attention and support.
- Participant satisfaction with the group was high with retention between 75% to 95% in the groups. "They all show up."
- Learning happens for both the staff and the patients as they share perspectives and learn from each other. "I love the connections between the women . . . and we learn things from them that you don't learn in textbooks."
- Logistics are more difficult with two patients, often two credentialed providers, and possible involvement of two clinics. There is definite need for a team approach and considerable system redesign.
- Enrollment was enhanced when the same clinician carried the group seamlessly from pregnancy to parenting. This was easiest with clinicians credentialed for care of both mother and baby (Bloomfield & Rising, 2013).

Writing in Pediatrics, *Edward L. Schor noted, "The nation's system of preventive pediatric care requires major revisions if chronic health problems and unmet behavioral and developmental needs among American children are to be addressed" (2004, p. 210).*

A randomized controlled trial of CenteringParenting was conducted by an interdisciplinary research team at Yale University. Ninety-two mother–baby dyads were randomized either to individual or to group care. Outcomes documented significantly more anticipatory guidance for mothers in group and more visits during the 12-month period. There also was better adherence to the immunization schedule (Fenick et al., 2011). A follow-up study of this population at age 2 showed a trend to less overweight children who were randomized to the group model (Shah, Fenick, & Rosenthal, 2016). Another longitudinal study of babies receiving well-baby group care showed significantly less obesity at age 2 in children who received care in groups rather than traditional care (Machuca et al., 2016).

A research team in Calgary, Alberta, completed a 2-year feasibility study in 2015 of a CenteringParenting model piloted in two Calgary clinics. The primary research question was: "Does the CenteringParenting model meet the needs of parents, nurses, and decision makers?" The data supported this research question with several outcomes demonstrating improvement for mothers and babies in the group model. Mothers expressed high satisfaction with the model (see Appendix A for more outcomes of the Calgary Study).

This model provides an excellent way for residents to learn. In one setting, a resident commented that he liked the opportunity to see many children together who were the same age. Also, having the attending physician right there with him gave him confidence in his skill building. A survey of physicians involved in group well-baby care documented improvement in most areas of skills and knowledge. One commented, "It is such a privilege to get to learn from our patients about the range of normal, and even more exciting to see how empowered they feel teaching each other" (Mittal, 2011, p. 41).

Social workers are ideal co-facilitators because of their training in group skills and their understanding of attachment. Gillian Fynn is a social worker who has worked as a co-facilitator of Centering-Parenting for many years. Here, she shares thoughts about why CenteringParenting is so important to her.

CenteringParenting provides the opportunity for me to:

• Watch the development of the relationship between mother–baby

- Lead a discussion that helped the parents to look more deeply at their babies, personality and cues. Things they might have missed in the daily routine of diapers, and so forth. Time to sit and wonder.
- Have relaxed conversation around parenting styles, dreams for the future that gave appreciation for cultural values/traditions. Many of the participants are graduate students separated from their extended family.
- Watch the women develop community. So many are socially isolated. The closing circle at the end of the CenteringParenting year is very emotional. If they haven't done so before, the women share contact information to help them continue to build their community.
- Monitor the emotional health of the mother. Spanish groups are very strong. Many women came over with coyotes, undocumented, no family, other children left in Guatemala with grandparents. They are just grateful to connect.

Gillian Finn, LCSW, Psychosocial Services Manager, LifeLong West Berkeley, Berkeley, California

Reflections From a Community Health Worker

Jocelyn de Sena

The relationships built in Centering are one of the most striking (and hardest to quantify) outcomes of the model, and what I love most about working in this model. The team approach to staffing allows those who are not medical or mental health providers to develop their skills, be recognized for their expertise, and act as collaborators with those who, in other settings would be considered "superiors." Working together over the years has built trust and camaraderie across disciplines, and it feels like we are all "comrades" in nurturing our program.

In addition, the relationships of mutual respect and trust that are built over time with the patients are simply beautiful. There are many times moms have reached out to me when they were in a rough spot, whether it is something as simple as being the one person the mom knows will return her call and help her get an appointment for a sick baby/deal with MediCal issues/talk through birth control options. Sometimes it is something as profound as having a mom walk in to clinic between groups asking to speak with you because she is in crisis/

depressed/being abused/has an unplanned pregnancy and knows she can trust you to not judge her and to empower her to access whatever resources she needs. I believe that kind of relationship with support staff is fostered by creating a kind of sanctity in group and sustaining it over time. Moms know that the group coordinators hold their care with consistency and accountability.

To see the friendships between the moms grow over time is the best part. The fact that group is a safe place to not only give every mom a chance to be the expert, but to ask silly questions and share challenges, builds social support for moms who often have no other support system. I remember the final session of one group which consisted of an African American mom, moms from Ethiopia, Nepal, Mexico, the Philippines, and Indonesia, who had all gone through both pregnancy and parenting groups together. In doing the closing activity with the yarn, the moms said that they had been both surprised and grateful by how they had been able to find a community of friends, and that although they were all from such diverse cultures, they felt like sisters.

Jocelyn de Sena, CenteringParenting Coordinator, LifeLong, West Berkeley, California

Bergman and colleagues summarize key issues thus: "We need a high-performing system of well-childcare designed to optimize the development of young children. New technologies and innovative clinical practices can provide the tools needed to create it. This will require transformational change; we will not be successful through efforts at the margin" (2006, p. vi).

The postpartum year is a particularly intense one for a woman due to the many physical and emotional adjustments, effort needed to care for the new baby and her family, and possible conflicting roles around motherhood, partner relationships, and need/desire to work outside the home. Health-promoting skills revolve around her ability to mobilize a social support system, to use her own real resources, and to have realistic expectations (Fahey & Shenassa, 2013). To be successful navigating this time period, a collaboration between community agencies, public health services, businesses and advocacy groups is essential to help provide the external resources needed.

The model, with its emphasis on relationship-centered care and extensive patient engagement mirrors the focus of a *Health Affairs* issue in which editor Susan Dentzer comments, "wherever engagement takes place the emerging evidence is that patients who are actively involved

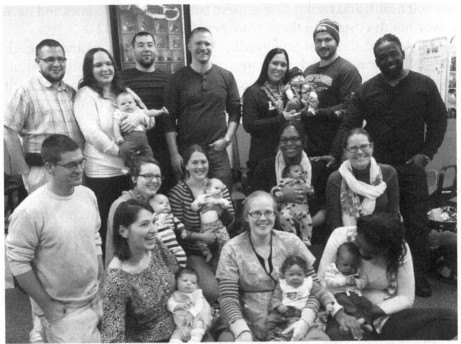

Group postpartum celebration.

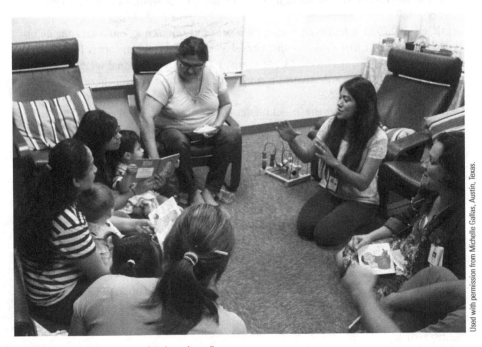

Encouraging mother–baby interaction through reading.

in their health and health care achieve better health outcomes and have lower health costs than those who aren't" (2013, p. 202).

Michael Lu and Neal Halfon add, "It is our belief that women's health care holds greater promise of improving pregnancy outcomes and eliminating disparities than prenatal care alone . . . the nation will be well served by making a commitment to advance women's health care to a similar extent as it has prenatal care" (2003, p. 25).

I'm continuing to see some of my CenteringParenting moms and children every year. In fact, some of them [the children] are 8 years old and still coming as a group. I love it!—Misae Vela Brohl, Nurse Practitioner

Yes, this model is complicated by caring for two patients and a circle of babies who eventually will want to crawl around the space. But this model also is fun and energizing for all participants. It's worth the effort!

References

Bergman, D., Plsek, P., & Saunders, M. (2006). A high-performing system for well-childcare: A vision for the future. *The Commonwealth Fund*, 1–58.

Bloomfield, J., & Rising, S. (2013). CenteringParenting: An innovative dyad model for group mother-infant care. *Journal of Midwifery & Women's Health, 58*(6), 687–688.

Brink, S. (2013). *The fourth trimester: Understanding, protecting, and nurturing an infant through the first three months*. Berkeley: University of California Press.

Brumley, J., Cain, M. A., Stern, M., & Louis, J. (2016). Gestational weight gain and breastfeeding outcomes in group prenatal care. *Journal of Midwifery & Women's Health, 61*(5), 557–562.

Dentzer, S. (2013). Rx for the 'blockbuster drug' of patient engagement. *Health Affairs (Millwood), 32*(2), 202.

Editorial: Screening for perinatal depression: A missed opportunity. [Editorial]. (2016). *The Lancet, 387*, 505.

Fahey, J., & Shenassa, E. (2013). Understanding and meeting the needs of women in the postpartum period: The perinatal maternal health promotion model. *Journal of Midwifery & Women's Health, 58*(6), 613–621.

Fenick, A., Gilliam, W., Leventhal, J., Rising, S., Gilliam, A., & Rosenthal, M. (2011, April 30–May 3). *Health care utilization in infants receiving group pediatric care*. Abstract presented at Pediatric Academic Society, Denver, CO.

Frayne, D. J., Verbiest, S., Chelmow, D., Clarke, H., Dunlop, A., Hosmer, J., . . . Zephyrin, L. (2016). Health care system measures to advance preconception wellness: Consensus recommendations of the clinical workgroup of the national preconception health and health care initiative. *Obstetrics & Gynecology, 127*(5), 863–872.

Fynn, G. (2009). Social worker at West Berkeley Family Practice clinic shared these results which also are referenced in Centering Parenting Program Final Evaluation Report. *LifeLong Medical Care.*

Hagan, J., Shaw, J., & Duncan, P. (Eds.). (2008). *Bright futures: Guidelines for health supervision of infants, children, and adolescents.* Elk Grove Village, IL: American Academy of Pediatrics.

Hale, N., Picklesimer, A., Billings, D., & Covington-Kolb, S. (2014). The impact of CenteringPregnancy® group prenatal care on postpartum family planning. *American Journal of Obstetrics & Gynecology, 210*(10), 50.e1–50.e7.

Harris, A., Chang, H., Wang, L., Sylvia, M., Neale, D., Levine, D., & Bennett, W. (2015). Emergency room utilization after medically complicated pregnancies: A Medicaid claims analysis. *Journal of Women's Health, 24*(9), 745–754.

Ickovics, J., Earnshaw, V., Lewis, J., Kershaw, T., Magriples, U., Stasko, E., . . . Tobin, J. (2016). Cluster randomized controlled trial of group prenatal care: Perinatal outcomes among adolescents in New York City health centers. *American Journal of Public Health, 106*(2), 359–365.

Kershaw, T., Magriples, U., Westdahl, C., Rising, S., & Ickovics, J. (2009). Pregnancy as a window of opportunity for HIV prevention: Effects of an HIV intervention delivered within prenatal care. *American Journal of Public Health, 99*(11), 2079–2086.

Lu, M. C., & Halfon, N. (2003). Racial and ethnic disparities in birth outcomes: A life-course perspective. *Maternal and Child Health Journal, 7*(1), 13–30.

Machuca, H., Arevalo, S., Hackley, B., Applebaum, J., Mishkin, A., & Shapiro, A. (2016). Well baby group care: Evaluation of a promising intervention for primary obesity prevention in toddlers. *Child Obesity, 12*(3), 171–178.

Magriples, U., Boynton, M., Kershaw, T., Lewis, J., Rising, S., Tobin, J., . . . Ickovics, J. (2015). The impact of group prenatal care on pregnancy and postpartum weight trajectories. *American Journal of Obstetrics & Gynecology, 213*(5), 688.e1–688.e9.

Mittal, P. (2011). CenteringParenting: Pilot implementation of a group model for teaching family medicine residents well-childcare. *The Permanente Journal, 15*(4), 40–41.

Schellinger, M. M., Abernathy, M. P., Amerman, B., May, C., Foxlow, L., Carter, A., . . . Haas, D. (2016). Improved outcomes for Hispanic women with gestational diabetes uring the CenteringPregnancy® group prenatal model. *Maternal and Child Health Journal.* doi:10.1007/s10995–016–2114–x

Schor, E. L. (2004). Rethinking well-childcare. *Pediatrics, 114*(1), 210–216.

Shah, N., Fenick, A., & Rosenthal, M. (2016). A healthy weight for toddlers? Two-year follow-up of a randomized controlled trial of group well-childcare. *Clinical Pediatrics.* doi:10.1177/0009922815623230

Siu, A. (2016). US Preventive Services Task Force (USPSTF) screening for depression in adults: US preventive services task force recommendation statement. *The Journal of the American Medical Association, 315*(4), 380–387.

Tanner-Smith, E., Steinka-Fry, K., & Gesell, S. (2014). Comparative effectiveness of group and individual prenatal care on gestational weight gain. *Maternal and Child Health Journal, 18*, 1711–1720.

Tanner-Smith, E., Steinka-Fry, K., & Lipsey, M. (2013). Effects of CenteringPreg-nancy® group prenatal care on breastfeeding outcomes. *Journal of Midwifery & Women's Health, 58*(4), 389–395.

Trotman, G., Chhatre, G., Darolia, R., Tefera, E., Damle, L., & Gomez-Lobo, V. (2015). The effect of CenteringPregnancy versus traditional prenatal care mod-els on improved adolescent health behaviors in the perinatal period. *Journal of Pediatric and Adolescent Gynecology, 28*(5), 395–401.

Westdahl, C., Milan, S., Magriples, U., Kershaw, T., Rising, S., & Ickovics, J. (2007). Social support and social conflict as predictors of prenatal depression. *Obstetrics & Gynecology, 110*(1), 134–140.

6 Facilitation: The Art and the Power

Facilitating takes a certain fearlessness . . . sufficient awareness of yourself to realize you don't know how to do it and a willingness to go with the flow of the group. It requires tapping into the group mind and creativity.

—*Hunter, Bailey, & Taylor (1995, p. 34)*

Facilitation is the heart of the Centering model. Facilitation defined, includes such concepts as acute listening skills, ability to "hold" the discussion threads and incorporate them into a summary, willingness to put one's own biases aside, and genuine curiosity about the group members and what each is bringing to the circle. The traditional hierarchy present within the health care setting is modified as clinicians, facilitators, patients, and support people all sit together without the usual attention to status. This new dynamic encourages each member to engage and contribute.

Facilitative leadership is built on a foundation of acute listening skills where facilitators bring out the wisdom of the group members and then join the conversation fibers into a meaningful whole. The result is a different model from that found in the didactic classroom where an "expert" provides the majority of the content to a more passive group of listeners. Facilitative leadership results in a dynamic interchange among facilitators and other group participants and encourages interactive learning among all members.

In a successful group, the facilitator helps members build confidence in their own knowledge and ways of knowing. Participants thrive in an atmosphere that encourages them to raise issues, test assumptions, and solve problems. The skilled clinician realizes that there is little evidence for most of what we tell patients and that we have only limited knowledge of the context of our patients' lives. For any degree of group success, it behooves us to listen well.

> *My physician colleague said to me that she didn't want to do groups because she really wanted to get to know her patients. I replied, "When I see women in the clinic they are just a blur to me. But when I see them in Centering groups, I really know them."*

Demystifying the Work of the Facilitator

In its ideal form, facilitation involves a balance of sharing and discussion of new material and ideas. The appropriate cultural context for facilitation involves all of the group members as equals. Each facilitator draws on his or her ability to listen to what is being shared and to let the group members respond from their own personal experiences. Years of schooling and conditioning make it difficult for most clinicians and staff to learn not to speak, to wait for the group wisdom to emerge. Facilitators may worry about losing control of the content or the group dynamics. Facilitators need to be aware of their own limitations; they need to be ready to follow the group's leadership and creativity. Crucial to effective facilitation is the ability to hold on to genuine curiosity about each group member while nurturing the ability to listen.

> *A mentor was observing a resident facilitating a discussion of old wives' tales and noticed that she was sitting on her hands, jaw clenched, trying not to say anything. When asked afterward how it felt to listen to the discussion she said, "Oh, it was SO hard."*

The Facilitator's Road

A young resident asked, "How do I learn to be facilitative?" The answer: "Start by not answering questions."

How does a clinician who has always done care in a closed door exam room move into the more open group space, sitting in the circle without

---

Scenario 1

Paul is the physician handling clinic today. The schedule lists 25 women for the morning, and he knows that at least some of them won't come or will be late. A nursing assistant helps him with flow and follow-up. Although his first patient arrives on time, he falls behind his schedule due to tie-ups at the intake desk and delayed arrival of some patients. When he brings a patient into the room and closes the door, he asks her how she is doing, looks at her chart on the computer, does a brief exam, refills her vitamin prescription, asks her a couple of questions and hopes that she doesn't have any for him—because already he has two to three women waiting for him. Paul opens the door, telling her that she is doing well and he'll see her again in a month. He knows he didn't give her much time to talk, and hopes he didn't miss any important issues.

Scenario 2

Paul looked at his schedule first thing and confirms that he has Centering group this morning. He remembers that this is his third session with the group of 11 women and wonders what issues will surface today. His co-facilitator will join him in the group. They work together well, helping the group conversation flow and attending to issues that emerge in the discussion. Paul likes the fact that women often answer one another's questions and that he doesn't always need to come up with a solution. Part of the joy of group care, Paul believes, is that he is learning more about differing cultural beliefs and values. Some strategies he has suggested in the past wouldn't work culturally. For a moment, he thinks about his productivity requirements. In this group, he sees 11 patients in a 2-hour time period, and he is confident that almost all health outcomes and patient satisfaction are going to improve, which may be reflected in his pay for performance.

---

a lab coat or stethoscope, listening with interest to what the participants are sharing. The accompanying scenarios contrast two approaches.

What does it take for a clinician like Paul to change the way he or she delivers care? It may take a growing dissatisfaction with the way things are and exposure to new methods of care. Following a CenteringPregnancy® workshop, one obstetrician commented, "I feel as if I've just come out of a tunnel after 12 years and seen the light!" This and many similar comments seem to say that Centering is tapping into some deep yearning sensed by many health workers in their search for more satisfaction and joy.

One young midwife wrote in her evaluation of the Centering workshop: "I came here ready to leave my profession because I was so unhappy, but this experience has given me new hope."

Listening: An Essential Skill

Andrew Wolvin, an expert in oral communication, proposes that listening is the most underdiscussed and underresearched of the communication process. Critical listening is the foundation for successful communication (1999).

Learning to listen is a difficult skill for many clinicians and staff members who have worked hard to gain knowledge and now are eager to share expertise with their clients. "I want my patients to know everything that I know," said one seasoned midwife. Facilitation requires a different kind of listening. The better we listen, the freer women are to tell us their stories. It means being present in a totally different way. A staff nurse became teary when she shared, "No one has asked women to tell their stories. We aren't the same after we have listened to the depth of their experience."

"I've worked for 2 years to learn everything so I could take care of patients and now you are telling me to sit and listen!" said a student midwife on the second day of a CenteringPregnancy workshop. Yet listening, she needed to realize, is at the core of the Centering model, with other elements there to support the interactive learning and resulting empowerment experienced by group participants because they have listened to one another.

Listening helps the facilitator identify when and how members of the group are open to learning. Learning is most apt to happen when information is presented in a culturally appropriate way—when the receiver has identified a need to know and when peers positively reinforce the content.

Ernestine Wiedenbach, the gifted nurse-midwife, who started the Maternal Newborn Educational program at the Yale School of Nursing wrote extensively on "meeting women's needs." She defined "a need for help as anything the person feels will be helpful to assist in functioning capably." Until a person identifies that she has a need, intervening won't be that helpful. Emphasis on listening is inherent in this basic philosophy (Wiedenbach, 1964).

Becoming a good listener is hard work. As professionals, our minds are pretty cluttered with "stuff": problems with the last patient visit, a call from school about our child, or plans for an upcoming vacation. Amid this list of concerns, how do we get centered enough to be truly present to the group?

A midwife says, "I used to do groups from 5:30 to 7:30 in our private office after seeing 25 women in a clinic across town. When I got to the office, I would lock myself in the bathroom, the only really private space, and spend a short time focusing. Which group is coming; what session; where did people sit last time; what concerns were surfaced by the group that we didn't get to talk about; what concerns do I have about the individuals and about the group dynamics? What materials might I need to use during the session; who do I want to sit by; what issues do I need to discuss with my co-facilitator? By the time the group arrived, I was ready and eager to meet them."

Being focused is essential for effective listening and leadership. There are many ways to get yourself and others focused: a brief meditation, which could be done with the group; taking a short walk; listening to some appropriate music; and so on. Each facilitator decides what will work best for this important preparation.

Listening is also predicated on curiosity. Curiosity makes possible authentic, caring, group conversations about individual concerns. The facilitator's internal monologue might go something like this: "I wonder what Ada is going to say?" "What has happened in her life since the last session?" "What new ideas will grow from today's discussion?"

When group members feel the facilitators' energy, they will respond to affirmation by paying attention and becoming engaged. Staying focused for an hour or more is hard work for everyone, and mind-wandering leads to missing something quite important. "I think I just missed something important . . . who can share that issue with me?" may be the best way to recoup lost conversation threads. The phrase "watch, wait, and wonder," seems applicable to this for all participants. Facilitators learn from what is said, from what members ask each other, from their silences, their body language and where they sit, how they engage . . . just what is happening to them. To do this has meant a clearing of the noise in the facilitators' own heads.

Understanding and Responding to What Is Heard

Otto Scharmer, as part of his Matrix of Social Evolution, has identified four types of listening that resonate with the work of facilitative leadership: habitual listening, factual, empathic, and generative (Scharmer & Kaufer, 2013, p. 154).

- Habitual Listening or Downloading. "My mother refuses to let me try new ways of cooking" and *you think*, "I've heard her say this before . . . it's an old story." It's easy to identify old judgments about the person or topic and be closed to new learnings.
- Factual Listening. This level allows movement from habitual thinking to putting the content into context. It is possible to input new data that starts to shift the response. "My mother refuses to let me try new ways of cooking . . . because she thinks that it is important to have a fried meat at every meal." Now there is a cultural issue that is surfacing that sheds new light on the issue.
- Empathic Listening. Now it is possible to see the person and her issue through her reality and understand why this is such an important discussion for her. "My mother grew up learning to cook in this way because that is what she learned from her mother and now wants to pass on those methods to me." Understanding of cultural beliefs and values grows as does insight for why former patterns of response may not have been helpful.
- Generative Listening. Being open to the wider issues, the listener now is able to imagine the possibility of inviting the mother to come with her daughter to a session or even to arrange for a nutrition/cooking class that might involve others in the group. These insights require the listener to move out of the center and hold the circle space so that new possibilities can emerge.

Group Facilitation: Focus on the Process

Getting to generative listening can be challenging. For example, when a woman states that raising her hands above her head will cause the baby's cord to wrap around its neck, the facilitator might want to respond, "No, that's not true." That response will bring other members of the group in defense of the group member, marginalizing the facilitator. At that time, the facilitator may use other resources, such as pictures and models to go through the learning process. For example: "Does your baby move a lot?" or "Can you imagine how the cord wraps around the baby?"

Parker Palmer in his book, Healing the Heart of Democracy, *states:* "*. . . presenting facts that contradict deeply held beliefs is more likely to reinforce those beliefs than compel people to change them." (p. 51)*

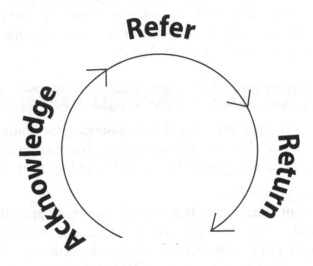

Group process may take many twists and turns, but at the heart there is a consistent way of managing what has been heard. The process of group facilitation relies on three steps: *acknowledge, refer, return.* Here is an example of how the process works:

Group member: "I have been having lots of low backache and I'm wondering how I can make it go away."

Facilitator (*acknowledge*) to the person: "I hear that you are uncomfortable with your backache."

Facilitator (*refer*) to the group: "I'm guessing that others in the group may also be dealing with backache. Am I right?"

Facilitator (*return*) to the person: "Several other women have shared their strategies for dealing with their back pain. Has this been helpful to you? Do you have any other concerns to share?"

To a general comment brought up by one of the members, the facilitator might say: "That's an interesting idea. Would you tell us more?"

or "We used to think that but we have some new information that is encouraging us to think about that differently. Can you think of some other ways to handle that?"

A recent study of data from the first Yale randomized trial demonstrates that facilitation is the key to the success of the group process. After looking at all the possible indicators for preterm birth, the analysis of the process fidelity determined that the more facilitative (and the less didactic) the session was, the lower the odds of both preterm birth and intensive care for the infant. Facilitation is the key part of the model design, allowing for discussion and problem solving that may lead to behavioral change (Novick et al., 2013).

Group Facilitation: It Is the Process, Not the Content

Just as with honing listening skills, mastering facilitation skills will take time. Three skills are discussed here: trusting yourself, trusting the group, and hanging onto threads and hooking them into structure.

- **Trusting yourself**

  Trying something new often feels daunting. As one clinician commented about the thought of being a facilitator: "Sitting with a group of women and not answering questions is terrifying!" The clinician worries, "Will I know the answers? What if someone says something I don't believe?" Trusting that just sitting and waiting will encourage women to talk with each other and perhaps answer the question seems difficult. For example: How to counter a woman's dependence on smoking? A partial answer is provided by this anecdote from a CenteringPregnancy group dealing with smoking cessation.

  One woman in a Centering group pointed to another and said, "You know how that smoke goes through the placenta to the baby . . . how can you continue to put that stuff into your body? I smoked two packs before I got pregnant and stopped. If I can do it, you can too. And I'll help you." With this interaction, the facilitator realized that others in the group could respond to issues and that their responses are even more powerful than what the clinician could say.

- **Trusting the group**

  For centuries, people have gathered in circles to share stories and to provide support for one another. Today, isolation grows as people are

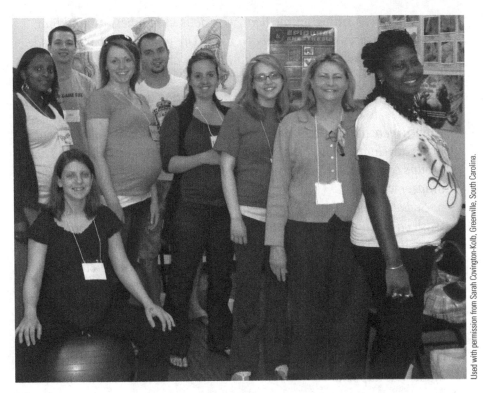

A Centering group.

more mobile, streets seem less safe, and distrust of others transforms even our own neighborhoods. In contrast, Centering groups allow trust to develop and women to share personal concerns that they may never have shared before, particularly not with a provider. "I thought I was the only one who had this problem, but I found out that other women in the group also had this problem, shared one group member."

In a group, women will share their concerns and strategies, most of which reflect their cultural beliefs and values. Facilitators report feeling enriched by new understanding. Imagine being part of this group:

It was the seventh session, so the group felt comfortable with the check-in and the discussion process. Several male partners participated dressed in jeans and cut-off shirts with tattoos covering much of their available skin. During the check-in time, they had gathered around the food table, casually teasing each other. The clinician, a young male physician, was sitting on the floor with dolls in blankets around him, ready for a discussion of newborn care. The group members started talking about what they knew/didn't know about babies. For some, it was very little. Then one of the men said, "Doc, I heard that if I'm sitting near my old lady on the couch and toking up, my kid gets a hit inside her. Is that true?" The men looked at each other startled, the women were at full attention, and the physician facilitator talked about brain development and the possible impact of drugs and alcohol. The group's comments—"no way," "you gotta be kidding"—indicated their amazement.

Suddenly, one young man got up, walked to the corner, retrieved a trash basket and came back to the circle where he went from one man to another. "Throw it in here," he said. "All of it." "We aren't doing this anymore." Man after man emptied his pockets of glassine envelopes, pipes, and paraphernalia. When he put the basket down, he proceeded to give the men his cell phone number. "Call me and I'll call you. We can do this for our kids' brains."

This facilitator sat in awe of the power of this interaction led by one of the men and realized that even a skilled clinician could not have made that happen.

The open sharing of content, concerns, and strategies leads at times to fragmentation. Conversations may get cut off for interactive learning. Parts of the discussion will be important to revisit. When time is up, or when another topic takes precedence, it is good to have a "container" available to keep track of topics. Perhaps a white board could be used to record these discussion areas, which could then be reviewed at the end of the session. For example, in the midst of discussion on nutrition, someone raises question about anesthesia. That topic could be put in the container so it isn't lost; there is a plan to talk about anesthesia later. The group can be reassured that the topic will surface again.

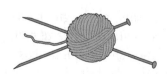

Hanging onto threads and hooking them into structure.

Organizing content before the group ends will enhance learning. Before the final closing, it helps to say, "Today we have talked about . . . and we didn't get back to the question of . . . we'll be able to spend time on that next session. Is everyone okay with that?" This process becomes one of knitting together threads of conversation from session to session, so that the facilitator is reassured that the participants have discussed the information that is important. Almost always, the underlying question regarding a health concern is, "When do I need to worry?"

Give It Time

On the surface, it is hard to believe that sitting in a group and talking together over the course of many sessions can actually affect preterm birth outcomes or breastfeeding outcomes. What is it about a group of people gathered for a similar purpose that actually leads to behavioral change? The data support stress reduction and empowerment as two outcomes of group (Heberlein et al., 2015; Ickovics et al., 2011; McNeil et al., 2012; Novick, Sadler, Knafl, Groce, & Kennedy, 2012). A new empowerment scale may help with studying the extent of empowerment felt by women through their care model (Klima et al., 2015). In group, women and their clinician have 10 times more time together than in traditional individual care, and most of the time is spent talking about what matters to them.

Margaret Wheatley says, "We are hungry for a chance to talk. People want to tell their story, and are willing to listen to yours. People want to talk about their concerns and struggles. Too many of us feel isolated, strange, or invisible. Conversation helps end that." (2002, p. 24)

Centering groups address the hunger to talk from people who are new parents. They also build community and trust at a critical time in life when people are open to change. Group members will continue discussion of issues and new learnings at home with other family members. The pregnant woman now has creative thoughts and strategies to share that influence her activities during pregnancy as well during parenting and childrearing.

We are having so much fun . . . I'm learning that it doesn't matter what we don't talk about because we are talking about what matters to the group.—A group facilitator

As the group session continues, both content and process issues emerge. It is important to remember the difference between a class and a

Centering group. In traditional care during pregnancy, we often encourage the attendance at classes for childbirth preparation, breastfeeding, car seat use, parenting skill development, and so forth. These are episodic events for the patient and usually require separate appointments. Unlike the more typical content-focused classes, Centering is a process model that encourages a focus on the interaction among the members, thus allowing the content to flow from this process. It incorporates the provision of care, using standards designed to have optimal health outcomes supported by the active involvement of the participants in this care. This structure provides for a dynamic of cooperation between the provider/facilitators and the participants, leading to a demonstration of personal empowerment exhibited by the women.

The discussion content evolves like a web, with concepts that connect into a meaningful form. Content may surface as a thread: a narrow band of content that is woven into the fabric of discussion and surfaces periodically. Examples of threads that surface often during the 10 sessions are: nutrition, exercise, stress management, breastfeeding, preterm labor, birth preparation, 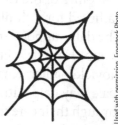 parenting skills, and gestational diabetes. Other threads include such areas as safe sex, smoking, or other substance abuse. The ability of the facilitator to identify potential threads is a skill that requires careful listening, knowledge of the group and its needs, and a familiarity with the common threads that fill the container.

Used with permission, Freestock Photo.

 "It was very educational and empowering. Someone would bring up a topic, which would trigger another person to discuss a related idea. And sometimes someone would bring up an issue that I was too embarrassed to ask about."

Looking at the content items in this model could reinforce for the facilitators the need to get didactic to "cover" all the items. This can lead to a discussion that turns into a "coil." It also is possible to have a discussion area turn into a "coil" of fairly inflexible content. It is apparent

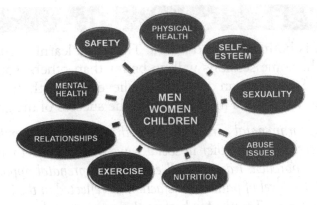

This model shows the several content areas discussed through the 10 sessions in CenteringPregnancy.

when the facilitator takes over with a didactic style of group leadership. This could happen when a facilitator feels that the group needs to be "educated" about a topic, puts a video on without a discussion plan, or when a guest comes to the group and does a presentation. It can also happen with research studies when a particular content area has been added to the session. The group usually responds with passive listening and the energy present during facilitation may diminish. The facilitator needs to be aware of this and move the group back to a more dynamic discussion.

To sit in circles with my patients, colleagues, students, volunteers and know that we can begin to heal each other and our communities gives me hope every day.—A group leader

Mindy's Musings

Really remembering who is sitting there and what their experience is. I could say, "Does anyone have any thoughts about this" or "What has been other people's experience? What are other people doing about nausea, vomiting in pregnancy?" Just remembering not to be the consummate teacher, or seeing myself as the expert on the group. Drawing the expertise out of the group was probably the hardest thing to learn. And that I was not in charge of answering every question, just making sure that the information is true and good and . . . hanging wallpaper does not cause a fetal cord death . . . that kind of stuff.—Mindy Schorr, MSN, CNM

Summary

Facilitation is both an art and a skill. There is a learning curve, but it isn't smooth. Some sessions will go better than others; some groups are easier to facilitate than others. We believe it is worth the effort and, indeed, may well be the major factor in the success of the group.

> *Centering for prenatal care resonates with today's young families who are connected to each other in social ways that fit perfectly with the centering approach. I don't recall ever having prenatal appointment scores at this level of patient satisfaction as reflected in the incredible MPS scores. . . . Thanks for having the passion and energy to try something completely different than we have ever done. I look forward to these patients being our ambassadors in the community as we have already seen from some new members who joined because they heard good things about centering from our patients.—An administrator*

Improving our listening skills is both energizing and humbling. As our facilitation skills grow so will our satisfaction with our relationship with our patients and coworkers. As one clinician said, "This is the one thing in my week that brings me joy."

> *A physician who was resistant to leading groups commented that for a year he had watched his colleague come out of his Centering group with a big smile on his face and walking 2 inches off the floor. "I decided that I wanted some of that joy for myself."*

Group facilitation is a lesson in *humility* . . . just when you think you have learned to listen well, you'll find yourself talking much too much. The important piece is to recognize that a momentary slip into didactic teaching has occurred . . . and then resolve to try again! This is the art of self-facilitation.

References

Heberlein, E., Picklesimer, A., Billings, D., Covington-Kolb, S., Farber, N., & Frongillo, E. (2015). The comparative effects of group prenatal care on psychosocial outcomes. *Archives of Women's Mental Health, 19*(2), 259–269. doi:10:1007/s00737-015-0564-6

Hunter, D., Bailey, A., & Taylor, B. (1995). *The art of facilitation: How to create group synergy.* Tuscon, AZ: Fisher Books.

Ickovics, J., Reed, E., Magriples, U., Westdahl, C., Rising, S., & Kershaw, T. (2011). Effects of group prenatal care on psychosocial risk in pregnancy: Results from a randomised controlled trial. *Psychology and Health, 26*(2), 235–250.

Klima, C., Vonderheid, S., Norr, K., & Park, C. (2015). Development of the pregnancy-related empowerment scale. *Nursing and Health, 3*(5), 120–127.

McNeil, D., Vekved, M., Dolan, S., Siever, J., Horn, S., & Tough, S. (2012). Getting more than they realized they needed: A qualitative study of women's experience of group prenatal care. *BMC Pregnancy and Childbirth, 12*(17).

Novick, G., Reid, A., Lewis, J., Kershaw, T., Rising, S., & Ickovics, J. (2013). Group prenatal care: Model fidelity and outcomes. *American Journal of Obstetrics & Gynecology, 112*, e3.

Novick, G., Sadler, L., Knafl, K., Groce, N., & Kennedy, H. (2012). The intersection of everyday life and group prenatal care for women in two urban clinics. *Journal of Health Care for the Poor and Underserved, 23*, 589–603.

Palmer, P. (2011). *Healing the heart of democracy*. San Francisco, CA: Jossey-Bass.

Scharmer, O., & Kaufer, K. (2013). *Leading from the emerging future: From ego-system to eco-system economics*. San Francisco, CA: Berrett-Koehler.

Wheatley, M. (2002). *Turning to one another*. San Francisco, CA: Berrett-Koehler.

Wiedenbach, E. (1964). *Clinical nursing: A helping art*. New York, NY: Springer Publishing.

Wolvin, A. (1999). *Listening in the quality organization*. Ithaca, NY: Finger Lakes Press.

II Centering Healthcare™: Transformative Change

7 Implementing Centering Group Care

All organizations [and systems] are designed, intentionally or unwittingly, to achieve precisely the results they get.
—R. Spencer Darling, Business Expert

It is one thing to come up with a bright idea, but it is quite another to implement the idea. It takes time and effort to realize the many difficulties of introducing a new model. Getting support and funding, encouraging clinicians to imagine the satisfaction of facilitating a Centering group, recruiting women to trust a new care alternative, and even finding appropriate space for group meeting all take commitment and ingenuity. Each task requires genuine enthusiasm for improving the care women receive, a dedicated leader/champion, and a strong steering committee. This chapter outlines (a) foundational work in the field of implementation science, (b) initial steps for site planning, (c) important guidelines for site leadership, and (d) an innovative use of telemedicine.

The popular phrase: "Change Is Hard; You Go First." may be an apt expression of champions who are imagining change but don't know how to begin.

Implementation Science: Foundational Work

A major component of success rests on the implementation team's ability to provide leadership with system and service changes: knowledge sometimes is not enough to fuel success. Even the most obvious change principles must be repeated, explained, moved forward, and coached in a manner that supports the strength of the providers and facilitators all while striving to create a welcoming and encouraging environment (Blase, Fixsen, Naoom, & Wallace, 2005; Heifetz, Grashow, & Linsky, 2009).

Requirements of the organization's team charged with implementing the Centering model include the following:

- In-depth knowledge of the Centering Healthcare™ model
- Ability to promote the model and articulate the stages of implementation
- Ability to provide technical assistance to various stakeholders as needed
- Provision of appropriate support to staff based on the culture of the institution
- Development of long-term relationships with key staff, who will be available when problems or questions arise

In each of these areas, competence must be developed and sustained. Through the selection of staff, training and coaching measures, when implemented, will help change and support new practitioner behaviors and skills. This focus on competence also supports maintenance of fidelity to the model, a crucial component to implementation success (Novick et al., 2013).

Fixsen and colleagues, experts in implementation from the National Implementation Research Network, state "Research that focuses specifically on implementation will be useful, to the extent that it improves practice and advances our conceptual and theoretical understanding" (Fixsen, Naoom, Blase, Friedman, & Wallace, 2005, p. 74). In their monograph, *Implementation Research, A Synthesis of the Literature*, Fixsen and colleagues recognized early that "what is known is not generally what is adopted and what is adopted is frequently not used with fidelity and good effect" (p. 2). The researchers in this mandate noted that what is newly implanted disappears over time. Research is clear: planning requires a 2- to 4-year process of implementation of a new model. Even exploring the introduction of a new model requires thoughtful discussion, reality-based thinking about barriers, the engagement of stakeholders at every level, and intentional and inviting introductions of all changes to the community (Blase et al., 2015; National Implementation Research Network, 2013).

Stages of Implementation for Centering Groups

1. **Exploration stage**
   New sites will benefit from outside consultation during this initial period. The Centering Healthcare Institute (CHI) has developed a

plan to assist systems to be successful in navigating each step of the process. From initial readiness through training and consultations over time, sites are guided through the process of implementation.

2. **Installation stage**
   This stage requires obtaining institutional support and a firm commitment to provide the necessary resources. Training for clinicians and support staff is key, as are designated space, equipment, staff, access to medical records, patient notebooks, and equipment for monitoring mothers, availability of snacks, and appropriate teaching materials for successful implementation.

3. **Initial implementation**
   a. This stage involves calling the first circle. This can be an awkward phase, with everyone trying out new skills, and patients wondering what they are getting into, making this a fragile and challenging stage. Ensuring success at this stage requires consultation and moral support.
   b. Data suggest that without a strong support team/consultation, "going it alone" means a prolonged and difficult road, with only 14% reaching implementation, and taking 17 years to get there. With effective implementation assistance, however, 80% of innovations reach effective implementation in 3 years (Balas & Boren, 2000; Blase et al., 2005).

4. **Full implementation**
   a. This stage is reached when most of the intended practitioners, staff, and team members are using the Centering model with fidelity and quality outcomes.
   b. This model has become the standard of care with 60% or more of eligible patients receiving care in groups.

These stages are not mutually exclusive, nor do they happen in a linear way. Staff turnovers, new students, and changes in the patient populations, for example, require leaders to reevaluate their process on a regular basis (Heifetz et al., 2009). "To diagnose a system or yourself, while in the midst of action, requires the ability to achieve some distance from those on-the-ground events. We use the metaphor of 'getting on the balcony'" (Heifetz et al., 2009, pp. 7–8). The ability to move away from the action and view it from a distance makes it easier to figure out what is happening in and among the multilayered departments by finding funding sources, conducting data analysis, analyzing cost centers, and evaluating staff. Changing from traditional one-on-one care to group health care is daunting. The "balcony" also provides some time to shed light on which changes are "technical" and which changes are "adaptive." If what needs fixing is a technical problem, such as reconfiguring a room for Centering groups, that change might be fixed by a work team at the institution—the change is relatively simple. However, if the change upsets the intrinsic way things have been done, or challenges deeply held beliefs of staff, this type of change is adaptive work and requires attention to the culture of the institution. Introducing a new model of care obliges staff and clinicians to change what they do and how they do it, and to alter well-entrenched beliefs and habits (Heifetz et al., 2009). The more that staff can be involved in the planning and implementation, the smoother the transition will be. **Involvement = investment = ownership.**

There are multiple situations that arise in the process of adapting a new approach to health care that can create difficulties:

1. People in the system (staff, administrators, stakeholders) find many reasons to resist the change, for example, funding, space, redistribution of staff, and so forth.
2. Clinicians may balk at the change in how they will be asked to deliver care. If the clinicians believe in the new model, they will "drive" the change.
3. Ancillary personnel, (receptionists, schedulers, support staff) find changing the scheduling system to be complex, as is organizing the room for a group session.
4. The community, the patients, and their families wonder what this model is about and why they or their loved one is not receiving one-on-one care. Many people in the community might have a hard time imagining receiving care in such a nontraditional manner and may believe giving up the current familiar model means sacrificing quality of care.

Organizations often fail to pay attention to the stress engendered when staff is asked to give up their familiar work habits or job descriptions that they have enjoyed and do well. The change may not be their idea, making it important for the implementation team to work on the "why" of this change. Helping women achieve a healthy, well-informed pregnancy, preventing preterm birth and its consequences, and strengthening self-empowerment and a sense of community can be powerful motivators for staff when they have been included in the development of the new model of care. As one lead clinician said, "Centering isn't an easy model to communicate."

Here comes the Trojan Horse galloping into the institution. It appears to be one thing: it's got a system, it's got a name, it's got theories, it's got research, it's got shape and form. It gets into the system and then starts to unload little soldiers that come out and start creating all this change and havoc. It's not havoc, it's change . . . but it does feel like havoc to the system.

Getting Started With the New Model

Some essentials of implementation for Centering groups are as follows.

▓ A Champion

Almost all sites start with a "champion," a person at the site who either is familiar with the Centering model or who just knows that change must happen. "I heard a presentation on the CenteringPregnancy model and just knew I had to figure out how to implement it at our site." This champion becomes the driver for initial planning. Strategic planning may lead the administration to conclude that Centering will help them reach their stated goals. Or, the site may be prompted by a grant, such as the Strong Start or Healthy Start grants that can provide money for system changes or encourage a renewed focus on prenatal care.

In Ohio, increasing concern about infant mortality rates (Ohio ranks 46th in the nation) motivated a team of providers, policy analysts, government officials, and community workers to commit to reducing racial disparities in maternity care. One component of the solution is providing Centering Healthcare. A new film, *One Life*, documents the problem of infant mortality in Ohio and suggests that when people look for a good place to live, they look at the health of the children in that area.

▓ A Readiness for Change

The assessment of readiness for change will help determine whether the time is right to move forward. Asking difficult questions, such as: Where are we in relationship to where we want to be with our maternal infant outcomes? What is the disparity in our outcomes between Black and Latino babies and White babies? What problems exist that we need to address? Do we have a mutually agreed upon goal? are questions that help a team to build trust and create an attitude of determination. A Readiness for Change assessment tool, and one is available on the website (centeringhealthcare.org), will assist a team in understanding the requirements for implementation of the new Centering model. The items included on this assessment tool are: estimating administrative and clinician interest; determining availability of financial support for implementation expenses; checking for appropriate space and availability; and assessing sufficient volume of patients to form the recommended cohorts.

A Coordinator and a Steering Committee

Once the decision has been made to move forward, the CHI assigns a consultant to the site. With the help of the consultant, the site then designates a steering committee to guide the process. This committee includes representation from key work areas such as: scheduling, administration, clinicians, data, billing. In addition, the committee will relate to an implementation team composed of high-level administrators and representatives of appropriate community agencies such as Healthy Start, home visiting, parenting programs, and advocacy groups such as Safe Sleep. This group provides input as needed to the steering committee and serves as a resource for moving the work of Centering into the community.

Administrators with budgeting authority are essential to the process. Initial funding might come from such sources as March of Dimes, local hospital foundations or auxiliaries, and other grant opportunities. Current and former patients who represent the community should be invited to serve on the steering committee. These participants must represent the racial and ethnic demographics of the population being served by the health center.

The Training

This model requires high-quality training for clinicians and facilitators. These group leaders need to be encouraged to stretch their comfort levels with facilitation while relinquishing their roles as experts to make space for the women in the groups to find their own wisdom. After the training, staff will need consistent and competent coaching as they begin to implement the model in their system. Only when training was accompanied by coaching in the service setting did researchers find substantial implementation in the practice setting (Joyce & Showers, 2002). Offering a workshop for only part of the staff, or sending one or two staff members to a training session, will not produce desired results.

In a small study that described the feelings of six experienced midwives as they moved through the stages of exploration, training, and completion of their first CenteringPregnancy group, Baldwin and Phillips understood that midwives were deeply involved in a paradigm shift when moving to group care (Baldwin & Phillips, 2011). The focus of their study was to capture the lived experience of the midwives as they began doing these groups. Five themes emerged that are helpful in understanding the shifts required of providers:

1. My practice is just fine just the way it is (Precontemplation)
2. I'm thinking about giving it a try (Contemplation)
3. Anxiety and stress (Actively engaged in trying to do this)
4. Confident and engaged in new behavior (Action phase)
5. Committed to the model and wanting to sustain the change (Maintenance)

The midwives in the study experienced personal challenges and moved to a sense of accomplishment and began to enjoy a sense of accomplishment and renewed energy for their work (Baldwin & Phillips, 2011).

What are the problems this model can fix? There are several important benefits such as reduction in preterm birth, cohesion and community among the women, and joy for the group leaders as they watch women benefit from sharing, freed-up space for gynecologic appointments.

It is obvious to us that the power of the circle exists in many contexts, and it's been extremely rewarding to watch this new idea take shape and further extend the lessons we have already learned.—A midwife

Ongoing Leadership

The need for leadership continues to be critical at every stage to ensure fidelity to and sustainability of the model. Barriers will arise, people will think and say openly that this is more work than they expected. This is why it is important to have the members of the steering committee be respected in their work area. They need to bring their coworkers along with the change.

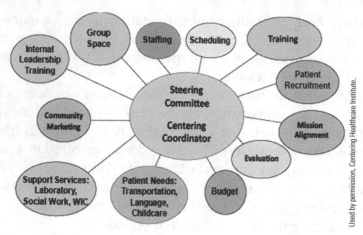

System redesign components.

Used by permission, Centering Healthcare Institute.

This model identifies the many system components that need attention during the planning period. The steering committee must meet at regular intervals during the initial months of implementation and then periodically to make sure that all issues are addressed and that enthusiasm is nurtured well beyond the initial stages of implementation. Perhaps the most difficult concept is that the Centering model is an alternative to individual/traditional care and not another educational or support program.

Identifying the institutional policy changes, challenges, recruitment processes, key staff, and protocols takes considerable consensus building by members of the steering committee. It takes time and effort for the organization to transform its ability to provide improved care, as well as to help families to a stronger appreciation of the role they play in self-determination, caring for their physical and mental health, relationships, and lifestyle. It also takes time to develop mechanisms for evaluation of multiple variables such as patient and provider satisfaction, health outcomes, feedback processes, and fidelity to the model. All of these tasks take time and team work but are the keys to success. Data collection is a time-intensive process but also necessary to ensure that care is improving. Sites assess their own outcomes and then set benchmarks focused on improvement; for example: increased numbers of women initiating and sustaining breastfeeding, better attendance at visits, numbers of women returning for postpartum care, depression screening (Heifetz et al., 2009; Ickovics et al., 2007; Novick, Sadler, Knafl, Groce, & Kennedy, 2013).

RAMONA

A few months after her delivery, Ramona was asked by the Centering coordinator if she would be willing to be part of the steering committee. On the committee, she would be joining a woman from a previous group to help ensure that the model was working well. The steering committee is composed of about eight people representing administration, clinicians, front desk and support staff, social work, and the current patient population. Early in the development of the Centering model, the group met twice a month, but now they are meeting once a month for 1 hour. Ramona was encouraged to bring her partner Dave whenever he could join and was assured that her small baby also could attend. The coordinator said that the group felt it important to have the voice of women and partners who had experienced care through Centering groups. Some of the specific issues with which they could help included ways to encourage women to seek group care, community messaging, and ideas for childcare resources.

Ramona was pleased to be asked, and she talked with Dave, who readily said he thought this would be a good thing for them and a way to give back to the clinic for what both of them considered to be an excellent way to get care. When she mentioned that she would need to take the bus, the coordinator said the clinic could arrange reimbursement for that expense.

The Challenges of Implementation

Experience over several decades and with more than 400 CenteringPregnancy sites has reinforced the knowledge that there are several common implementation challenges: finding dedicated space for group sessions; providing sufficient support for schedulers as they learn to shift from one-on-one appointments to scheduling eight to 12 women for a series of appointments at the same day and time; consistently enrolling sufficient numbers of women who have received information about the model's strengths; and encouraging providers and support staff to learn facilitation skills as the key ingredient of successful group sessions. To be successful at enrolling women in groups, it is important for all staff to provide a consistent, positive message. Some sites have held the intake visit in the group space for new women entering the system. One study looked at two different ways of scheduling the group assignment (Hackley, Applebaum, Wilcox, & Arevalo, 2009). Once a woman comes to a group session she very seldom doesn't come back. Additional challenges such as providing healthy snacks, figuring out electronic charting for a group, and difficulties planning for childcare are among the issues that continue to surface as the model takes hold. The Steering Committee's attention to all of these issues is crucial to the initial and ongoing success of this group model.

Mindy's Musings

Recruitment is also a significant problem. Systems are getting better and they can still be worked out better. If it could be *opt out for first-time moms, it would be a societal boom.* There is something about Centering patients when they come into the hospital for their births. They have been open to group prenatal care. There is something about their outlook by definition that is already different. Some staff members really embrace the opportunity to do something different and be a part of the Centering circle. There are many people who want the opportunity to be co-facilitators. But, then there are those who say they'd rather die than do that.—Mindy Schorr, MSN, CNM

More than 20 years of documenting the Centering experience underscores the importance of attention to each of the steps in implementation. While most major changes require an in-house champion who will steer the work, this person alone cannot suffice, yet too frequently this champion is expected to carry the responsibility for all the implementation. The steering committee, by committing to the Centering model, must continue to dialogue with the staff about successes and difficulties they are having. As the stories of the women in successful Centering groups emerge, sharing the stories with all the staff continues to strengthen the purpose of the program.

Fidelity to the Model: Key Predictor

Unless consulting and support is provided to the teams until they develop competence, the implementation is not ensured. Human nature being susceptible to drift means that it is easy to relax standards; vigilance is crucial. Clinicians may feel they are too busy to review the session each time, or attention to detail such as early room set-up may seem less important. Experience has shown fidelity to the model helps to ensure success and sustainability. In their work on this subject, Novick and colleagues documented that greater process fidelity to the model was significantly connected to reduction in preterm birth (2013).

Xaverius and Grady conducted a project in Missouri to inform clinicians and staff at 17 prenatal sites about the CenteringPregancy model. A pre-/posttest was used to assess understanding of the model before and after the presentation. To assess uptake of content, the 223 respondents were asked to respond to questions related to the content presented. Greater than 91% of the responders could provide a descriptive paragraph of Centering after the seminar, compared to 34% before the seminar. Of the 15 sites in the study eligible to adopt the model, eight sites moved ahead with training and implementation. There were significant differences between adopters and nonadopters including leadership support, appropriate space, and funding for sustainability. Difficulties for patients included what have become recognized barriers for sites contemplating implementation: childcare, transportation, and language barriers (Xaverius & Grady, 2014).

Ongoing consultation in the first few years allows the system to build capacity and change the model of delivery for health care. This consultation requires hands-on and frequent positive reinforcement to address the ambitious objectives of increasing parents' knowledge of pregnancy, birth, and childcare; of taking providers who have spent years learning to deliver information and ask them to listen and facilitate the women's own wisdom; and of converting traditional health care systems into circles of learning. As Gary Oftedahl (personal communication, April 28, 2016) notes:

> Participant fatigue with implementation can be costly. It is easy for people to begin to drift back to doing things the way they have always done them. Hospitals and clinics are stocked with the carcasses of well-designed projects that were not nurtured into an adaptive change.

It is naïve for leadership to expect that staff will maintain their initial enthusiasm after the new model has taken root. Perhaps another new program has been presented diverting energy and attention. Complacency takes hold, and so new habits fade into the background. It is important to watch for signs of drift. The relationships developed as staff begins the new model need to be encouraged and supported by the project leaders. The steering committee needs to stay the course in order to remember why they are doing this: to improve the outcomes and experience of care for their patients (Duhigg, 2014; Heifetz et al., 2009).

When difficulties arise, it is important to remember the comments of a CenteringPregnancy team in South Carolina. Sarah Covington-Kolb, a social worker and Centering coordinator, shares these comments, "Centering has changed the women. They are different women . . . they have come out of their shell. You can see that you are doing something that has real meaning. We have so many stories. . . a patient was having surgery and had no family so a mom in the group took care of her baby while she had surgery."

After several groups have experienced their care through Centering-Pregnancy there will be initial data for the staff to assess. Word of mouth will begin to spread in the community that a new model of care has been implemented. At the checkout counter in one city, the clerk was wearing an "Ask Me About Centering" button and a woman said, "Oh, I know all about that model. That's how I got care and I loved it!" Facilitators may be vying with each other for doing the next group.

I looked at my schedule and saw that I was starting a new group and I felt happy. Being in group was so much better than spending a morning seeing patients in the clinic.

Once the implementing site has gained confidence in the model through participant feedback and reinforcing data, it may be time to scale up across a health center or a community, introducing the model in more and more sites.

South Carolina Scale-Up Project

An example of system-wide successful implementation and what it took to get there comes out of the South Carolina scale-up project. Much of the content referenced here is from the work of Sarah Covington Kolb and the doctoral work of Kristin Van De Griend.

The first CenteringPregnancy site in South Carolina started in Greenville in 2009. Amy Picklesimer, an MD at the Greenville site, shared the maternal–infant outcome data collected in Greenville from 2009 to 2010 with the director of South Carolina Medicaid. During this same time, state health care officials, providers, and organizations focused on the well-being of women and infants and were increasingly concerned about perinatal outcomes in the state. South Carolina had the fourth highest rate of preterm births in the country. The March of Dimes had begun issuing its premature birth report card in 2008, helping to call attention to the health problems associated with early elective deliveries, among other issues. The South Carolina Birth Outcomes Initiative (SCBOI), an effort by the South Carolina Department of Health and Human Services (SCDHHS), the South Carolina Hospital Association (SCHA), March of Dimes, BlueCross BlueShield of South Carolina (BCBSSC) and more than 100 other stakeholders, came together in 2011 to work on improving health outcomes for newborns in the Medicaid program and throughout the state (Van de Griend, 2015). These providers, administrators, and funders have continued to meet in work groups once a month. CenteringPregnancy is one of their recommended strategies for improving birth outcomes.[1]

In 2013, based on the outcomes from the Greenville CenteringPregnancy site (Kolb, Picklesimer, Covington-Kolb, & Hines, 2012), the March of Dimes and the South Carolina Department of Health and Human Services put out a call to sites indicating the availability of funding for expansion of the CenteringPregnancy network. An important criterion for funding included readiness for change as demonstrated by the willingness of sites to create steering committees. These committees addressed challenges, brainstormed solutions to the concerns, and made plans for sustaining CenteringPregnancy at their sites. As the team continued their data collection and publications documented continued reassuring outcomes, more funding was made available. Politically influential people from within their clinics and from associated departments or organizations outside of the clinics were brought together on the steering committees. At one site, patients were included on the steering committee, and members of the committee found patient insights particularly helpful in planning and problem solving.

South Carolina's demonstrated commitment to improving birth outcomes through CenteringPregnancy was implemented in 12 health care settings across the state from 2013 to 2015. The findings in the South Carolina CenteringPregnancy expansion evaluation study showed that support from key stakeholders and strong leadership at the state level created windows of opportunity for start-up funding and enhanced reimbursement. Within individual practices, collaborations and strong leadership were essential

---

[1] B. Z. Giese, the director of South Carolina Birth Outcomes Initiative, has provided expert leadership to this initiative and continues to spread this expertise to other states interested in expansion and enhanced reimbursement for CenteringPregnancy.

for the adoption of the model into their complex health systems. During readiness assessments, sites demonstrated that they had support from administrators, clinic staff, and direct health care providers. In sites that were part of larger health systems, hospital administrators, public relations officers, and other decision-makers also influenced the process.[2]

▮ Consortium Building

As compared to traditional prenatal care, there were substantial logistical, time, and financial demands for CenteringPregnancy implementation. While sites are strongly encouraged to have a Centering coordinator in place as part of the application process, some sites continue to try getting by without one. The coordinators manage logistical and administrative demands, and these positions are largely unfunded ones except when enhanced reimbursement funds are made available. The March of Dimes and DHHS then funded Sarah Covington-Kolb, the coordinator at Greenville, to do state coordination of the expansion project. She visited sites, held webinars, wrote a blog, and provided technical support to the developing sites. There continue to be challenges with this consortium work. In the fall of 2015, Sarah brought Centering leaders from all of the South Carolina sites together at the Birth Outcomes Initiative state meeting. Sites shared their challenges and successes, and Sarah led interactive continuing education exercises (S. Covington-Kolb, personal communication, 2016).

This statewide consortium provides an active venue for ongoing communication, cross-site collaborations, information sharing, and brainstorming. Most sites agreed that ongoing training should be made available at no or low cost due to staff turnover. Overall, successful implementation of CenteringPregnancy throughout South Carolina was made possible through collaborations among stakeholders, strong leadership, commitment of enhanced reimbursement from the state, and ongoing technical training and assistance.

This was the first coordinated statewide scale-up of CenteringPregnancy and the first thorough process evaluation to describe the work of implementation. The findings highlight the critical importance of continuing political and financial support.

---

[2] Additional discussion on this project and the efforts for enhanced reimbursement may be found in Chapter 10.

When practices get together, they share their experiences, ideas, and challenges. Just as in a CenteringPregnancy group. This is incredibly valuable and helpful to them.—Sarah Covington-Kolb

Nationally, the development of networks of communication in several states continues. Often there is a particular task to be addressed, such as payment reform. It is clear that resources, both in terms of professional time and money, are essential to the successful development of viable consortiums. CHI hosted four major national conferences in the past decade, inviting researchers, clinicians, program administrators, payers, students, and educators to come together for learning and networking. These meetings provided opportunities to learn from public and private consultants with expertise in funding, expansion, implementation, and research (Massoud et al., 2006).

Telemedicine and CenteringPregnancy

It is difficult to form group cohorts with patients who are living in rural or isolated areas. Telecommunication and electronic information have increased the ability of sites to provide care that is time sensitive and easily accessed by many. One telehealth simulation model predicted a national savings of $4.3 billion with appropriate telehealth models (Piñeiro et al., 2014). Telehealth is used for primary care and specialist referrals as well as for patient monitoring, or for communicating with patients over the Internet. Consumers search daily for information on drugs, diseases, and pregnancy health data. Connecting with their health care providers on a dedicated portal makes getting this information easier. In addition, the decreased number of maternity providers in remote areas, created by smaller populations and skyrocketing malpractice rates, create real and potential crises for women living far from the nearest hospital or clinic (Lapolla, Chileli, & Dalfra, 2011).

Reflections From a Clinician: Telemedicine in Southern Georgia

Jacqueline Grant, MD, MPH

Imagine having a circle of six to eight women and a computer screen in place of one of the chairs. This is the reality of the telemedicine initiative spearheaded by Jackie Grant, a board-certified obstetrician gynecologist. "Two high-volume

---

physicians were no longer practicing in the area, and as a result many low-income women had difficulty accessing prenatal care early and experienced disparate birth outcomes. We had no idea that we would be providing care to 16 counties starting out—there were providers in the Albany area, but many of them did not accept Medicaid. So it was our intent to provide Medicaid-eligible women with early access to patient-centered care and improve birth outcomes and reduce disparities. The question was, What can we do to improve prenatal care access and improve birth outcomes for our most vulnerable?"

The March of Dimes provided initial funding for Jackie to set up the first Centering site in 2009, utilizing women's health nurse practitioners who worked under her guidance. A second site was added in 2011 at one of the district's farm worker clinics. The first site was at a local health department where care was provided by nurse practitioners trained by Jackie; the second site used certified nurse–midwives, donated in-kind by local hospitals, who practiced under Jackie's protocols. In 2012/2013, telemedicine technology was available to the health departments, and Jackie saw this as an opportunity to provide even better care for the women in the Centering groups. Through the telemedicine connection, a maternal–fetal medicine specialist joined the group at selected sessions for a few minutes of discussion around any medical issues. Across the hall from the group space was a perinatal suite where ultrasounds could be done and reviewed. The response of the women was positive.

Although Jackie left her clinics to enter a maternal fetal medicine program in another state, she set up the system so well that it is continuing without her. She reflected, "We are helping women with poor access to the health care system and providing them with the skills to better navigate the system to optimize their care; for some patients, this is their first continuity relationship with a provider." Community partners provided lots of help including donations of books, midwife provider time, and incentives from the pregnancy resource center.

Jackie concluded, "This is more than just about birth outcomes. It's changing the culture of communities. We're teaching patients what they should expect from their health care providers . . . how to ask questions. I loved everything about Centering and I could not imagine leaving until I was sure CenteringPregnancy would stick after I left."

Implementation in Action

Following is an overview of the development of a midwifery practice that incorporated CenteringPregnancy from the very beginning.

Profile of a CenteringPregnancy Clinician

Paula Greer, CNM, MS

Three years ago, Paula Greer was recruited to start a new midwifery service at Baltimore-Washington Medical Center, affiliated with the University of Maryland. Two years earlier, an obstetrician from Boston started the obstetric service at the medical center. His goal was to employ midwives and he wanted the care model to be CenteringPregnancy.

Paula brought with her a strong background in wellness and health. She was intrigued by this model because it paralleled her previous work. She believed in getting people involved in their care and saw the CenteringPregnancy model as a way for participants to learn from one other and to provide motivation and support for behavioral change. She had no experience in grant writing or fundraising, but she caught the interest of the March of Dimes chapter, which gave her $25,000 for 3 years. Another potential funder, Anthem BlueCross and BlueShield, also approached her with funds to increase their outreach for Hispanic women and women with risk issues, particularly diabetes.

Nine midwives now lead Centering groups with Paula. Centering group leadership is a condition of hire. The practice midwives attend 400 of the system's 600 births each year. To be a successful promoter, Paula says, "You must believe in it to sell it." After Paula returned from family medical leave, she noticed that enrollment was down. She talked with each clinician to encourage them to do "what we know is the best for our patients."

Paula's site expanded time offerings for CenteringPregnancy to include dinner. These dinner groups are the most popular group time options. Centering+Dinner runs from 5:30 to 7:30 p.m. and the women bring their partners. Some nights there may be 24 people to feed. Paula said she enjoys introducing healthy foods; one young woman told her, "I've never had spinach or a green vegetable in my life, and now I really love spinach!" Paula gathers her personal friends together to make scented rice socks that are used during the "stress management session" which now is labeled, "spa night." The groups have women from varied backgrounds including a wide age range, education level, and ethnicity. Paula said, "I would never want to do it any other way." "These mixed groups are so interesting and the women really support each other." Combined Medicaid and private insurances cover the clinical costs of these sessions.

One young woman in a group had a cerclage procedure at 18 weeks. When it was removed at 36 weeks because she was contracting, she really wanted to deliver. The group rallied around her, encouraging her to get to 39 weeks and promised her an ice cream sundae if she did. She did make it to 39 weeks. Paula said she knows she will have to remember to bring ice cream to the postpartum reunion. Paula works hard to keep the dads involved. One night, one of the women had to leave right after the belly check but her husband stayed, "to be sure I don't miss any of the content." It was breastfeeding night, and Paula talked about the breastfeeding props and there were many laughs as the dads worked at positioning the dolls for breastfeeding. They also use an empathy belly so the dads can get a better idea of how it feels to be carrying around lots of baby weight.

One night, a 70-year-old grandfather came to the group. He was newly diagnosed with diabetes and the group took him under their wing, giving him dietary information and encouraging him to do his best to have a healthy lifestyle. He left the group that evening with solid advice and a whole group of young people sending him off with positive messages.

"Centering is my passion," Paula said, "so I don't find it a burden to do extra things to make the groups special." The practice is expanding. There are now three sites, and their primary office has been renovated. There is administrative buy-in, which helps to ensure continued support for the groups. Paula is continuing to work with the March of Dimes in Maryland and Virginia and hopes to participate in efforts to get enhanced reimbursement for Centering.

Paula and her practice were honored with the Minogue Award by the Maryland Patient Safety Center for solutions that improve quality and patient safety.

Keeping the Vision Alive

Changing paradigms in health care takes a strong commitment to making things better. The endeavor to implement Centering Healthcare can be, and frequently is, in competition with other projects and goals in the organization. The tensions that arise are normal. It is crucial that CenteringPregnancy champions maintain a sense of optimism, determination, and realism. To implement successfully, it takes engaging, negotiating, and documenting benefits to mothers, babies, and the communities. Caring deeply for mothers and their infants means *listening* from the heart to their stories and *speaking* from the heart as we change the system of care.

The benefits of the program have the potential to be enormous. We believe it is time to start thinking of group prenatal care as the default model for prenatal care.—Diane Garretto, MD, and Peter S. Bernstein, MD (2014)

References

Balas, E. A., & Boren, S. A. (2000). Managing clinical knowledge for health care improvement. In J. Bemmel & A. T. McCray (Eds.), *Yearbook of medical informatics 2000: Patient-centered systems* (pp. 65–70). Stuttgart, Germany: Schattauer Verlagsgesellschaft.

Baldwin, K., & Phillips, G. (2011). Voices along the journey: Midwives' perceptions of implementing the CenteringPregnancy model of prenatal care. *Journal of Perinatal Education, 20*(4), 210–217. doi:10.1891/1058-1243.20.4.210

Blase, K., Fixsen, D., Naoom, S., & Wallace, F. (2005). *Operationalizing implementation: Strategies and methods.* Tampa: University of South Florida, Louis de la Parte Florida Mental Health Institute.

Blase, K., Fixsen, D., Sims, B., & Ward, C. (2015). *Implementation science: Changing hearts, minds, behavior, and systems to improve educational outcomes.* Paper presented at the Institute's Ninth Annual Summit on Evidence-Based Education, Berkeley, CA.

Duhigg, C. (2014). *The power of habit: Why we do what we do in life and business.* New York, NY: Random House Trade Paperbacks.

Fixsen, D. L., Naoom, S. F., Blase, K. A., Friedman, R. M., & Wallace, F. (2005). *Implementation research: A synthesis of the literature.* Tampa, FL: University of South Florida, Louis de la Parte Florida Mental Health Institute, the National Implementation Research Network (FMHI Publication #231).

Garretto, D., & Bernstein, P. (2014). CenteringPregnancy: An innovative approach to prenatal care delivery. *American Journal of Obstetrics & Gynecology, 210,* 14–15.

Hackley, B., Applebaum, J., Wilcox, W., & Arevalo, S. (2009). Impact of two scheduling systems on early enrollment in a group prenatal care program. *Journal of Midwifery & Women's Health, 54*(3), 168–175.

Heifetz, R., Grashow, A., & Linsky, M. (2009). *The practice of adaptive leadership: Tools and tactics for changing your organization and the world.* Boston, MA: Harvard Business Press.

Ickovics, J., Kershaw, T., Westdahl, C., Mariples, U., Massey, Z., Reynolds, H., & Rising, S. (2007). Group prenatal care and perinatal outcomes: A randomized controlled trial. *Obstetrics & Gynecology, 110*(2), 330–339.

Joyce, B., & Showers, B. (2002). *Designing training and peer coaching: Our needs for learning.* Alexandria, VA: Association for Supervision and Curriculum Development.

Kolb, K., Picklesimer, A., Covington-Kolb, S., & Hines, L. (2012). CenteringPregnancy electives: A case study in the shift toward student-centered learning in medical education. *Journal of the South Carolina Medical Association, 108,* 103–105.

Lapolla, A., Chileli, N., & Dalfra, M. (2011). Telemedicine in pregnancy complicated by diabetes. In G. Graschew (Ed.), *Advances in telemedicine: Applications in various medical disciplines and geographical regions.* New York, NY: InTech.

Massoud, M., Nielsen, G., Nolan, K., Nolan, T., Schall, M., & Sevin C. (2006). *A framework for spread: From local improvements to system-wide change.* Cambridge, MA: Institute for Healthcare Improvement.

National Implementation Research Network; Frank Porter Gramham Child Development Institute; nirn@unc.edu (2013). Retrieved from http://fpg.unc.edu

Novick, G., Reid, A., Lewis, J., Kershaw, T., Rising, S., & Ickovics, J. (2013). Group prenatal care: Model fidelity and outcomes. *American Journal of Obstetrics & Gynecology, 209*(2), P112.e1–P112.e6.

Novick, G., Sadler, L., Knafl, K., Groce, N., & Kennedy, H. (2013). In a hard spot: Providing group prenatal care in two urban clinics. *Midwifery, 29*(6), 690–697.

Piñeiro, M., Graterol, J., Sood, S., Rhyu, J., Cheng, J., Tse, P.-K., & Wei, D. (2014). *Center for Information Technology Leadership, 2007–2008.* In a presentation, "Telehealth for New Hampshire Medicaid," at the Geisel School of Medicine, Hanover, NH.

Van de Griend, K. (2015). *Statewide scale-up of group prenatal care in South Carolina* (Doctoral Dissertation). The Norman J. Arnold School of Public Health, University of South Carolina, Columbia, SC.

Xaverius, P., & Grady, M. (2014). CenteringPregnancy in Missouri: A system level analysis. *Scientific World Journal, 2014*(2014), 1–10. doi:10.1155/2014/285386

8 Transformative Change

> *Why would we stay locked in our belief that there is one right way to do something, or one correct interpretation to a situation, when the universe demands diversity and thrives on a plurality of meaning?*
> *—Margaret Wheatley (2006, p. 73)*

What is meant by transformative change? And what does it take to transform care from the current norm to a new culture informed by evidence indicating better care, better health, and lower cost? This chapter explores three themes: the need for exposure to the CenteringPregnancy® model for interprofessional students, implementing a group model with an extraordinary prenatal population, and, finally, an in-depth look at the process of change for one clinician.

Centering and Student Experience

To change the fundamentals of how care is delivered, student health professionals must be exposed to alternative care models while at school. A medical resident at a recent Centering Healthcare Institute training workshop commented, "Everything you are telling us makes so much sense and it is the opposite of what we are being taught."

Creating opportunities for students to imagine a different way to provide care, particularly a way that is relationship-centered and mutually satisfying, is an essential step in making sustainable change. The initial article on the CenteringPregnancy model was subtitled, "An Interdisciplinary Model of Empowerment" (Rising, 1998). Centering groups provide the opportunity for diverse providers such as physicians, midwives, advanced practice nurses, social workers, physical therapists, community health workers, and nutritionists to work together in harmony with patients in a way that maximizes health care, learning, and community building. Training workshops provide a rich learning environment for increasing collaboration among members of the team.

> It is clear that our interprofessional educational objectives should include the preparation for team-based and collaborative practice. (Kaplan, Shaw-Battista, & Stotland, 2015)

Recently, the American College of Obstetricians and Gynecologists (ACOG) issued a task force report titled, *Collaboration in Practice: Implementing Team-Based Care*. They define team-based care as the provision of health services by at least two professionals working collaboratively with patients and their families and engaging patients as full participants. The report includes guiding principles along with implementation guidelines. "This report will be most useful for those who are charged with developing new practice models based on the changing demographics of health care practices and financial reimbursement structures" (ACOG, 2016).

One of the benefits of team-based interprofessional education is the input made possible from teachers and learners coming together from across the health care spectrum. A solid understanding of the social determinants of health (SDOH), which frame the health of a community, is crucial to improving health of individuals and to focusing on population health. In the 1970s, Bill Walczak, former executive director of Codman Health Center in Dorchester, Massachusetts, was a 20-year-old college dropout working as a spray painter. He looked around his community, which was trying to recover from devastating racial tension, and he saw a need for improved health care. As he worked on the design of the health center he stated, "It was clear to me that a health center alone does not make a healthy community." He went on to seek money for a community center, a health club, and a high school academy focused on preparing inner-city youth for college.

Regardless of the specific focus of individual health professionals, all "need to develop an understanding during their foundational education and training of the outside forces that impact a person's, community's or population's health and well-being" (Committee on Educating Health Professionals to Address the Social Determinants of Health et al., 2016, p. 15). It is hard to imagine a more dynamic learning opportunity than that available in Centering groups where participants share from the depths of their own lived experience.

The following sections explore the use of the CenteringPregnancy model in educational programs for midwives, medical students, and residents through the self-told reflections of three health professionals: Sage, the student midwife perspective; Amy, a nurse-midwife mentor in a large university setting; and Sung Chae, a family medicine residency director.

Midwifery Education

A short survey sent to the midwifery educational programs that are accredited by the American Midwifery Certification Board (AMCB) asking about student involvement with CenteringPregnancy yielded a 74% response rate from the 39 total programs. Ninety-three percent of the programs have Centering content in the curriculum and all of the students have opportunity to participate in Centering groups as part of their educational experience. Only 18% of the programs provide the students training in leading Centering groups prior to their participation and only 41% of the programs indicated that half or more faculty were trained. It is encouraging to have the majority of student midwives exposed to the model; more work is needed to provide training in the development of facilitation skills (correspondence with Carrie Klima, chairperson of the Directors of Midwifery Education, 2015).

Reflections From a Student Midwife

Sage Berman, CNM, MSN

The first Centering group that she participated in had a medical student as co-facilitator. They were able to process each session together, so that Sage gained real insight about how the Centering model contradicted the usual medical model. This was an excellent introduction to interprofessional collaboration.

Her second CenteringPregnancy group was with a low-income population with more social challenges. Sage worked with a midwife and included some experience for the participants with mindfulness, which brought additional useful skills to the women, especially as they dealt with such difficult issues as verbal assault. The women in the group found community in the CenteringPregnancy groups despite their ethnic diversity and socioeconomic differences, finding they were united by commonality of being pregnant.

"This experience is an opportunity to really learn about pregnancy from the woman's perspective and gain important listening skills. Each student should have this opportunity. When you are a student, you want to look as if you know a lot; but in CenteringPregnancy you don't need to have all the answers. You learn not to fill the space with your own voice; wisdom from the group is more real. This experience was a huge gift to me."

Physician Education

Several academic sites are involving students in CenteringPregnancy and CenteringParenting®.

Reflections From a Faculty Clinician

Amy MacDonald, CNM, MSN

A nurse-midwife, Amy MacDonald, is responsible for the obstetrics rotation for the Primary Care Leadership Track (PCLT) for medical students at Duke University School of Medicine. This is a special program for students interested in primary care that takes eight students a year.

The students receiving training in CenteringPregnancy spend 2 days in a regular clinic to gain skills and see what traditional prenatal care is like and then move into their group. They meet ahead of time with the midwife who is facilitating the group. The students work with the facilitator and get to know the women and how Centering works. They help greet and orient new patients to the group and assist with vital signs for the first two to three sessions. By the fourth session, students begin doing the mat assessments. The patients who need the most time and attention are seen for their assessment in the latter half of the Centering session.

The students voluntarily take initiative by creating private Facebook pages with the patients' permission, setting up group texts, and sending out appointment reminders to the patients. Recently, there was a serious weather problem and the medical students were calling the women, talking with Amy about rescheduling or combining two groups, and so forth. The women have the medical students' numbers and call them with concerns. The students then call the midwife for any issues needing more follow-up. The show rates for the sessions have increased. This is the students' favorite rotation.

Amy states: "Clearly the students involved in CenteringPregnancy are MUCH MORE invested in their patients. The quality of this connection is so different from what I see happen with medical students not in this track. Just today a former CenteringPregnancy medical student asked to set up a 1-year birthday party with her former Centering patients."

A medical student commented, "My patients really appreciated my being present during their prenatal care and delivery. For example, one of my patients wanted me to help her with positioning during labor and was comfortable with me delivering her child, with the CNM [certified nurse-midwife] in the room. As a student, I do not feel I could have established such rapport and gotten such hands-on experience with a patient I had just met the day they came to the L&D [Labor and Delivery] floor. This was my favorite part of second year; I wish my peers could experience something similar."

One Duke student commented:

It can be difficult to be a male student on the Labor and Delivery ward. It was different when my three Centering patients delivered their babies. We saw each other more and more as the due dates approached. They texted me on their way to the hospital to say they were on their way in, and then when I knocked on their door, I wasn't greeted with an awkward pause. I was greeted by a whole family glad to see a familiar face and excited about a baby on the way.

Reflections From a Faculty Clinician

Sung Chae, MD

Sung Chae, MD, is a faculty member who directs the Centering model at the JFK Family Medicine residency program. She read an abstract about CenteringPregnancy, attended a training workshop, and then started groups, always with resident involvement. Sung said that the initial pilot groups were hard, especially since it was difficult to get buy-in from the staff and patients, which led to challenges with recruitment. Despite this, gradual growth occurred.

The hospital foundation helped to secure a March of Dimes grant that provided Centering training for all of the residents and also provided money to hire a part-time Centering coordinator. Recruitment still was difficult, but Sung said she made time in her schedule to make the first visits for the targeted/eligible moms to reinforce the benefits of the model and to "put a face" to the facilitator for the group. This increased enrollment.

Now, residents know that at some time in their training they will co-facilitate a group and that their rotation schedule is set over a year ahead. A nurse, social worker, and the coordinator are involved in the groups. Sung feels the success of the group is dependent on the skill of the facilitator.

When asked if only interested residents should be involved in co-facilitating the groups, Sung answered, "Even if they aren't interested in group leadership, they still learn so much. I see a huge difference in how they counsel patients once they've been through Centering. They have had time to listen to patients' stories and learn how to address the practical aspects of the pregnancy experience. They would lose a lot and wouldn't have the vision of how groups could be used with other populations. Almost everyone who does a group thinks it's a great way to provide prenatal care. Their experience with the model also has been an asset in their job search."

"Groups are great but you never know what will happen," commented Sung. "In one group a mom started crying and shared how alone she felt. Other

(continued)

members had partners but hers wasn't involved and they were having issues at home. I wondered, now what do I do? I just sat there . . . it was so hard not to respond immediately . . . then one of the other women looked at the distressed woman and said, 'You are so great. You are caring for your children, keeping things going at home, etc.' Then the group started to rally around the woman. The mom said it felt like group therapy, and was wonderful support."

More Benefits

Involvement in CenteringPregnancy or CenteringParenting groups provides students with a holistic approach to childbearing and parenting. It can fulfill the continuity requirement for learning objectives outlined for OB/GYN residents for their basic experience of the childbearing process. Both preceptors and students appreciate the ability to observe each other in their patient interactions that happen within the group setting. A pediatric resident commented: "I wanted to do CenteringParenting because it gave me direct contact with my attending preceptor. It was so much easier just to ask her a question or have her give me feedback on my baby exam without needing to seek her out in a busy clinic." Since Centering brings together a cohort of patients of the same gestation or baby developmental stage, there is maximal imprinting for the student of normal and deviant findings.

One site that had OB/GYN residents involved in facilitating groups with an attending physician or nurse practitioner found that their rotation design allowed for the residents to attend all of the sessions . . . 100% continuity . . . and the average satisfaction level was 7.9 out of 10 contrasting with 5.75 out of 10 for residents not involved in Centering groups.

The design for student involvement varies depending on the rotation template of the institution and the overall commitment to group care. One of the essential elements of the Centering model is continuity of the clinician throughout the 10 sessions. In the Centering model, content emerges through the process. Because discussion evolves in varied ways in the groups it is essential for the facilitators to carry the group process from session to session. One preceptor commented that students must commit to all 10 sessions, even if it means being present at the group during vacations.

A report titled *A Framework for Educating Health Professionals to Address the Social Determinants of Health* recently was released from the Institute of Medicine and published by the National Academies Press (March 2016). The study posits that health professionals need awareness of the potential causes of ill health and understanding of the importance of addressing them in their work and in their communities. Recommendations in this extensive report include creating lifelong learners "who appreciate the value of relationships and collaborations for understanding and addressing community-identified needs and for strengthening community assets" (Committee on Educating Health Professionals to Address the Social Determinants of Health et al., 2016); preparing health professionals to take action on the social determinants of health; and encouraging organizations, governments, and community groups to include the SDOH in their mission and culture.

Using the lens of Centering groups provides learners with "real-life" interaction with women and families who are struggling with issues stemming from a lack of social justice and demonstrating the need for inclusivity in our framing of care. Centering groups and workshops provide an ideal opportunity for students to learn team-based care and further understand the basic competencies outlined for interprofessional practice (Committee on Educating Health Professionals to Address the Social Determinants of Health et al., 2016). One of the strengths of the Centering model of care is its appropriateness for physicians, midwives, and advanced practice nurses as well as social workers, nurses, nutritionists, and others credentialed to provide care to engage in this model. The Centering Healthcare Institute workshops have attracted people from all of these disciplines, creating a dynamic atmosphere for interprofessional learning. OB/GYN residents from Yale were involved in the early groups that were part of the initial matched cohort study and the randomized controlled trial (Ickovics et al., 2007). One of the residents commented:

> Every resident should have the opportunity to participate in a CenteringPregnancy group. We learn things about the women and about pregnancy that we won't learn through the traditional rotations and we need that knowledge too.

Kolb and colleagues noted,

> It may seem more efficient to have an expert quickly answer a question and move on. . . . Instead, in the CenteringPregnancy model, medical students are able to watch as patients gain confidence in their peers'—and their own—ability to locate the answers to their questions. (2012, p. 103)

One site reports that third-year family medicine residents were involved in co-facilitating CenteringPregnancy groups. They developed skills in facilitation and also learned new information from the patients about pregnancy, breastfeeding, birth, parenting, and basic needs. All of the residents reported 100% satisfaction saying that pregnancy issues were normalized with less attention on medical aspects. This also provided an excellent opportunity for team collaboration (McLeod, LaClair, & Kenyon, 2011).

One family medicine residency reports on their patient care outcomes when residents learned maternity care through their participation in groups. "The process of learning prenatal care through group visits impacted how residents viewed and treated all their patients" (Committee on Educating Health Professionals to Address the Social Determinants of Health et al., 2016). They comment that patient outcomes are directly affected by how well the residents are trained, and by involving residents in group care they documented significant decrease in cesarean sections and a strong trend toward a lower rate of low birth weight and preterm birth (Barr, Aslam, & Levin, 2011).

This chapter concludes with two in-depth profiles. The first highlights the work of Lisa Kugler and Mari-Carmen Farmer, who introduced an innovative adaptation of the CenteringPregnancy model for pregnant mothers and the powerful Healing Circle for the care providers. The second is an interview with Carrie Klima, one of the earliest adopters of the Centering model.

"Mama Care": A Centering-Like Prenatal Model for Women Carrying Babies With Congenital Birth Defects

Lisa Kugler, CNM, MSN and Mari-Carmen Farmer, RN
Children's Hospital of Philadelphia

Children's Hospital of Philadelphia (CHOP), starting in 2008, was the first freestanding children's hospital in the world to provide comprehensive perinatal care for families with prenatally diagnosed birth defects. The interdisciplinary team includes seven midwives who provide prenatal care and attend many of the births. Women are referred from around the world, but the greatest number come from states surrounding Pennsylvania. Depending on the distance from the hospital and the nature of the medical issues, they may commute from home or move to Philadelphia and stay for several months with or without their partners or other family members.

A key goal for the inclusion of midwives in this care model was to normalize the birth experience for these women and their partners. Recognizing that the prenatal period was often one of isolation and stress for families expecting a baby with a birth defect, one of the team members who had been trained in CenteringPregnancy suggested that might be an ideal model of care. The team began offering groups in 2014.

Most women are in their last trimester when they arrive and are invited to join a group based on their gestational age. A new group starts every 4 to 6 weeks. Sometimes women in the group have babies with the same diagnosis which makes for an especially powerful relationship. There are a total of four sessions lasting 2 hours that are offered for each group. The format follows the components and elements of the CenteringPregnancy model. Twelve groups with four to six women in a group met during 2014 and 2015. The groups are facilitated, have involvement from other team members, and are very participant centered.

For women carrying a fetus with a prenatally diagnosed birth defect, connecting with other pregnant women is not easy. Finding joy in a pregnancy characterized by uncertainty and fear is difficult. The weeks that these expectant mothers spend participating in "Mama Care" Centering groups offer each the chance to have a normal experience as a pregnant woman. These experiences are so powerful that if they deliver early they often come back to the group postpartum to share their experience and stay connected. Between 50% and 60% of the babies born at CHOP have cardiac anomalies and go to the cardiac intensive care unit where moms still can stay in contact with each other. Often, the dads attend the group sessions and appreciate the opportunity to bond with each other.

Lisa and Mari-Carmen state, "We have created our own way of honoring the connection between our special mamas. Each of the mothers receives a bracelet that is hand-beaded to look very much like the baby ID bracelets of old. These bracelets come to mean a great deal to the mothers as a symbol of their solidarity and unique transition into parenthood." In 2014, PBS aired a documentary called *Twice Born* about the Center for Fetal Diagnosis & Treatment and the Garbose Family Special Delivery unit at CHOP. There are many stories to share.

In one group each of the couples was greeted with a large gift bag at their seat. One of the mothers, after the previous meeting, was feeling so thankful for the support she found in the Mama Care group that she had crocheted each of the babies a beautiful individualized blanket. She expressed the sentiment of feeling that although the diagnoses and specifics

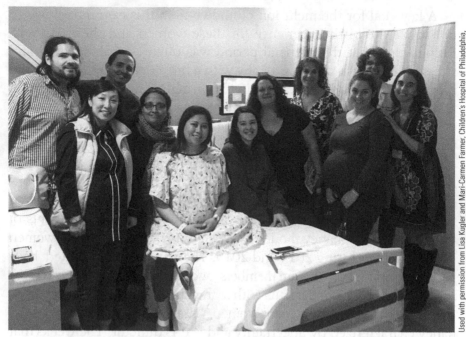

Used with permission from Lisa Kugler and Mari-Carmen Farmer, Children's Hospital of Philadelphia, Pennsylvania.

A Mama Care group supporting one of their members in the labor unit.

of treatment might be different, they represented a community of parents who felt isolated from the norm. As one mom expressed so eloquently, Mama Care helped her "walk through a very dark and scary place.

And then there was the amazing day when three of our Mama Care patients were laboring on the Special Delivery Unit at the same time. One of the mothers took it upon herself to become a one-woman welcoming committee, greeting the other two couples at the door when they arrived, checking on them and sharing encouragement throughout her own labor, and then ensuring they continued to look out for each other during their hospital stay.

The Healing Circle

Lisa and Mari-Carmen continue their story by talking about the Healing Circle. The Healing Circle evolved in great part because of our experience in Mama Care and our partnership as facilitators. We were struck by the parallels between the two experiences and wanted to continue to explore them further. It was obvious to us that the power of the circle exists in many contexts, and it has been extremely rewarding to watch this new idea take shape and further extend the lessons we have already learned through Mama Care.

As members of our unique team, we are asked to provide compassionate support and tireless care for our patients. However, often we don't take time to care for each other and share our thoughts on how to nurture resilience in a work place where we often come face-to-face with loss, heartbreaking choices, and unspeakable suffering.

The Healing Circle was organized to be an inclusive experience that would give us all a chance to listen, to reflect, and to share our stories and collective wisdom about the most challenging aspects of our work. We wished to create a space of shared support and connection. An invitation was sent out to all staff with instructions that by accepting this invitation, the person simply expresses commitment to be a nurturing presence in the group and bear witness to the struggles that are shared that evening. Participation could be by talking or just by listening—in both ways we would be supporting each other.

We hoped to see all of the disciplines represented on our team at the Healing Circle, since each of us brings different perspectives and has insight into varying aspects of the patient experience. Our hope was that our Healing Circle would be helpful for all of us.

Sixteen team members from all disciplines come to the inaugural Healing Circle. The circle opened as Mama Care does, with the setting of ground rules and expectations. Participants were offered the opportunity to speak or to pass as they preferred. As the talking piece moved around the circle, participants grew more comfortable and shared more and more. As people spoke, it became obvious that the power of the circle had something to offer providers and caregivers as we had seen happen with our patients. The Healing Circle provided a facilitated opportunity to transcend hierarchies of the workplace and allowed participants to be vulnerable and share their own emotional response to caring for families facing the birth of a child with an anomaly. There was a strong sense of connection that was forged among the participants. We plan to continue holding the healing circles several times a year.

An Interview With Carrie Klima, CNM, PhD

We interviewed Carrie Klima about her personal journey with the CenteringPregnancy model. She first became acquainted with the model while on the Yale School of Nursing faculty, which quickly led to her assuming a major role in the Centering training workshops. Her engagement with Centering continued when she joined the faculty at the University of Illinois, Chicago, where she led groups, did research, and led national trainings for the Centering Healthcare Institute. Here is her story.

It makes sense, really. CenteringPregnancy highlights what midwives do best.

I remember excitement among students, nurses, and obstetricians about the model. There was a *New York Times* article about CenteringPregnancy that came out in 1999 and then came a brief presentation by Sharon in the School of Nursing followed by a workshop in New Haven. I thought, "This is a midwifery model of care" and was excited that the OB/GYN residents and the director of the obstetrics and gynecology department all expressed interest. The workshop was a real turning point for me and was clear that, this model brings together all the things that should be part of prenatal care.

As we began to do groups, the entire team was filled with passion for making health care better for pregnant women. The OB/GYN chair, the nurses, receptionists . . . everyone had reached a point that the system we were using wasn't working for anyone anymore, providers or patients, so they were all willing to jump in.

But, in the early days of Centering development, before it became the national model that it now is, a few midwives were meeting to discuss the new model, what should be included, what should be included in the training. Do we need a business plan? Strong bonds were created among the founding mothers. Assembling manuals on the kitchen table at Sharon's house, the excitement of being invited to talk about the model, the surprise of the eager responses was infectious. Soon we were worrying about how to respond to so many requests. We just jumped in and tried many strategies to make the groups work. I was also part of the early research on the model that was led by Jeannette Ickovics and her team at the Yale School of Public Health.

It was the perfect storm . . . the current care system wasn't working. This was just the right time to try a new model. The mantra was: it can't be worse, maybe it will be better, and it isn't harmful. It also was a wonderful model for resident education.

Early on, the chair of the department of obstetrics and gynecology was supportive, providing the residents were included and there was research. In the beginning, we had to move a very heavy table out and then back in the room for every group. Evening groups were very popular and we were soon over-subscribed.

There is, however, a cautionary tale. Staff began to turn over, normal in a very large medical center. A research grant paid for much of the original expense. When the grant ended, provisions had not been made to assume the tasks of paid research assistants who had been doing the recruiting of patients. Staff who had become used to others doing this work became resentful. New staff had to be included in the training. We need to remember to be attentive . . . to do a better job with sustainability once the initial enthusiasm dissipates.

I became more committed to the model and joined with Sharon in leading some of the first workshops and also thinking through the structure for a nonprofit. We had annual retreats for midwives, researchers, and others interested in supporting a design for this work. An annual retreat circle became a time for us to exchange the wonderful stories that were beginning to accumulate by those leading groups/workshops.

There was a real sense of purpose and renewal in these retreats. We shared our love of Centering and realized that it was an internal flame for each of us that needed regular rekindling.

I was part of the incorporating group for the Centering Pregnancy and Parenting Institute, later the Centering Healthcare Institute. In those early days, we got together and made notebooks, paid attention to what we saw happening with the model, and shared our own experiences with group leadership. Sharon and I became a seasoned team doing workshops together.

I had completed my dissertation and moved to Chicago where research mentors quickly saw the value of continuing work with Centering. It was a wonderful model for student midwives and received continued support from the midwifery practices. I continued to provide guidance at a national level to hone workshops and increase support to sites. It has allowed me to pursue something I'm passionate about; I'm proud of this work and what I've contributed to the movement.

Now I've been able to bring the model to Africa and have seen that pregnant women the world over have similar needs. Women excel at sharing together in circles. The challenge is to make the model culturally appropriate and sustainable within a variety of systems.

I believe with all my heart that this is the best way to provide prenatal care.

—Carrie Klima

References

American College of Obstetricians and Gynecologists. (2016). Collaboration in practice: Implementing team-based care. *Obstetrics & Gynecology, 127*(3), 612–617.

Barr, W., Aslam, S., & Levin, M. (2011). Evaluation of a group prenatal care-based curriculum in a family medicine residency. *Family Medicine, 43*(10), 712–717.

Committee on Educating Health Professionals to Address the Social Determinants of Health; Board on Global Health; Institute of Medicine; National Academies of Sciences, Engineering, and Medicine. (2016). *A framework for educating health professionals to address the social determinants of health.* Washington, DC: National Academies Press. Retrieved from http://www.nap.edu/21923

Ickovics, J., Kershaw, T., Westdahl, C., Magriples, U., Massey, Z., Reynolds, H., & Rising, S. S. (2007). Group prenatal care and perinatal outcomes: A randomized controlled trial. *Obstetrics & Gynecology, 11*(2, Pt. 1), 330–339.

Kaplan, R., Shaw-Battista, J., & Stotland, N. (2015). Incorporating nurse-midwifery students into graduate medical education: Lessons learned in interprofessional education. *Journal of Midwifery & Women's Health, 60*(6), 718–726.

Kolb, K., Picklesimer, A., Covington-Kolb, S., & Hines, L. (2012). CenteringPregnancy electives: A case study in the shift toward student-centered learning in medical education. *Journal of the South Carolina Medical Association, 108*(4), 103–105.

McLeod, A., LaClair, C., & Kenyon, T. (2011). Interdisciplinary prenatal group visits as a significant learning experience. *Journal of Graduate Medical Education, 3*(3), 372–375.

Rising, S. (1998). CenteringPregnancy: An interdisciplinary model of empowerment. *Journal of Midwifery & Women's Health, 43*(1), 46–54.

Wheatley, M. (2006). *Leadership and the new science: Discovering order in a chaotic world.* San Francisco, CA: Berrett-Koehler.

9 Spread of the Model to Other Health Populations

A family physician cared for a patient with type 2 diabetes for 10 years. "I saw that he was getting sicker and sicker and desperately needed to start insulin, which he steadfastly rejected. I finally got him to attend one of the diabetes groups and at the group session he agreed to start insulin. I tried for 10 years, and the group experience did it in 1 hour!"

Early in the development and implementation of the Centering model for prenatal care, it was evident that the three components—health care, interactive learning, and community building—and the defining essential elements would fit any health population except for those needing acute or emergency intervention. Carmen Strickland, MD, comments:

Simply put, group medical visits using the Centering model promote the development of relationships between patients and their care teams. Through Centering, patients become better patients; they are empowered to partner with their care team and learn to trust that health goals can be achieved. These individuals can then carry these skills beyond their participation in the group. Through Centering, clinicians are reminded that listening to patients leads to more effective problem solving. There is joy in practice that comes from establishing healing relationships with patients and their communities. This model belongs in all of primary care.

During the past decade, there have been many Centering-like models that have developed for use with other populations. At a recent Society for Teachers of Family Medicine conference, residency programs shared successes obtained using this model for metabolic syndrome/obesity, chronic obstructive pulmonary disease (COPD), and chronic pain including suboxone therapy. This chapter provides a brief overview of the history of the development of chronic group care, one design for CenteringPregnancy® for women with diabetes, and vignettes describing the use of the Centering model for populations across the spectrum of health care.

Brief History of Group Care

A review of the general group literature outside of the abundant Centering literature revealed several important publications. The first known reference to the use of groups was published in 1907 regarding group care for the treatment of people in the Boston area diagnosed with consumption. Dr. Joseph Pratt, an internist, noted the improvement in the emotional state in patients getting care in groups and later promoted the use of groups for psychiatric patients (Pratt, 1907). The next mention of group care in the literature was in 1974 with a description and evaluation of a model created by Marie Feldman for groups of parents and children receiving well-childcare (Feldman, 1974). This work was followed by that of Lucy Osborne and James Taylor in the 1980s (Osborn & Woolley, 1981). Besides demonstrating that the groups led to better patient/physician satisfaction, they were able to show better health outcomes as well as efficiency for the system.

During the 1990s, besides the piloting of CenteringPregnancy, there was an increase in the development of other group models specifically for chronic care. The Cooperative Health Care Clinic (CHCC) model was developed by Dr. John Scott, an internist in Colorado, and promoted especially for chronically ill, older health maintenance organization (HMO) patients (Scott et al., 2004). He conducted workshops with Marlene McKenzie, RN, and also collaborated with Dr. Ed Noffsinger in his work to develop DIGMAs (Drop-In Medical Appointments) and Physician Shared Medical Appointments (PSMAs), both of which brought people together for one-time consultation and/or physical examination.

A qualitative review of current research on group visits was published by Jaber, Braksmajer, and Trilling (2006). This work concluded that "group visits are a promising approach to chronic care management for the motivated patient" (p. 289). These visits provide an opportunity for combining education with medical care while also allowing for productivity and adequate revenue generation.

There is considerable data about the effectiveness of these models. In chronic care, the most common model cited in the literature is for the diabetic population, but articles also discuss group care for patients with dementia, obesity, cancer, asthma, HIV, stress, women's health, and so forth. In general, the data supports improved health outcomes and high patient satisfaction for patients getting care in groups. There is also evidence of greater efficiency of care provision, including access to care.

Centering Healthcare™

The combination of evidence-based effectiveness, efficient use of personnel, and well-defined core components that can be replicated make this model attractive for adaptation to new settings and for other health concerns (Rising, Kennedy, & Klima, 2004).

The following vignettes illustrate how the Centering model is being used to provide care for specific populations. These examples of the use of the Centering model have developed from specific interest of clinicians who already were caring for the population and who, upon training in the Centering model, then realized the applicability to their specific patient groups. For each extension of the model, the vignette description includes details on the population served, desired outcomes, and, to the extent possible, the actual outcomes in answer to the question: How is this model working for the women?

Centering for Special Prenatal Populations

The first two vignettes focus specifically on the use of Centering with special prenatal populations, including those identified as having diabetes or being at risk for gestational diabetes and for women who are pregnant and obese.

CenteringPregnancy Diabetes

Kathleen Dermady, LM, CNM, DNP
Regional Center in Central New York

CenteringPregnancy Special Care Women With Diabetes, at the Regional Center in Central New York, to date, has involved 88 women of similar gestational age in groups with an average of five to six women per group. This woman-centered perinatal care facilitates assessment, education, and shared decision making that promotes a healthy pregnancy for women with diabetes. Women are responsible for complex self-management decisions such as balancing food intake, activity, blood glucose levels, and medication use, often insulin. A healthy pregnancy outcome is dependent on maintaining near-normal glucose levels at all times during the pregnancy. Diabetes education and knowledge of the needs of the growing fetus help mothers understand how blood glucose control affects and is affected by the pregnancy.

Group size, due to the complexity of management, is six to eight women of similar gestational age. Reviewing blood glucose records is done during the individual assessment time within the group space. Although the blood glucose challenges and trends in blood glucose control and insulin resistance are discussed in the group setting, the individual nature of insulin management by injections or pump adds additional time to the assessment. Perinatal Center Maternal Fetal Medicine (MFM) providers participate in the management planning and review of diabetes management with the group's facilitators, but group facilitation is the responsibility of the certified nurse-midwives and nurse practitioners, nurses, nutritionists, social workers, and lactation consultants working at the Perinatal Center.

Women are scheduled every 2 weeks for three visits, every 3 weeks for the next three visits, and every 2 weeks for the remaining sessions. Women attend the groups as scheduled and have asked to have group care continue for their entire pregnancy. The options for testing are discussed, and usually the nonstress test (NST) is conducted in the group space during the discussion time with the permission of the participant.

> "I had never known anyone who really took good care of their diabetes, and I had never known any other pregnant women who had diabetes and had to do all the things that I had to do. In the group, it was great to watch other women pulling out their glucometer to test. I always thought I was the only one in the world who had to do that. I like hearing and seeing that other people were going through the same thing I was going through. It made me try harder."

At the first visit, the group began with introductions and discussion of their journey with diabetes, discussing challenges and triumphs with management. Three of the members shared difficulties with management of previous pregnancies. One of them expressed an interest in knowing more about the insulin pump. Two members of the group who were pump users offered to show this mother their pumps and discuss how using the pumps had changed their management. The facilitator supported the discussion to provide clarity and medical information. This young woman began using an insulin pump and found that her glycemic control significantly improved over the pregnancy.

How is this model working for the women? At the final session, one woman noted that the experience of Centering was a new beginning for her. There is growing support at the health center for the model, and the next steps may be seeing women with other medical problems in the CenteringPregnancy groups.

CenteringPregnancy for Obese Women—An Opportunity to Meet Gestational Weight Gain Goals

Michelle A. Kominiarek, MD, MS

Northwestern University Feinberg School of Medicine

Trends in adult weight over the past several decades highlight the escalating role that obesity plays in women's health: 31.8% of reproductive age women (20–39 years) were obese in 2011 and 2012 (Ogden, Carroll, Kit, & Flegal, 2014). The combination of obesity and pregnancy introduces additional complications such as birth defects, preeclampsia, gestational diabetes, stillbirths, and cesarean deliveries.

Most programs addressing gestational weight gain for obese women are individual-level interventions (e.g., one-to-one nutrition consults and exercise advice). Few have used a group approach, and these are non-pregnancy-related, for example, Weight Watchers. However evidence has suggested that socialization through groups can help people achieve goals that would not be reachable by individuals alone and that support from attending meetings enhances feelings of control and confidence.

To investigate the perceptions of pregnant women about obesity and gestational weight gain and to explore strategies on how to improve the management of obesity in pregnancy with an emphasis on group prenatal care, 16 primarily non-Hispanic Black pregnant women with a prepregnancy body mass index ≥ 30 kg/m^2 participated in focus groups at an inner-city teaching hospital (Kominiarek, Gay, & Peacock, 2015). Women frequently stated that their gestational weight gain goal was more than 20 pounds and described a body image not in line with clinical recommendations—"weighing 200 pounds is not that big." They wished that their providers would not use the term "obese," but also admitted there really wasn't a "nice way to say it."

They were interested in learning about nutrition and culturally acceptable healthy cooking. They also wanted to learn about how to build exercise into their daily routine. Women viewed the group setting as an environment that could provide support as evidenced by the following quote: Family members could help them reach their goals, but

 "It could be people in a group going through the same thing you are going through, so you don't feel that it is just you. Once you get out into these groups or you talk—you start talking and then your family starts listening."

generational differences posed challenges as many of their mothers and grandmothers thought they needed to "eat for two" and that exercise was harmful during pregnancy.

In CenteringPregnancy, group leaders promote engagement of both women and their support person by employing participatory group activities, by referring questions raised during discussions back to the group, and by encouraging women to share information with one another. All these features closely mirror what obese women in the focus group study said they were searching for. A group prenatal care setting would also fit the needs of these women because obesity is multifactorial in nature and requires an integration of health care services that can occur when nutritionists, exercise physiologists, and social workers co-facilitate these sessions.

Preliminary data suggests that culturally tailored programs that use acceptable terms for obesity, provide education regarding healthy eating and safe exercise, and encourage support from social networks may be effective in addressing gestational weight gain in obese minority women. Because CenteringPregnancy has its roots in social support and group problem solving, these women, already at high risk for adverse pregnancy outcomes including excessive gestational weight gain, may have an opportunity to improve their own and their offsprings' health with the intervention of Centering care. Funding is being sought for a formal study building on this preliminary work.

Centering Healthcare for Chronic Care Populations

The following models are used for provision of chronic care with a variety of populations including those with chronic pelvic pain, sickle cell disease, breast cancer survivors, healthy hearts, and diabetes.

Centering and Chronic Pelvic Pain

Priscilla Abercrombe, PhD, NP, AHN-BC
Women's Health and Healing, Healdsburg, California

Maria Chao, DrPH, MPA
University of California, San Francisco, California

This model was offered by the University of California, San Francisco Osher Center for Integrative Medicine and San Francisco General Hospital Women's Health Center. The program was developed and studied by a holistic nurse practitioner and a researcher interested in health disparities.

Women with chronic pelvic pain (CPP) suffer from a variety of complex conditions involving many different organ systems. CPP can severely impact a woman's quality of life, including the ability to participate in normal activities of daily living, sexual functioning, and emotional well-being. The Centering model was chosen for this work because it provides assessment, education, and support in a group environment that is empowering and gives a sense of belonging to women who often feel very isolated. It was also a natural fit with an integrative health approach where the patient–provider relationship, caring for the whole person, and the use of a broad range of conventional and complementary treatment strategies are central to health care.

The women served with this model received either public or private insurance, were English-speaking, multiethnic, and ranged in age from 20 to 70. Many of the women were on disability because of their pain. The 10-session program was developed from a review of the literature and from clinical practice and was modeled after the Centering Diabetes groups. The session topics included understanding CPP, easing pain and symptoms, myofascial pain, medications, nutrition, managing stress, setting goals, communication, sexual pain, and spirituality. The program sought to reduce barriers to pain care, especially for underserved women, foster self-management of symptoms, and improve quality of life (Chao, Abercrombie, & Duncan, 2012).

Preliminary research was conducted and found that the groups:

- Improved health related quality of life
- Improved sexual health
- Decreased number of unhealthy days
- Decreased depressive symptoms

In addition, participants found that as a result of the groups:

- They learned about how to reduce pain
- They used the information from the groups in their daily lives
- They found emotional support in the groups
- The groups were a safe place to discuss issues
- They were treated with respect by the leaders
- They would recommend the group to other women with CPP (Chao, Abercrombie, Santana, & Duncan, 2015)

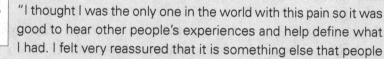

"I thought I was the only one in the world with this pain so it was good to hear other people's experiences and help define what I had. I felt very reassured that it is something else that people have, and I've come to terms with the fact that it might never go away."

Group Care for Adolescents With Sickle Cell Disease Transitioning to Adult Care

Crystal Patil, PhD
University of Illinois at Chicago

CenteringPregnancy is now a well-established and efficacious example of group prenatal care. The combination of evidence-based effectiveness, efficient use of personnel, and well-defined core components that can be replicated make this model attractive for adaptation to new settings and for other health concerns (Rising et al., 2004). Sickle cell disease is an inherited blood disease that affects nearly every system in the body. It is associated with acute and chronic pain, increased risk for infection, and progressive damage to organs.

Individuals with sickle cell disease have an increased risk of early death, but the advent of newborn screening, early entry into health care, and use of preventative drugs have increased life expectancy. Prior to newborn screening, life expectancy was about 14 years of age. Today, more than 90% of individuals reach 18 years of age, and the average life expectancy is closer to 50 years (Claster & Vichinsky, 2003; Quinn, Rogers, McCavit, & Buchanan, 2010). The increased life expectancy has created a need for the development of programs that prepare adolescents and young adults (AYAs) with sickle cell disease for transitioning from pediatric to adult health care. Unfortunately, AYAs do not always receive successful preparation for the transition to adult care, leading to more emergency department visits, rehospitalization, and an increased risk of death. This highlights the need for successful transition programs, yet no ideal transition program for individuals with sickle cell disease has been identified (Jordan, Swerdlow, & Coates, 2013).

Our review of the CenteringPregnancy model led us to consider this type of group care as a promising innovation to address the challenges associated with living with a chronic disease and transitioning. This process-driven model did not require new technologies or huge budgetary demands, so we designed and pretested a CenteringPregnancy-based model and content through an adolescent social support group. We determined that the model had acceptability among adolescents.

We are now conducting a complete pilot of the program with a single group of AYAs to assess acceptability and feasibility within a health care setting—the Pediatric Sickle Cell Clinic. We expect this transitioning model will make a significant contribution to efforts to improve outcomes for those living with this ever-changing chronic disease. Our team includes a medical anthropologist, social worker, medical doctor, and pediatric nurse practitioner so we can draw on our collective research and practice experience to fully develop and assess the value of group care for adolescents and these young adults.

Based on our collective experience, we designed an eight-session program to cover the following major topics: dispelling myths about sickle cell disease, healthy living (nutrition, hydration, and keeping active), effective health care communication and coping, navigating the health care system, employment and education, reproductive health, and the adult clinic. The objectives of the pilot are the following:

1. Produce a final first draft of the facilitator's guide
2. Determine the acceptability of group care as a health care model for transitioning among AYAs with sickle cell disease
3. Complete a pilot to determine whether sessions can be conducted with fidelity to the core processes of this well-established group care model and whether or not patients and providers see value in this model

Centering Heart Circles: The Healthy Heart Project

Sally Lemke, DNP, WHNP-BC
Former Program Manager, Healthy Heart Project for Women

Heart Circles, a collection of group care sessions, was developed over the course of 2007 to 2008 as part of the Healthy Heart Project, focused on reducing cardiovascular risk in women. The session ran from 2007 to 2011.

Heart Circles consists of 12 core sessions of group care based on the Centering model. Sessions were developed as part of a funded program aimed at reducing cardiovascular risk in adult women. Sessions were conducted by two facilitators, one nurse practitioner and one peer leader who was hired by the program and trained in the basics of facilitated group leadership and core content of the sessions. The health care provider and peer leader worked closely together throughout the program. Group participants were residents of an agency that provides housing and social services to homeless women with histories of addiction. The women involved in Heart Circles were aged 30 to 65, with the average age being mid-40s. The majority were African American. All had some sort of cardiovascular risk, with obesity, hypertension, and smoking predominating. Several women had hyperlipidemia and/or diabetes.

Groups were conducted onsite at a residential facility where health care services were provided to residents. Sessions were intended to be held once a month but typically ran every other week in the residential setting because there were no restrictions on frequency of care for the participants. Services were not billed but designed to be billable.

Group format was modeled after Centering sessions. Prior to circle-up, participants performed self-care activities such as blood pressure (BP) check, weight check, and glucose monitoring when indicated and self-assessment forms on session topics, followed by a face-to-face encounter with the nurse practitioner. Sessions began with an opening, contained experiential learning activities, and ended with a closing. Content focused on healthy lifestyle adoption and support. Participants were provided with a binder containing session content in addition to food and activity journal sheets.

A series of six sessions focusing on the use of art and artistic expression as a way to achieve personal change for improved cardiovascular health was also incorporated into the program during the weeks between the core sessions.

Funding for the health care component of the program expired, and so the groups, as designed, are no longer running. Also, I moved into a new role at my job site. However, ongoing educational and peer support groups targeting heart health that are organized and run by a group of health care volunteers have continued. Heart Circle provided the foundation for these groups.

Approximately 120 women participated in some or all of the group sessions over the course of 4 years. Women indicated high satisfaction with the groups. In addition, the program evaluation showed improvements in BP, improved nutrition for things such as numbers of fruits and vegetables, fried-food reduction and take-out food consumed each week, and minutes of moderate and aerobic activity performed in each week. There were no changes for smoking. Body mass indexes (BMIs) were tracked and showed inconsistent change.

Breast Cancer Survivorship Groups

Kathryn J. Trotter, DNP, CNM, FNP-C
Duke University School of Nursing

In 2007, this nurse practitioner saw a need for women survivors of breast cancer to meet together for follow-up care. She brought together six to eight women who were 3 years or more from diagnosis and free of metastatic disease for care and discussion. The session design was patterned after the Centering Healthcare model. These groups provided an avenue for the provision of psychological support and health-promotion activities, as well as surveillance for recurrence of the cancer or late effects. Each woman was asked to prepare a written breast cancer survivorship care plan for her own use. This plan also was shared with her primary care provider. The women were asked if they wanted to stay in the cohort and then were scheduled for their yearly appointments in the same time block. Over the years, about 60% to 85% of the women made the cohort appointments. Having six to eight in a group provided strong group dynamics, timely visits for the women, and adequate reimbursement for the system.

Over the years, some adaptations have been made to increase the efficiency of the visits, for example, mammogram, bloods, bone density, complete physical exam, but the basic design of the sessions remained the same. Women took their own blood pressure, completed a self-assessment sheet, and had a quick check-in with the clinician. The discussion revolved around their prioritized issues. The clinician noted that because of her contact with the women during the group time, she spent less time doing the extensive physical exam that happened after the group.

Groups for women at high risk for breast cancer based on genetic carrier syndromes or strong family history of breast or ovarian cancer continue. Over 300 patients have been followed in this model since the start of groups in 2007. One evaluation of 122 women showed high satisfaction with receiving care in the group visit, and 86% of these women continued their follow-up in the group.

Male partners are asking why there isn't a group model for prostate cancer survivors. "We have questions too that need time to discuss!" People with a variety of health issues could benefit from receiving care in groups. This is an ideal model for teaching nurse practitioner students and other clinicians about meeting the needs of people in the cohort (Trotter, 2013; Trotter, Frazier, Hendricks, & Scarsella, 2011; Trotter, Schneider, & Turner, 2013).

Centering and Diabetes: A Chronic Care Model

Monte Wagner, RN, DNP
Community Health Center, Inc., Danbury, Connecticut

After a long afternoon seeing adult patients with diabetes at a federally qualified health center in Connecticut in 2013 and answering similar questions about diabetes over and over, the idea of creating a group visit program was developed. After trying out several models, from drop-in groups to a cohort-style program, we realized that just talking about diet, exercise, medications, and preventative care would only scratch the surface of what our patients needed. They had difficulties with putting into action what many of them already knew. The biggest hurdles were coping with the chronic disease, solving problems as they presented, and managing the tasks of caring for themselves under challenging psychosocial circumstances. The Centering Healthcare model offered a program-based approach combining sharing information about the disease and its care with an effective approach to motivate and engage individuals in a safe group environment.

Currently, groups meet monthly and follow an eight-session program using the seven talking points for adults with diabetes developed by the American Association of Diabetic Educators. The co-facilitators are a nurse practitioner and either a nurse or a behavioral health clinician. In addition to the 2-hour monthly groups, a nurse and a behavioral health clinician also offer weekly 45-minute self-management support groups that focus on goal setting and management. This was found to be a helpful addition to the medical groups because many previous participants struggled with achieving even basic goals like checking their blood sugars or taking their medicines regularly. It also integrates in the interprofessional care model of the community health center, where professionals from medicine, nursing, behavioral health, dentistry, podiatry, and pharmacy closely collaborate to manage the often complex needs of this population.

Since starting in January 2013, about 100 patients have attended the groups, and many return to the groups because they enjoy the extended time with the clinical team, the engaging group discussions, and the additional support received from other group members and staff. The program has become a regular component of medical care at the community health center, and it is planned that multiple groups are run concurrently throughout the year. One nurse practitioner has created a formal program and evaluation, including institutional review board approval, as part of his doctoral project, which should be completed by March 2016.

"I don't have a lot of friends, and I'm a shy person, and I don't like to share my stuff and I've realized being in this group how important it is to talk about what's going on in my life and to share with the others in my group about my diabetes. There's a lot of stress . . . it's made a difference for me. I think now I'm going to be able to share more, and I've learned a lot more about my diabetes and how what I do affects my family, my children."

CenteringPregnancy and Adolescents

Despite the fact that adolescent pregnancy has declined over the past decade, the United States continues to have a higher rate than other industrialized countries. The majority of these pregnancies are unintended and add stress to the significant social and health issues faced by young women at a time when they are moving into adult roles and struggling with developmental issues. The rapid adoption of social media and the availability of information on blogs and websites often lead to a dizzying array of messages, many conflicting. An early study of the teen CenteringPregnancy model at Barnes Jewish Hospital in St. Louis, Missouri, found that teens in CenteringPregnancy had better attendance at visits, low rates of preterm birth and low-birth-weight infants, and high satisfaction. One teen commented, "It's really fun to come to a program that teaches you a lot of things you thought you knew until you came here" (Grady & Bloom, 2004, p. 415).

A retrospective chart study of 150 pregnant adolescents receiving care between 2008 and 2012 was conducted by the MedStar Health Research Institute (MHRI/MedStar) Washington Hospital Center. Fifty patients were included in each of three groups: CenteringPregnancy care, traditional single-provider or traditional group-provider arms. A review of the results from January 2008 to June 2012 demonstrated a positive effect on compliance with prenatal visits, the uptake of long-acting contraceptive methods, adequate weight gain, and increased rates of breastfeeding compared to the traditional-care groups (Trotman et al., 2015). Their conclusion states, "Our study supports CenteringPregnancy as a viable option to encourage healthy behaviors in a high-risk adolescent population" (Trotman et al., 2015, p. 400).

TAPP Program at MedStar

The Teen Alliance for Prepared Parenting (TAPP) is an adolescent secondary pregnancy prevention program based at MedStar Washington Hospital Center in Washington, DC. TAPP provides clinical and psychosocial services to young mothers and fathers with a primary goal of preventing second births in adolescence. TAPP adopted CenteringPregnancy in 2012 because mothers younger than the age of 20 are more likely to experience a preterm birth, are less likely to regularly attend prenatal care, and are less likely to breastfeed.

TAPP CenteringPregnancy groups are facilitated by a certified nurse-midwife and a licensed social worker. Since 2012, TAPP has made CenteringPregnancy standard of care and has facilitated 23 CenteringPregnancy groups, which average six participants per group. Every medically eligible youth is automatically enrolled in Centering. Since adopting Centering, only 4% of TAPP participants have experienced preterm delivery and just 6.5% of TAPP participants have delivered a low-birth-weight newborn. The preterm delivery rate for the district is 11% and 12.7% of infants born to teen mothers are low birth weight. Additionally, the percentage of participants who initiate breastfeeding increased from 73% in the first year to 90% last year. Overall, 98% of participants are highly satisfied with their prenatal care, emphasizing support and education as key program benefits. A TAPP participant said this about Centering: "It is actually helpful because you feel less alone and it gives you a lot of support if you did not have any during your pregnancy." Another client noted educational benefits, stating "Centering is a nice place to enjoy and discuss things about you and your baby and a place you can learn from."

Our health care providers are also more satisfied with providing care in the group setting. Centering offers more time with patients and allows for more in-depth discussion about important health education topics. Centering visits occur in a group and are 90 to 120 minutes, compared to 15- to 30-minute traditional prenatal appointments (personal communication, Elysia Jordan and Loral Patchen, 2016).

CenteringPregnancy and the Military

The CenteringPregnancy model of prenatal care has been used by all branches of the military. With approximately 1 million prenatal visits and

90,000 births to military families each year, there is great opportunity for Centering to be a mediator for the stress felt by these families.

Researchers have found that when women's lives are intensely stressful, they have a 44% greater chance of having a preterm birth (Christopher, 2014). It is logical to assume with a population that has experienced more than 2 million deployments in the past 14 years, there is an increased stress factor for the pregnant military families (Tarney et al., 2015). Resultant preterm birth and postpartum depression rates in a population of deployed and nondeployed spouses documented the increased risk to families serving in the military (Tarney et al., 2015). The early history of the development and strengths of the model in the armed forces are reviewed by Foster and colleagues (2012).

A multisite randomized controlled trial of CenteringPregnancy conducted from 2005 to 2007, demonstrated improved satisfaction, more knowledge of pregnancy and birth, and documented that women in groups were six times more likely to receive adequate prenatal care (Kennedy et al., 2009; Kennedy et al., 2011).

The armed services continue to increase the number of Centering-Pregnancy sites on their bases. The Centering Healthcare Institute has formalized a contract with the Army to establish a service-wide contract to maximize this model to its beneficiaries.

Summary

Two pioneers in the development of chronic care groups, Edward Noffsinger and John Scott, write, "Various types of proven group visit programs will be used increasingly in the delivery of health care because of their ability to provide better, more efficient care at reduced cost and to create high levels of both patient and provider professional satisfaction" (2000, p. 87). The pressures on systems to meet the triple aim—better health, better care, and lower costs—continue to stress an already overburdened system. There are insufficient financial resources available to meet all of the demands, and hence groups are seen as one way to increase efficiency and patient engagement with improving health outcomes (Edelman et al., 2012; Noffsinger, 2009; Noffsinger, 2013; Schmucker, 2006).

The models highlighted in this chapter discuss just a few of the populations that can be well-served by group care. The Centering Healthcare model with its three components of care, interactive learning, and community building provides an excellent framework for the implementation and evaluation of group care for almost any population.

References

Chao, M., Abercrombie, P., & Duncan, L. (2012). Centering as a model for group visits among women with chronic pelvic pain. *Journal of Obstetric, Gynecologic, & Neonatal Nursing, 41*(5), 703–710. doi:10.1111/j.1552-6909.2012.01406.x

Chao, M., Abercrombie, P., Santana, T., & Duncan, L. (2015). Applying the RE-AIM framework to evaluate integrative medicine group visits among diverse women with chronic pelvic pain. *Pain Management Nursing, 16*(6), 920–929. doi:10.1016/j.pmn.2015.07.007

Christopher, G. C. (2014). The future is born every day. *American Journal of Public Health, 104*(Suppl. 1), S7.

Claster, S., & Vichinsky, E. (2003). Managing sickle cell disease. *British Medical Journal, 327*(7424), 1151–1155. doi:10.1136/bmj.327.7424.1151

Edelman, D., McDuffie, J., Oddone, E., Gierisch, J., Naagi, A., & Williams, J., Jr. (2012). Shared medical appointments for chronic medical conditions: A systematic review. *Evidence Based Synthesis Program.* Retrieved from www.ncbi.nlm.nih.gov/books/NBK99785

Feldman, M. (1974). Cluster visits. *American Journal of Nursing, 74*(8), 1485–1488.

Foster, G., Alviar, A., Neumeier, R., & Wootten, A. (2012). A tri-service perspective on the implementation of a CenteringPregnancy model in the military. *Journal of Obstetric, Gynecologic, and Neonatal Nursing, 41*(2), 315–321.

Grady, M. A., & Bloom, K.C. (2004). Pregnancy outcomes of adolescents enrolled in a CenteringPregnancy program. *Journal of Midwifery & Women's Health, 49*(5), 412–420.

Jaber, R., Braksmajer, A., & Trilling, J. (2006). Group visits: A qualitative review of current research. *Journal of the American Board of Family Medicine, 19*(3), 276–290.

Jordan, L., Swerdlow, P., & Coates, T. (2013). Systematic review of transition from adolescent to adult care in patients with sickle cell disease. *Journal of Pediatric Hematology/Oncology, 35*(3), 165–169.

Kennedy, H. P., Farrell, T., Paden, R., Hill, S., Jolivet, R., Willetts, J., & Rising, S. S. (2009). "I wasn't alone"—A study of group prenatal care in the military. *Journal of Midwifery & Women's Health, 54*(3), 176–183.

Kennedy, H. P., Farrell, T., Paden, R., Hill, S., Jolivet, R., Willetts, J., & Rising, S. S. (2011). A randomized clinical trial of group prenatal care in two military settings. *Military Medicine, 176*(10), 1169–1177.

Kominiarek, M., Gay, F., & Peacock, N. (2015). Obesity in pregnancy: A qualitative approach to inform an intervention for patients and providers. *Maternal and Child Health Journal, 19*(8), 1698–1712.

Noffsinger, E. (2009). *Running group visits in your practice.* New York, NY: Springer.

Noffsinger, E. (2013). *The ABCs of group visits: An implementation manual for your practice.* New York, NY: Springer.

Noffsinger, E., & Scott, J. (2000). Potential abuses of group visits. *The Permanente Journal, 4*(2), 87–98.

Ogden, C., Carroll, M., Kit, B., & Flegal, K. (2014). Prevalence of childhood and adult obesity in the United States, 2011–2012. *Journal of the American Medical Association, 311*(8), 806–814.

Osborn, L., & Woolley, F. (1981). Use of groups in well-childcare. *Pediatrics, 67*(5), 701–706.

Pratt, J. (1907). The class method of treating consumption in the homes of the poor. *Journal of the American Medical Association, 49*(9), 755–759.

Quinn, C., Rogers, Z., McCavit, T., & Buchanan, G. (2010). Improved survival of children and adolescents with sickle cell disease. *Blood, 115*(17), 3447–3452. doi:10.1182/blood-2009-07-233700

Rising, S., Kennedy, H., & Klima, C. (2004). Redesigning prenatal care through CenteringPregnancy. *Journal of Midwifery & Women's Health, 49*(5), 398–404.

Schmucker, D. (2006). *Group medical appointments*. Boston, MA: Jones & Bartlett.

Scott, J., Conner, D., Venohr, I., Gade, G., McKenzie, M., Kramer, A., . . . Beck, A. (2004). Effectiveness of a group outpatient visit model for chronically ill older health maintenance organization members: A 2-year randomized trial of the cooperative health care clinic. *Journal of the American Geriatrics Society, 52*(9), 1463–1470.

Tarney, C., Berry-Caban, C., Jain, R., Keely, M., Sewell, M., & Wilson, K. (2015). Association of spouse deployment on pregnancy outcomes in a U.S. military population. *Obstetrics & Gynecology, 126*(3), 569–574.

Trotman, G., Chhatre, G., Darolia, R., Tefera, E., Damle, L., & Gomez-Lobo, V. (2015). The effect of CenteringPregnancy versus traditional prenatal care models on improved adolescent health behaviors in the perinatal period. *Journal of Pediatric Adolescent Gynecology, 28*(5), 395–401.

Trotter, K. (2013). The promise of group medical visits. *The Nurse Practitioner, 38*(5), 48–53.

Trotter, K., Frazier, A., Hendricks, C. K., & Scarsella, H. (2011). Innovation in survivor care: Group visits. *Clinical Journal of Oncology Nursing, 15*(2), E24–E33.

Trotter, K. J., Schneider, S. M., & Turner, B. S. (2013). Group appointments in a breast cancer survivorship clinic. *Journal of the Advanced Practitioner in Oncology, 4*(6), 423–431.

The Centering Healthcare™ Model: Making Change Sustainable

10 Making Change Sustainable: The Role of Policy and Advocacy
Lisa Summers

Our capabilities for groundbreaking research, innovative technology and communications tools are unprecedented today and can be leveraged to influence health in multiple ways.—Gail Christopher

This chapter focuses on the role of policy and advocacy in the scale, spread, and sustainability of Centering Healthcare™. Why a chapter on policy and advocacy? The U.S. health care system is undergoing significant change and, as earlier chapters have made clear, Centering has remarkable potential to lower preterm birth. The potential for significant cost savings alone is of interest to policy makers. The transformation of service delivery from the individual model to group care is a significant undertaking which can be facilitated by advocates working together toward the improvement of maternal and child health.

The chapter provides a brief background and framework for considering Centering within the context of a reforming health care system, describes what policy makers have already done to facilitate the scale and spread of Centering, particularly with regard to reimbursement, and provides suggestions for what advocates can do moving forward.

Why the Time Is Right: A Reforming Health System

Efforts to establish national health insurance in the United States date to the New Deal of the 1930s. The establishment of Medicare and Medicaid in the 1960s stands out as one successful effort in a long history of failed attempts at reform (Christopher, 2014; Kaiser Family Foundation, 2009). An analysis of how policy makers might learn from the failure of the 1993 Clinton Health Security Act ends with the observation that,

> *"Clinton was the not the first president to fail at health care reform: he was following in the footsteps of Franklin Roosevelt, Harry Truman, and Richard Nixon. Ultimately, the demise of the Clinton plan says less about the administration's mistakes than it does about the extraordinary difficulty of adopting comprehensive health care reform in the United States." (Oberlander, 2007, p. 1679)*

Despite this history, the skyrocketing costs of health care made the need for reform a top issue of the 2008 presidential campaign, and so Barak Obama launched his presidency with a vow to make health system reform a top priority. As the White House Office of Health Reform was established and advocates and members of Congress readied proposals and strategized, there were concerted efforts to learn from the history of failed attempts (Alliance for Health Reform, 2008).

In Crossing the Quality Chasm: A New Health Care for the 21st Century, *the Institute of Medicine (IOM, 2001) outlined 10 rules for health care redesign. Table 10.1 compares those 10 rules with elements of Centering Care Models.*

In keeping with those lessons learned—"Don't try to put everything into one bill," and "Be willing to deal,"—the Patient Protection and Affordable Care Act (ACA) that was signed on March 23, 2010, was not the sweeping reform sought by some advocates. It did, however, usher in an era of significant, broad insurance reforms: denial of coverage for pre-existing conditions (which had included pregnancy) and lifetime limits on coverage were eliminated; key preventive services were mandated cost-free for many Americans; coverage was extended to young adults who were allowed to stay on their parents' plan until they turned 26 ("Key Features of the Affordable Care Act," 2010).

The ACA contains numerous provisions intended to move toward "value-based purchasing," with less emphasis on payment for procedures and more emphasis on primary and preventive care. The Act established the Center for Medicare and Medicaid Innovation (CMMI or "The Innovation Center") within Centers for Medicare and Medicaid Services (CMS) to test payment and service delivery models. Strong Start is a CMMI initiative that has significantly raised awareness of both birth centers and CenteringPregnancy®.

TABLE 10.1 IOM Rules and Elements of Centering Healthcare

IOM Rules for Health Care Redesign	Elements of Centering Care Models
Care based on continuous healing relationships	✓ Stability of group participants and care providers, establishing trust
Care customized according to patient needs and values	✓ Educational content allows emphasis to vary with group needs ✓ Facilitative leadership encourages exploration of cultural values
The patient is source of control	✓ Participants are involved in self-care activities
Knowledge is shared and information flows freely	✓ Participants share their own knowledge and experience
Decision making is evidence based	✓ Sites continually evaluate outcomes
Safety is a system priority	✓ Group process promotes trust and openness
Transparency is necessary	✓ Participants have access to and track their own health information
Needs are anticipated	✓ Skilled facilitation supports the process
Waste is continuously decreased	✓ Health assessment occurs in the group space
Cooperation among clinicians is a priority	✓ Interdisciplinary collaboration is fostered

IOM, Institute of Medicine.

Used with permission from Centering Healthcare Institute.

ACA-Funded Initiative Raising Awareness of Centering

The visibility of Centering, particularly among administrators of state Medicaid programs, was raised significantly with the announcement in 2012 of the Strong Start for Mothers and Newborns initiative. Funded through the CMMI, Strong Start aims to reduce preterm births and improve outcomes and serves as a catalyst for midwifery-led innovation: the American Association of Birth Centers received a Strong Start grant to convene a group of 45 birth centers from 19 states, and 15 awardees are implementing group visits across 54 sites.

Strong Start has, however, created some challenges for Centering, since sites are not required to avail themselves of facilitation training or materials from Centering Healthcare Institute (CHI), although CHI is working closely with the sites implementing group visits. As noted in the year 2 evaluation, "Strong Start awardees implementing group prenatal care are not required to adopt a particular curriculum, but most have an affiliation with Centering" (Strong Start, 2016). Given the importance of model fidelity and the design of Strong Start, it may be difficult to draw meaningful conclusions about Centering versus "group visits." On the other hand, this may be an opportunity to expand the important but limited research on the impact of modifying Centering: "These non-Centering versions of group prenatal care may still improve outcomes over individual care, and studying these versions may help us understand which elements of group prenatal care truly improve outcomes" (Strong Start, 2016). The final evaluation of Strong Start is expected in 2018.

▉ Essential Health Benefits

One key component of the ACA is the establishment of essential health benefits (EHBs), a set of comprehensive health care service categories that certain health plans were required to cover beginning in 2014. States expanding Medicaid coverage must provide these benefits to people eligible for Medicaid, and insurance policies must cover these benefits in order to be offered in the health insurance marketplaces. EHBs is an example of "the devil in the details": "maternity and new-born care" are mandated EHBs, but how are they defined? As policy makers, particularly at the state level, answer this question, Centering advocates have an opportunity to work with other stakeholders and leverage an opportunity to demonstrate how maternity and newborn care have been redesigned in CenteringPregnancy (American College of Nurse-Midwives, 2013; National Partnership for Women & Families and Childbirth Connection, 2012).

Medicaid Expansion

Opposition to the ACA has taken many forms, but perhaps most significant in terms of implementation was the legal challenge to increase coverage through Medicaid expansion. With Medicaid as the source of payment for about half of all births in the country (Medicaid and

CHIP Payment and Access Commission, 2013), this is a particularly important issue for Centering advocates. The ACA expands Medicaid up to 138% of the federal poverty level for most low-income adults, but the June 2012 Supreme Court decision left the decision of whether to adopt Medicaid expansion up to the states (Kaiser Family Foundation, 2013). The status of state action on the Medicaid expansion decision is constantly changing, highlighting the need for advocates to be aware of trusted nonpartisan resources for finding current information, such as the Henry J. Kaiser Family Foundation (Kaiser Family Foundation, 2016).

Despite partisan challenges, there is an agreement that the U.S. health care "system" is unsustainable. There is a growing understanding of the need to pursue "the triple aim": improving the individual experience of care; improving the health of populations; and reducing the cost of care (Berwick, Nolan, & Wittington, 2008). Centering advocates can leverage this national conversation to ensure that policy makers understand Centering and support policy changes to facilitate the scale and spread of Centering. A story from California illustrates the importance of relationship building and the long view required when affecting policy change.

Reflections From a Clinician: Time and Relationship Building

Margy Hutchison, CNM, MSN

My policy work in my state had to do with helping our state's perinatal Medicaid program (called CPSP, or Comprehensive Perinatal Services Program) to understand Centering, and figure out how it could fit the CPSP program.

When I wanted to start the first CenteringPregnancy site in California in 1999, my clinic participated in CPSP and I knew there might be challenges to providing Centering within the confines of the CPSP model. CPSP provides enhanced MediCal (Medicaid) reimbursement if the site provides care according to their structure and was designed to make sure that Medicaid dollars went to providers and sites who did more than quick medical visits—who attended to the important education, nutrition and psychosocial needs that are so much a part of supporting healthy pregnancy outcomes. CPSP and Centering share many goals, but take very different approaches to achieving these goals. Centering is based on group interaction, and CPSP on periodic one-on-one assessments of women's needs in these areas.

In anticipation of starting Centering, I arranged a meeting with the state director of the CPSP program and our CPSP county coordinator. I introduced *them to Centering, and together we brainstormed about how CPSP sites could implement CP and stay in compliance with CPSP. We left that meeting with a clear understanding that first, the state CPSP office was supportive of the implementation of Centering and second, what aspects of care had to be included/maintained to stay in compliance. My site and our San Francisco CPSP coordinator then became the resource for almost every one of the next 20 or so CPSP sites that rolled out Centering in California in the state. It was not unusual for me to get an e-mail from a provider in another county who wanted to implement Centering, but had met confusion or resistance from the county CPSP coordinator. As you can imagine, what worked well in these situations was not for me to talk to the coordinator, but for their San Francisco peer to do so. I also presented about Centering at a couple of statewide CPSP meetings to continue working on awareness and buy-in by coordinators all across the state.*

So it's all about building relationships and finding your partners to support change.

I also have invested a fair amount of time over the years in trying to influence what the CPSP program actually looks like in our state—restructuring it so that one of the options for participation in CPSP was use of the Centering model. We're not there yet, but 17 years is but a moment in such a tremendous change endeavor!

Margy Hutchison, CNM, MSN, Clinical Professor, University of California, San Francisco, Department of OB/GYN.

Health Information Technology and Telehealth

The ACA contains a number of provisions intended to spur the adoption of electronic health records and increase utilization of telehealth. The shift from a paper chart to electronic records has required Centering sites to think creatively about how women can continue to engage in their care by documenting their weight, blood pressure, and the like. The case study from Georgia included in Chapter 7 is an illustration of how one provider adapted to a changing environment by using telehealth to bring CenteringPregnancy to more women.

Transformation to More Patient-Centered, Team-Based Care

Despite a lot of conversation about the need to fix our fragmented system that serves the industry and providers before patients, there are few examples of significant system transformation to bring about *truly* patient-centered, team-based care. In the words of one policy maker introduced to Centering, "Centering is an example of the real deal." Centering is a model that transcends provider groups.

Patient-centered care. On first exposure, policy makers might view Centering as an "efficiency model" with potential loss of the patient-centered, individualized care assumed to be found in traditional one-on-one visits. Descriptions of the model should stress how Centering fits the Institute of Medicine (IOM) definition of patient-centeredness: "providing care that is respectful of and responsive to the individual patient preferences, needs and values, and ensuring that patient values guide all clinical decisions" (IOM, 2001).

The Patient-Centered Outcomes Research Institute (PCORI) is an independent, nonprofit, nongovernmental organization created by the ACA to "improve the quality and relevance of evidence available to help patients, caregivers, clinicians, employers, insurers, and policy makers make informed health decisions." PCORI is interested in research that explores what models of perinatal care lead to better birth and patient-centered outcomes for patients at risk for experiencing disparities in care and included Centering among those models (Patient-Centered Outcomes Research Institute, 2013).

Team-based care. There is also an increasing focus on improving health care delivery by facilitating team-based care. In 2012, the IOM, acknowledging that each health care team is unique, described five core principles of team-based care: shared goals, clear roles, mutual trust, effective communication, and measurable process and outcomes (Institute of Medicine of the National Academies, 2013). They also described five values that describe effective members of high-functioning teams: honesty, discipline, creativity, humility, and curiosity. A number of specialty societies from cardiology (Brush et al., 2015) to obstetrics (American College of Obstetricians and Gynecologists, 2016) have used this work as a springboard, describing their view of team-based care.

There is general agreement that patients, providers, and the health care system will all benefit from a shift to team-based care, and these values and principles provide common reference points to guide efforts, but they remain relatively abstract and difficult to apply in many traditional models of health care delivery. Centering, by its very structure, is a model that drives each of the principles of team-based care: Centering groups are designed to helps teams articulate goals for care; clear roles have been spelled out for the functions and responsibilities of team members, and the model optimizes efficiency; facilitation training can help build mutual trust and refine communication skills; and CHI's CenteringCounts data system provides a framework for measuring processes and outcomes. Indeed, the first article published on CenteringPregnancy was titled, "CenteringPregnancy: An Interdisciplinary Model of Empowerment" (Rising, 1998).

■■■ The Importance of Maternal–Child Health (MCH)

For decades, the limited attention paid to the health care system focused on chronic care and the impact aging baby boomers would have on Medicare. That has changed dramatically in the recent past and provides an important opportunity for Centering advocacy.

There is a growing realization among policy makers of the importance of MCH care and the lifelong costs of *not* providing better care at the beginning of life. Among the organizations "waking up" to MCH, the National Governors Association (NGA) launched a Learning Network on Improving Birth Outcomes (National Governors Association, 2013), Catalyst for Payment Reform (CPR) has developed resources on payment alternatives that can "align incentives for providers and hospitals to adhere to evidence-based practices," and CPR teamed up with Childbirth Connection and the Center for HealthCare Quality and Payment Reform to produce "The Cost of Having a Baby in the USA" (Truven Health Analytics, 2013). Within the U.S. government, the Maternal and Child Health Bureau (MCHB) within the Health Resources and Services Administration (HRSA) has long administered programs designed to improve MCH, including the Title V Maternal and Child Health Block Grant program and Healthy Start. In 2012, MCHB launched the Collaborative Improvement & Innovation Network (CoIIN), a public–private partnership that aims to leverage this growing awareness. The CoIIN has identified six strategy areas: (a) improve safe sleep practices; (b) reduce smoking before, during, and/or after pregnancy; (c) pre/interconception care: promote optimal women's health before, after, and in between pregnancies, during postpartum visits and well-adolescent visits; (d) social determinants of health: incorporate evidence-based policies/programs and place-based strategies to improve social determinants of health and equity in birth outcomes; (e) prevention of preterm and early term births; and (f) risk-appropriate perinatal care: increase the delivery of higher risk infants and mothers at appropriate level facility. The National Institute for Children's Healthcare Quality (NICHQ) leads the teams and provides the data infrastructure, online community, and continuing expert technical assistance needed to support their efforts.

Collaborative Improvement and Innovation Network: The Power of Collective Impact

Art James, MD

Art James, MD, offered the following reflection on what "collective impact" can look like in one region of the country.

At the initial meeting of the Region V CoIIN (Collaborative Improvement & Innovation Network), which began during March of 2013, representatives from Illinois, Indiana, Ohio, Michigan, Minnesota, and Wisconsin met with representatives from the HRSA, the Association of State and Territorial Health Officials (ASTHO), March of Dimes, CityMatCH, National Institute for Children's Health Quality, (NICHQ), and the Association of Maternal & Child Health Programs (AMCHP) to adopt region-wide infant mortality reduction strategies. These region-wide meetings often represent the first time that individuals from various states get to come together and compare strategies and form alliances that allow all of us to improve at a faster pace.

"An example of something that is emerging from this collective impact model is that, at this meeting, we elected to work on the social determinants of health because Region V has the highest Black infant mortality rate of all regions in the country. Since working on this effort will take longer than the 2 years allocated to CoIIN projects, Dr. Ed Ehlinger (Department of Health for Minnesota) had the idea of engaging the CIC (Committee on Institutional Cooperation) of the Big 10 in this work. Funding from the Kellogg Foundation and the Robert Wood Johnson Foundation supported developing a proposal to the CIC, and during February of 2016 representatives from the 15 Big 10 universities and representation from the Departments of Health from the 11 states that make up the Big 10 met to discuss drafting proposals to support longer-term work to decrease racial disparities within the Big 10 states."

Arthur James, MD, FACOG, Associate Clinical Professor, Ohio State University, Columbus, Ohio

---

These efforts are gaining traction in part because of a growing understanding of what has been called "The Life Course Perspective," an approach to examining racial and ethnic disparities in birth outcomes first proposed by Michael Lu and Neal Halfon in 2003 (Lu & Halfon, 2003) and addressed in Chapter 2. In a few short years, thought leaders in MCH policy were proposing a new agenda for MCH policy and programs, integrating a life course perspective (Fine, Kotelchuck,

Adess, & Pies, 2009) and the idea that we need to address "upstream" determinants of health and spending began to catch on.

It's All About the Money

Although Centering can dramatically lower health care costs through improved outcomes, the current payment system primarily benefits the payers, not the sites providing Centering, even though the process of redesigning care delivery from an individual to a group care model represents a significant investment for the practice sites. Fortunately for advocates of Centering, "payment reform" is a hot topic. Policy makers are certainly interested in enhancing access to care and improving quality, but the most significant driver of change is cost. The move away from fee-for-service payment models toward a variety of alternative payment models—in the private insurance market as well as government health care systems—provides opportunities for thinking creatively about support for new models of care.

The Centering Return on Investment

It has been noted in earlier chapters how difficult it is to change "the way we've always done it." Policy makers have been influenced by the acceptance of a new model among obstetrician-gynecologists. In an editorial in the influential *American Journal of Obstetrics & Gynecology* in January 2014, Garretto and Bernstein (2014) conclude, "We believe it is time to start thinking of group prenatal care as the default model for prenatal care."

From the early days of Centering, there has been interest in evaluating the return on investment (ROI) of Centering. In particular, the March of Dimes, having funded the startup of a significant number of Centering sites, was interested in evaluating "the business case for Centering." A final report submitted to the California March of Dimes in 2009 (French, Moini, Reyes, & Yonejura, 2009), found that CenteringPregnancy yielded a positive ROI, depending on group size and who the co-facilitators were. It concluded:

> CenteringPregnancy is an evidence-based and financially viable model of prenatal care that could address parity in perinatal services for low-income mothers-to-be and enhance the quality of perinatal care provided in Los Angeles County. That said, external funding to cover

the start-up costs for CenteringPregnancy training and consulting and policy change that support reimbursement for high-quality perinatal services will likely be needed for most organizations to consider implementing the model.

There have been other unpublished studies conducted to determine the impact of CenteringPregnancy on cost of care. In another report to the March of Dimes, providers at a county health department providing care to an uninsured and largely undocumented population found that "Centering enabled the clinic to provide prenatal care to up to twice as many women in the same time and at a much lower cost in terms of labor resources as compared to traditional model" (Cox, Obichere, Knoll, & Baruqa, 2006, p. 3).

Despite the difficulty of studying cost effectiveness of prenatal care, there have been several published cost studies that can be summarized for policy makers. Other than the first review that found no significant cost differences between group prenatal care and individual care (Ickovics et al., 2007), studies using a variety of methods have demonstrated cost efficiency. Providers at a small, nonprofit, critical access hospital created an economic model using volume, cost, and revenue estimates, with findings that underscore the importance of sufficient volume to realize financial benefit (Mooney et al., 2008; Picklesimer, Heberlein, & Covington-Kolb, 2015). One study from an urban practice largely reimbursed by Medicaid-managed care employed mathematical cost–benefit modeling using variables that included group size, payer mix, patient no-shows, staffing, supply usage, and overhead cost. They concluded that group prenatal care "can be not only financially sustainable but a possible net income generator for the outpatient clinic" (Rowley et al., 2016, p. 1). A study using quality-adjusted life years (QALYs) in a decision-analytic model found that CenteringPregnancy is less costly ($18,857 vs. $20,188) and more effective (26.4557 vs. 26.4508 QALYs) than traditional care in decreasing preterm births (Ohno, Rodriguez, Wiener, & Caughey, 2012). A study in South Carolina used propensity score analysis to study the difference in outcomes between CenteringPregnancy and individual prenatal care and concluded that because of the significant reduction in the risk of premature birth and the savings inherent in reduced risk of a neonatal intensive care unit (NICU) state, the state investment of $1.7 million saw an estimated return on investment of nearly $2.3 million (Gareau et al., 2016).

In 2013, UnitedHealth Center for Health Reform and Modernization released "100% of Our Future: Improving the Health of America's Children" (UnitedHealth Center for Health Reform & Modernization, 2013). In addressing the need to give children the best possible start in life by encouraging healthy pregnancy, the report describes group prenatal care as one of several "practical opportunities for improvement." The report references a Centering study (Ickovics et al., 2003) and used claims data for newborn costs and NICU to estimate potential savings that would result from widespread use of group prenatal models:

> Nationally, if half of pregnant women enrolled in Medicaid received care through a group model over a 5-year period, we estimate that net savings to the Medicaid program overall would be about $12 billion over the next decade. (United Health Report, 2013, p. 30)

In 2015, students in the MBA for Executives program at Yale School of Management won the annual National Healthcare Case Competition with "CenteringPregnancy: A Low-Tech, Patient-Centered Care Model to Reduce Preterm Birth." Noting the population health impact, high cost and poor ROI of maternity care, and the role of moms as "early adopters," the authors make a case for scaling up an underutilized, evidence-based solution: CenteringPregnancy. Among the recommendations offered to further develop a viable business model, some are particularly relevant to policy makers and payers:

- Hospitals and health systems should target CenteringPregnancy programs for possible payment innovation pilots, since they have a high likelihood of improving outcomes and patient experiences.
- Payers have the most at stake for reducing preterm birth and should absorb the operational and opportunity costs of CenteringPregnancy programs. Enhanced payments are one promising mechanism.
- Health systems should consider shared risk contracts with payers, linked to preterm birth rates, breastfeeding outcomes, patient experience, and other measures that may be improved with CenteringPregnancy.
- CHI should continue to focus policy efforts on Medicaid reimbursement, using data from CenteringCounts and ongoing research studies funded by CMMI (Romano & Ianelli, 2015).

While most published research has focused on pregnancy, in 2013 a team at Yale published a small cost analysis for group well-child visits. The study looked at three provider mixes—advanced practice nurses, pediatric residents/attendings, and attending pediatricians—as well as group size, length of contact, and salary level. The outcomes supported the ability of the model to be cost effective (Yoshida, Fenick, & Rosenthal, 2014).

South Carolina: A Case Study in Advocacy for System Change

South Carolina provides a case study in effective advocacy and system change. Concerned by very high rates of premature birth and infant mortality (ranking 47th for premature births and low birth weight, and 42nd for infant mortality) South Carolina care providers and policy makers were ready to invest in turning those statistics around. The commitment of clinical leaders and the relationships they built with policy makers have resulted in a dramatic growth of Centering in the state.

The Greenville Health System OB Center began offering Centering-Pregnancy prenatal care in 2009, and by 2012, published data documented an impressive reduction in preterm birth. There was also a growing appreciation of the role incentives could play in encouraging providers to adopt CenteringPregnancy, and so the South Carolina Department of Health and Human Services (SCDHHS) began to support the expansion of that program with a grant of $1.7 million over 4 years to fund implementation, provide consulting services, and provide incentivized payments. SCDHHS sponsored an expansion project for another 3 years, providing 10 additional practice sites with start-up funding, training, and technical expertise (Giese, 2015).

South Carolina leaders in both the clinical and policy arenas are committed to documenting and evaluating the Birth Outcomes Initiative to serve as a model for other states seeking to expand an evidence-based health care model within an existing health care framework. The expansion evaluation study showed that support from key stakeholders and strong leadership at the state level created windows of opportunity for start-up funding and enhanced reimbursement. (For more information on the South Carolina implementation and consortium building, see Chapter 7.)

Evidence-Based Policy

One might argue that the most important factor in driving interest and support for Centering was compelling data on the reduction in preterm births. The push for evidence-based practice is driving policy makers as well. Just as it was important early on to establish the business case for CenteringPregnancy, the March of Dimes and CHI were intent on developing a data system that would help Centering sites understand their impact. Today, CenteringCounts, a Microsoft Excel–based tool used by CHI, allows sites to maintain data on health outcomes (preterm births avoided, healthy birth weights, and breastfeeding rates), understand their impact on cost savings, as well as ensure model fidelity and track practice scale. A robust web-based version will be released during 2017.

■ Billing, Coding, and Reimbursement for Centering

Key to the initial success in adoption and spread of Centering is the fact that Centering sessions are billable health care encounters within the existing fee-for-service system. Each patient in the group care session receives an individual assessment with the provider within the group space. The assessment includes all the necessary components to meet the standard of care guidelines and constitutes a billable visit.

Although coding varies depending on the state and payer, there is no need to create a separate billing system, and Centering is billed within a site's existing billing system using routine Current Procedural Terminology (CPT) codes. CenteringPregnancy prenatal care is billed as a routine prenatal care encounter for each participant, and CenteringParenting® mother–baby dyad care is billed as a routine postpartum or well-woman encounter for the mother and a routine well-baby encounter for the infant.

Centering can dramatically lower health care costs through improved outcomes, but the current payment system primarily benefits the payers, not the sites providing Centering, even though the process of redesigning care delivery from an individual to a group care model represents a significant investment for the practice sites. CHI's major policy priority is to establish mechanisms for enhanced reimbursement for approved Centering sites. CHI is working with payers in states across the country to negotiate enhanced reimbursement as well as to encourage payers to help defray the costs of implementation.

Some payers are already offering enhanced reimbursements to providers or beneficiaries who chose Centering, including these two examples from Texas and South Carolina:

- Texas: Effective April 2011, Texas Medicaid provides enhanced reimbursement for CenteringPregnancy. Providers are reimbursed an additional $30 per visit for prenatal care provided in group visits.

The procedure code 99078 (group clinical visits) is used, and the benefit criteria are documented.

- South Carolina: As noted earlier, South Carolina has been a leader in establishing policies to incentivize innovate approaches to improve MCH. In 2011, South Carolina Medicaid announced the Birth Outcomes Initiative to support quality outcomes.

SCDHHS, through the Birth Outcomes Initiative, established a billing mechanism for enhanced reimbursement for CenteringPregnancy visits. Every site that is either approved or under contract for site approval with CHI is eligible to charge this enhanced reimbursement for their CenteringPregnancy visits. For every CenteringPregnancy visit charged with the unique billing code (established by SCDHHS), Medicaid reimburses $40 to the patient's managed care organization; of this, $30 must be passed on to the provider. There is a $200 per patient cap on these charges.

BlueCross and BlueShield of South Carolina and BlueChoice Medicaid of South Carolina both removed the cap on the charges, providing practices the enhanced reimbursement for all 10 Centering sessions, or up to $300 per patient to the practice. In addition, if the patient attends at least five Centering sessions, the practice can charge a one-time incentive payment of $175 per patient.

These payments are limited to sites either approved by CHI or under contract for site approval. A significant expansion of these payment policies occurred in 2014 when BlueCross BlueShield of South Carolina and BlueChoice implemented a payment incentive program, reimbursing $30 per member per session up to $300. In addition to this $300, once the patient has had at least five CenteringPregnancy visits, the provider can bill a one-time retention incentive of $175 per member.

Some Centering sites use multiple modifier codes to bill for prenatal care coordination, nutrition services, childbirth classes, parenting classes, and infant safety classes. While the additional reimbursement contributes to the sustainability of the sites, the administrative burden makes this a less desirable option. Another option being explored with payers is the use of codes for preventive medicine, counseling, and risk reduction (99402, 99403, and 99404).

Industry Support for Centering

Although mergers have changed their names over the years, a number of payers have made enduring investments to support CHI's work.

The Aetna Foundation has funded several research studies that focus on outcomes from the model. The Anthem and Amerigroup Foundations have provided significant startup funding for CenteringPregnancy, much of this money given to the March of Dimes and their state chapters for distribution to promising sites. In addition, the Anthem Foundation has provided a substantial grant to continue the development of the CenteringCounts data system at CHI. Getting data from approved Centering sites is critical to the continued evaluation of the model.

Forward-looking policy makers, in government as well as industry, have begun to realize the value of investing in Centering. Karen Shea, vice president, Maternal Child Health for Anthem, Inc. states, "The clinical outcomes alone are impressive but, we also appreciate the provider and patient satisfaction that is so apparent with the Centering model of care." She acknowledges that getting providers to support changing their care model is key to continued adoption of the model. Amerigroup in Louisiana is the convener for the Strong Start grant that involves five sites in CenteringPregnancy implementation and expansion. The plan offers sites an extra $40 per person per visit in Centering groups if the 99078 with the TH modifier is used. This is an incentive for the sites to implement and helps to cover additional expenses, for example, start-up costs, personnel, food, and materials that might be incurred due to model requirements.

The Potential for Policy "Levers" to Impact System Transformation and Sustainability

In addition to the support of industry and the federal government, there are a number of other ways in which advocates and policy makers can impact Centering.

New Mexico Senate Bill 69: African American Infant Mortality Program: Why Centering Fit the Bill

In 2013, CHI's director of policy and advocacy attended the congressional Tri-Caucus Health Disparities Summit in New Mexico and, through a chance encounter, met Sunshine Muse, the chair of the New Mexico Office of African American Affairs Health Advisory Committee. Learning of CenteringPregnancy and the potential to impact infant mortality,

Profile of Sunshine Muse

In September 2013, I was working in New Mexico as a health disparities consultant. At the time, I was chairing the New Mexico State Office of African American Affairs' Health Implementation Team. As a community advocate working to increase equity and decrease disparities in health access, experience, and outcomes, I worked alongside the Robert Wood Johnson Center at the University of New Mexico to ensure that African Americans, who experience the worst health outcomes in almost every facet of health in our county, were well represented as experts at the 2013 Robert Wood Johnson Health Disparities Summit. At that summit, I met Lisa Summers, the Centering Healthcare Institute policy director, who described CenteringPregnancy and my reaction was instant and soul resonant; the prenatal care took place in groups, in a circle, with providers as facilitators and women coming together as peers and experts in their own care, supporting one another and taking ownership of their own well-being and prenatal health care. This was what I'd seen in Africa and believed was inherent to all women before and beyond patriarchy, the circle, the sisterhood, the ownership of our bodies and care, the inherent and traditional ways of women's knowing.

Shortly after the summit, as the Health Team moved forward with its work, we partnered with our legislature to address African American infant mortality in New Mexico. I brought Centering to the team as a suggested model that could help. Centering has been proven to decrease preterm birth rates by up to 33% across ethnicities, with higher rates of success among African American women.

As a result of our team's efforts, during the 2014 legislative session, Senate Bill 69 directed the Office of African American Affairs to address this issue, and Governor Susana Martinez allocated funding for the office to pilot its efforts. The result of this legislation, which passed unanimously on the House and Senate floors, and the funding from our governor, resulted in the Office of African American Affairs being able to offer CenteringPregnancy and to work with a powerful team of experts to educate African Americans, multiethnic providers, and a host of community organizations about the disparate outcomes that African American women and their babies face and what we can do to change that.

The role of race/ethnicity in poor outcomes among African American women is thought to come from generational and personal experiences of racial discrimination and hardship over one's life, including psychological factors. Unlike most health disparity areas, when it comes to African American infant mortality, an increase in income and education in pregnant African American women's lives can actually increase the likelihood of infant mortality. Preterm birth and/or low birth weight are the primary causes of infant mortality for infants born to

> African American mothers. CenteringPregnancy and provider cultural humility
> and education can help to address these factors. Providers must keep in mind
> that African American mothers have an elevated risk, regardless of maternal
> report of stress, and therefore need to be monitored and listened to with extra
> care and kindness during pregnancy.

Ms. Muse decided "it was a natural fit" for the committee's work. Well
versed in the legislative process, Sunshine worked with a Senate champion
to get a bill passed and signed. A year later, physicians and midwives
at the University of New Mexico Health Sciences Center gathered with
state officials and community members to launch a project bringing
CenteringPregnancy to New Mexico.

◼ Ohio Community Health Centers Tap the Health Transformation Innovation Fund

As is the case in many states, Ohio's Federally Qualified Health Centers
(more commonly referred to as Community Health Centers) are advanced
primary care practices already located in areas of high-need, high poverty, and higher than average infant mortality rates. In an initiative led
by the Ohio Association of Community Health Centers (OACHC), in
collaboration with legislative champions state senators Shannon Jones
and Charleta Tavares and with strong support from Governor Kasich
and his administration, four Community Health Centers were selected
to participate in the 2-year CenteringPregnancy Demonstration Project.
The project was allocated $900,000 from the Ohio Health Transfor-
mation Innovation Fund awarded by the Governor's Office of Health
Transformation, which includes funding for fixed costs associated with
implementation of the CenteringPregnancy program, as well as a Pay
for Performance component based on outcomes.

"With a proven record of delivering high-quality, low-cost health
care, coupled with a strong presence in vulnerable/highest need
communities—including impoverished urban neighborhoods, small
towns and rural counties where poverty and unemployment are
historically high—Ohio's Community Health Centers are poised and
ready to use the CenteringPregnancy data-driven model with significant
success," notes Julie DiRossi-King, chief operating officer of the OACHC.

▆ Policy and Advocacy Are a Critical Component of the Centering Implementation Plan

CHI has decades of experience assisting sites in transforming care. CHI consultants have incorporated lessons learned into a Centering Implementation Plan that provides guidance for sites from start-up through site approval. Engaging stakeholders, financing and budgeting, and billing and reimbursement—all essential to creating a strong, sustainable Centering practice—are part of that implementation plan.

What Will It Take to Sustain Change?

From the early days of Centering, there has been an appreciation of the need to engage policy makers. A 2004 review of CenteringPregnancy and the current state of prenatal care concluded, "With further research as well as intensive activity in the policy arena, Centering may be recognized as a viable alternative to the current flawed system of prenatal care" (Novick, 2004, p. 410).

▆ The Importance of Coalition-Building: The "Case for Not Going It Alone"

Each of these initiatives addressed earlier (the NGA, CoIINs, etc.) offers Centering advocates an opportunity to engage with other stakeholders intent on improving maternal child health and addressing health inequities. Coalitions are a central component of advocacy work and have been particularly visible and, some would argue, successful in health care reform efforts. Involvement in a health care coalition offers advantages for busy clinicians and nonprofits with limited resources—leveraging the power of the group. At the same time, the growing number of coalitions poses a problem. What makes an effective coalition, and which ones are worth the investment of time and resources (The California Endowment, 2011)? One might argue that much of the success of the Birth Outcomes Initiative in South Carolina has been a result of the coalition building.

▆ Engaging Women and Communities

Just as women's voices are heard in the Centering circle, the needs of women and communities must be heard in the policy arena. Genuine consumer engagement is being sought as never before, and the sorts of dynamic partnerships between health centers, communities, and the business communities that helped launch Centering are crucial to sustaining group care. Centering is a model of care that provides women and communities a greater opportunity to take ownership of problems that impact maternal child health and work with stakeholders to bring about lasting change.

■ Payment Reform

Payers—be it the government programs that pay for about half of all births, or industry—have the most to gain financially from reducing preterm birth. Enhanced reimbursement and other forms of financial support to assist sites in the transformation from individual to group care should come from payers.

Centering is an innovation that holds significant potential to bring about substantial improvement in health care, but it requires continued advocacy on the part of providers and support from policy makers. Centering providers must collect and utilize data to document outcomes. Advocates must be able to present those data and frame the importance of Centering in language that policy makers will understand, translating data to cost savings. And policy makers—particularly payers—must be ready to invest in supporting system change with funding for implementation and help sustain this enhanced care with enhanced payment.

References

Alliance for Health Reform. (2008). Lessons learned: The health reform debate of 1993–1994. Retrieved from http://www.allhealth.org/publications/uninsured/health_reform_debate_of_1993-94_81.pdf

American College of Nurse-Midwives. (2013). Coverage for birth center and midwifery services under Medicaid and the health insurance marketplaces: A discussion of key questions. Retrieved from www.midwife.org/acnm/files/ccLibraryFiles/Filename/000000003595/CoverageforBirthCenterandMidwiferyServices-10-5-13.pdf

American College of Obstetricians and Gynecologists. (2016). Collaboration in practice: Implementing team-based care. *Obstetrics & Gynecology, 127*(3), 612–617.

Berwick, D., Nolan, T., & Wittington, J. (2008). The triple aim: Care, health and cost. *Health Affairs, 27*(3), 759–769.

Brush, J., Handberg, E., Biga, C., Birtcher, K., Bove, A., Casale, P., . . . Wyman, J. (2015). 2015 ACC health policy statement on cardiovascular team-based care and the role of advanced practice providers. *Journal of the American College of Cardiology, 65*(19), 2118–2136. doi:10.1016/j.jacc.2015.03.550

The California Endowment. (2011). What makes an effective coalition? Evidence-based indicators of success. Retrieved from http://www.tccgrp.com/pdfs/What_Makes_an_Effective_Coalition.pdf

Centering Healthcare Institute. (2015). Centering: A better way to get care. Retrieved from www.centeringhealthcare.org/uploads/files/FX_Fact-Sheet-Full -Set_NoCC.pdf

Christopher, G. (2014). Editor's choice: The future is born every day. *American Journal of Public Health, 104*(S1).

Cox, R., Obichere, T., Knoll, F., & Baruqa, E. (2006). *A study to compare the productivity and cost of the CenteringPregnancy model of prenatal care with a traditional prenatal care model.* Final report submitted to the March of Dimes, White Plains, NY.

Fine, A., Kotelchuck, M., Adess, N., & Pies, C. (2009). A new agenda for MCH policy and programs: Integrating a life course perspective. Retrieved from http://cchealth.org/lifecourse/pdf/2009_10_policy_brief.pdf

French, J., Moini, M., Reyes, C., & Yonejura, M. (2009). *The business case for CenteringPregnancy.* Final report submitted to the March of Dimes, White Plains, NY.

Gareau, S., Lopez-de-Fede, A., Lourdermilk, B., Cummings, T., Hardin, J., Pick-elsimer, A., . . . Covington-Kolb, S. (2016). Group prenatal care results in Medicaid savings with better outcomes: A propensity score analysis of CenteringPregnacy participation in South Carolina. *Maternal and Child Health Journal, 20*(7), 1384–1393.

Garretto, D., & Bernstein, P. (2014). CenteringPregnancy: An innovative approach to prenatal care delivery. *American Journal of Obstetrics & Gynecology, 210*(1), 14–15.

Giese, B. (2015). CenteringPregnancy: A successful model for group prenatal care. Retrieved from www.scdhhs.gov

Ickovics, J., Kershaw, T., Westdahl, C., Magriples, U., Massey, Z., Reynolds, H., & Rising, S. (2003). Group prenatal care and preterm birth weight: Results from a matched cohort study at public clinics. *Obstetrics & Gynecology, 102*(5), 1051–1057.

Ickovics, J., Kershaw, T., Westdahl, C., Magriples, U., Massey, Z., Reynolds, H., & Rising, S. (2007). Group prenatal care and perinatal outcomes: A randomized controlled trial. *Obstetrics & Gynecology, 110*(2), 330–339.

Institute of Medicine of the National Academies. (2013). Core principles & values of effective team-based health care: Best practices innovation collaborative. Retrieved from www.nationalacademies.org/hmd/~/media/75CD7BA7BF B14576931326A22AFCEC36.ashx

Kaiser Family Foundation. (2009). National health insurance: A brief history of health reform efforts in the U.S. Retrieved from http://kff.org/health-reform/ issue-brief/national-health-insurance-a-brief-history-of

Kaiser Family Foundation. (2013). Guide to Supreme Court decision on ACA Medicaid expansion. Retrieved from https://kaiserfamilyfoundation.files .wordpress.com/2013/01/8347.pdf

Kaiser Family Foundation. (2016). Status of state action on the Medicaid expansion decision. Retrieved from http://kff.org/health-reform/state-indicator/ state-activity-around-expanding-medicaid-under-the-affordable-care-act

Key Features of the Affordable Care Act. (2010). Retrieved from www.hhs.gov/ healthcare/facts-and-features/key-features-of-aca/index.html

Lu, M., & Halfon, N. (2003). Racial and ethnic disparities in birth outcomes: A life-course perspective. *Maternal and Child Health Journal, 7*(1), 13–30.

Medicaid and CHIP Payment and Access Commission. (2013, June). Report to the Congress on Medicaid and CHIP. Retrieved from www.macpac.gov/wp-content/ uploads/2015/01/2013-06-15_MACPAC_Report.pdf

Mooney, S., Russell, M., Praire, B., Savage, C., & Weeks, W. (2008). Group prenatal care: An analysis of cost. *Journal of Health Care Finance, 34*(4), 31–41.

National Governors Association. (2013). More states to focus on US birth outcomes. Retrieved from www.nga.org/cms/home/news-room/news-releases/2013--news -releases/col2-content/more-states-to-focus-on-us-birth.html

National Partnership for Women & Families and Childbirth Connection. (2012). Guidelines for states on maternity care in the essential health benefits packages. Retrieved from http://transform.childbirthconnection.org/wp-content/ uploads/2012/08/REPRO-Guidelines-for-States-on-Maternity-Care7-30-12.pdf

Novick, G. (2004). CenteringPregnancy and the current state of prenatal care. *Journal of Midwifery & Women's Health, 49*(5), 405–411.

Oberlander, J. (2007). Learning from failure in health care reform. *New England Journal of Medicine, 357*(17), 1677–1679.

Ohno, M., Rodriguez, M., Wiener. S., & Caughey, A. (2012). *CenteringPregnancy for the prevention of preterm birth: A cost effectiveness analysis.* Presented at the 34th Annual Meeting of the Society for Medical Decision Making, Phoenix, AZ. Retrieved from https://smdm.confex.com/smdm/2012az/webprogram/Paper6929.html

Patient-Centered Outcomes Research Institute. (2013). Perinatal care and outcomes workgroup: Topic brief. Retrieved from www.pcori.org/assets/2013/10/ PCORI-Perinatal-Care-Workgroup-Topic-Brief-102413.pdf

Rising, S. (1998). Centering pregnancy: An interdisciplinary model of empower-ment. *Journal of Nurse-Midwifery, 43*(1), 46–54.

Romano, A., & Ianelli J. (2015). *Healthcare delivery innovation: A low-tech, patient-centered care model to reduce preterm birth.* BAHM 2015 Case Competition, Denver, CO.

Rowley, R., Phillips, L., O'Dell, L., El Husseini, R., Carpino, S., & Hartman, S. (2016). Group prenatal care: A financial perspective. *Maternal and Child Health Journal, 20*(1), 1–10.

Strong Start for Mothers and Newborns Evaluation: Year 2 Annual Report. (2016). Retrieved from https://downloads.cms.gov/files/cmmi/strongstart -enhancedprenatalcare_evalrptyr2v1.pdf

Truven Health Analytics. (2013). The cost of having a baby in the U.S. January 2013. Retrieved from http://transform.childbirthconnection.org/wp-content/uploads/2013/01/Cost-of-Having-a-Baby-Executive-Summary.pdf

UnitedHealth Center for Health Reform & Modernization. (2013). 100 percent of our future: Improving the health of America's children. Retrieved from www.unitedhealthgroup.com/~/media/uhg/pdf/2013/unh-working-paper-10.ashx

Yoshida, H., Fenick, A., & Rosenthal, M. (2014). Group well-childcare: An analysis of cost. *Clinical Pediatrics, 53,* 387–394.

11 Growing Edge: Exploration of Innovation

"Leadership is an improvisational art. Everything you do in leading adaptive change is an experiment."—Heifetz (2009, p. 277)

This chapter documents the careful process being used in three research studies focused on adding content to the CenteringPregnancy® care model. The first focused on the integration of Mindfulness-Based Childbirth and Parenting (MBCP) into CenteringPregnancy, started in the early 2000s when Nancy Bardacke and Sharon Rising began discussing synergy between their two models. The second study, CenteringPregnancy Oral Health (CPOP), is conducted by a psychologist nurse researcher and a dentist at the University of California, San Francisco. This work evolved from the CenteringPregnancy Smiles initiative at the University of Kentucky College of Dentistry. And the third study on health literacy and CenteringPregnancy, while still in earlier stages of exploration, seeks to further our understanding of the potential of groups to increase health literacy of the participants.

There have been other studies that have added particular content to the Centering Healthcare model, most notably the CenteringPregnancy Plus work, which adds relationship building/communication skills and safe sex content particularly focused on young pregnant women. The study was funded by the National Institute of Mental Health with HIV/AIDS prevention dollars (Ickovics et al., 2007). Because of the team's interest in women's health reproduction issues, additional content was prepared related to women's sexual risk and added to the Centering-Pregnancy curriculum. These content areas included awareness of risk, assertiveness, partner negotiation, planning, and goal setting; content application was interactive and introduced in four of the 10 sessions. This model, tested by the Yale School of Public Health team led by Jeannette Ickovics, has been referenced extensively throughout the book.

Another promising model, CenteringPregnancyDads, developed by Doug Edwards, needs further testing, but initial work shows promise for purposeful inclusion of dads in the CenteringPregnancy and Parenting models.

Part A: CenteringPregnancy With Mindfulness Skills: Enhancing the Thread of Presence

Nancy Bardacke, CNM, MA, and Larissa G. Duncan, PhD

nancy@mindfulbirthing.org and larissa.duncan@wisc.edu

CenteringPregnancy With Mindfulness Skills (CPMS) is an initiative focused on integrating the life skill of mindfulness as taught in the MBCP program into the CenteringPregnancy group care model, both in the form of an enhanced prenatal care curriculum and an advanced professional training program for CenteringPregnancy providers. Through a partnership that respects the foundational principles and integrity of each program, CPMS brings into synergistic relationship two powerful health-promoting modalities in order to maximize the health and well-being of expectant mothers, their developing infants, and their social ecologies.

Mindfulness-Based Childbirth and Parenting

MBCP is a 9-week program offered prenatally that provides expectant parents an opportunity to learn the life skill of mindfulness—"the awareness that arises from paying attention, on purpose, in the present moment and nonjudgmentally" (Kabat-Zinn, 2005, p. 108)—for working with the stress of pregnancy, for meeting the pain and fear that are often a normal component of the childbirth experience, and to have these skills in place for parenting mindfully from the moments of birth. MBCP parents-to-be consistently report that as they practice mindfulness, they are able to live through this life transition with greater confidence, resilience, and joy. As a result, the practice of mindfulness becomes a lifelong resource for attuned parenting and living daily life with greater awareness, kindness, connectedness, and care, both for one's self and others.

The MBCP program (Bardacke, 2012) was developed by Nancy Bardacke, CNM, MA, in 1998. MBCP is a formal adaptation of the Mindfulness-Based Stress Reduction (MBSR) program (Kabat-Zinn, 2013) founded in 1979 by Jon Kabat-Zinn, PhD, at the University of

Massachusetts Medical Center. MBSR has been the subject of numerous clinical trials demonstrating its impact on health and well-being. Many other evidence-based mindfulness programs that are currently available to the general public in a wide variety of settings, such as Mindfulness-Based Cognitive Therapy (MBCT) (Segal, Williams, & Teasdale, 2012) for prevention of depression relapse, can trace their roots directly to the MBSR program or have been influenced by it.

Mindfulness practice facilitates bringing a nonreactive quality of attention to the full range of one's physical, emotional, and cognitive experiences. A universal capacity of the human mind, mindful awareness is cultivated through regular meditation practice. With consistent practice, a more self-aware and less reactive relationship to one's inner experiences develops, thereby increasing the ability to see external reality with greater clarity, make wiser decisions in the present moment, and bring more ease into everyday life.

More than three decades of published research shows that mindfulness practice can reduce stress and promote a perspective of open, nonjudgmental acceptance. Increased resilience, adaptability in the face of change, and compassion for oneself and others are often by-products of regular mindfulness practice. In addition, studies have shown that this self-regulatory approach to physical and emotional health challenges has been effective in reducing chronic pain, hypertension, insomnia, migraines, asthma, anxiety, depression, and stress in daily life.

Stress in the Perinatal Period

A growing body of empirical evidence in both animal and human studies indicates that stress and negative mood during pregnancy are risk factors for poor pregnancy and childbirth outcomes, such as preterm labor and low birth weight. Stress is also a factor in prenatal and postpartum depression and in the development of a less than optimal mother–infant attachment. In addition, data are accumulating regarding the effects of prenatal stress on the long-term emotional, cognitive, and social development of babies and children. By infusing mindfulness into CenteringPregnancy, the opportunity exists to harness this health-promoting modality, further strengthening the mental and physical health benefits for mothers, babies, and families already seen with the CenteringPregnancy model of care.

Foundational Attitudes of Mindfulness Practice

There are a number of attitudes that are cultivated in mindfulness practice that can become touch-points for both formal mindfulness practice and for when difficulties arise in daily life. These attitudes are beginner's mind, nonjudging, patience, nonstriving, inner trust, acknowledgment, "letting be," and kindness.

The Provider and the Client: A Win-Win

A foundational principle for anyone wanting to facilitate mindfulness skills in another is the grounding in one's own practice of formal mindfulness meditation and informal mindfulness practice (the application of mindfulness to activities and experiences in everyday life). While it is well documented that group care brings improved satisfaction and better health outcomes to pregnant women, their babies and families, as well as benefiting the health professionals through renewed satisfaction in their work, the benefits of training providers in mindfulness skills may further extend these benefits. Though group care may be a bright spot in the day or week of a Centering provider, health care professionals are still confronted with the daily stress of a seriously dysfunctional health care system. With training in mindfulness skills, CPMS facilitators not only learn a skill for reducing stress and bringing more ease into the lives of those they serve, they also cultivate self-care skills for their own physical and mental health and well-being, potentially bringing even greater presence and joy to their work of service (Warriner, Hunter, & Dymond, 2016)

Synergy Between Programs: Mindfulness Practice Supports and Strengthens the Core Components and Essential Elements of CenteringPregnancy

The inner attitudes cultivated through regular mindfulness practice (see MBCP section) support and strengthen the three core components of the Centering model of care—health care, interactive learning, and community building—as well as enhance the elements that are key to the success of the Centering model.

Health Assessment With Mindfulness

Mindfulness practice is consistent with the health care component occurring within the group space that is a hallmark of the Centering model of care. Given that one of the qualities often strengthened in a mindfulness practitioner is concentration and the ability to be in the present moment, the Centering health care provider may find that her or his ability to be more focused and present during the brief time allotted to physical assessment enhances the ability to serve an individual woman's health needs. In addition, this focus may help the provider make more accurate, appropriate, and compassionate decisions of care, even in the midst of what might appear to be chaotic external circumstances.

For the participant in CenteringPregnancy, the quality of beginner's mind cultivated in mindfulness practice promotes curiosity and openness to new learning. This curiosity and openness can deepen the impact of the active participation in self-care activities that is so essential in the Centering model. Learning self-care activities, such as to check one's own blood pressure and weight, promote an attitude of active participation and responsibility in caring for one's own body and health rather than being a passive recipient of care. Curiosity and active participation are vital qualities to encourage in those who already are or will become a parent, one who is responsible for overseeing a child's well-being. In addition, the quality of inner trust, a trust in oneself that is also cultivated in a mindfulness practice, promotes a kind of confidence in one's capacities and abilities, further enhancing the Centering model of care.

Interactive Learning and Mindfulness

Interactive learning, the second core component of the Centering model, is also core to supporting the development of mindfulness skills. Rather than learning from "an authority" in a top–down, hierarchical, information-based structure, the learning of mindfulness is fundamentally about persons coming to understand that they are the authority of their own experience. In this sense, there is no one right way, only finding, through turning one's attention inward, what is right or true for oneself. Mindfulness practice offers the opportunity to find and strengthen this inner knowing.

While recognizing that there is a need for giving guidance and instruction in formal meditation practice, much of the inner learning that can come through mindfulness practice happens during the process of inquiry. Through kind and skillful coinvestigation regarding a participant's experience during meditation practice, the group facilitator gently encourages an attitude of curiosity about the participant's inner experiences. Embodying the attitudes of mindfulness, a skillful mindfulness practice facilitator guides participants in a gentle and nonjudging way to investigate their own habits of mind and body, thereby learning together what might be discovered.

Essential to facilitating mindfulness skills is the understanding by the group participants that the facilitator is working at her or his own mindfulness practice and the common human experience we call "living a human life." A CPMS group facilitator does not ask of participants any more or less than they are asking of themselves. In this way, the group facilitator is a midwife of awareness, using the essential care-provider skills of kindness, presence, intelligence, and his or her own experience of mindfulness practice. With an unshakable belief in the participant's inner strength and capacity to meet and labor with whatever challenges may arise in this very life, the CPMS facilitator inspires and enhances this capacity for all participants.

One of the essential elements in CenteringPregnancy that is also true of the MBCP program is that while each session has a plan, the curriculum is not fixed. Emphasis may vary according to the needs of a particular group or population and, most importantly, to what is arising in the present moment during a particular session. For example, core to mindfulness practice is the importance of using the breath and body as an anchor to the present moment; how to work with the mind when it wanders; working with body sensations, thoughts, and emotions; and coming to understand the difference between reacting and responding, particularly in relation to physical pain as part of childbirth preparation. However, how to respond to a particular participant in the moment when a particular experience during a meditation practice is being shared in the group is where the creativity and skill of the facilitator lies. In this way, facilitating a CPMS group becomes a mindfulness practice in and of itself.

Flexibility, the ability to pay attention and to respond skillfully to whatever is arising in the present moment during the group, is key to the facilitative leadership of CPMS sessions. The group facilitator must not only balance the overall plan for the session and the core content, but also make the moment-to-moment decisions regarding staying with the core content of a session or allowing what is arising in the group to take center stage in the flow of the overall group experience. Process or content is often a key choice, and there is no one right way.

Community Building Through Mindfulness

As with health assessment, mindfulness practice enhances the essential elements of community building so elegantly interwoven and fundamental to the Centering model of care. Consistency of facilitators, group members, and support people; groups conducted in a circle; group size that is optimal for interaction; and opportunities for socializing among participants are essential elements of both the Centering model and the MBCP program.

Having consistent group members, support persons, and facilitators is essential for establishing an environment of trust, safety, and belonging. These are fundamental human needs that, when met, can deepen the joy and pleasure that can be found in the company of others who are engaged in a common experience. Further, when there is trust that each person will be met with the attitudes of mindfulness including kindness, respect, and nonjudging, group members feel enhanced freedom and trust to be more authentically themselves and speak what is true for them. This experience alone can be a healing one, one that a participant or perhaps many participants in a Centering group may not have experienced in the past. A nonjudging attitude toward oneself and others that is deeply embedded into mindfulness practice itself, and by extension the CPMS facilitator, enhances this sense of belonging and safety, allowing even more kindness to be manifest among group participants.

Further, the consistency of facilitators, group members, and support persons allows for deepening group cohesion and for a CPMS facilitator to track the learning of each participant in the ongoing conversation about becoming more aware in one's life through the shared condition of pregnancy and the shared experience of learning mindfulness practice. Session by session, as the learning of mindfulness as a life skill thread is woven into each Centering session, trust and understanding grows and deepens among participants. When the ability to see oneself as both unique and as one who shares the common human experiences of living in a body with physical sensations that can be both pleasant and unpleasant; living with a mind that thinks thoughts that can be observed; and experiencing human emotions such as fear, anger, and joy that are common to all—all within the common experience of bringing new life into the world—learning becomes both an individual and collective experience. Mindfulness is about respect for all things, and when the inner experience of all present is held in highest regard with an attitude that each participant is the expert of her own experience, insight and wisdom can emerge.

Ongoing Evaluation of Outcomes

Ongoing evaluation of outcomes is essential for CenteringPregnancy, MBCP, and CPMS. As data provides a powerful vehicle for demonstrating effectiveness and for promoting change, all of these programs share a strong commitment to being evidence-based. Ongoing evaluation of outcomes allows for these programs to be akin to living entities, built on a process of collective creative learning with adjustments being made when appropriate for the particular circumstances and populations being served, all the while maintaining model fidelity.

Process of Development of CPMS

When adapting a model with existing evidence supporting its efficacy, careful attention to maintaining adherence to its essential elements is needed, and this was fundamental to our approach from the very beginning. The project began in 2008 as a collaboration between Sharon Schindler Rising, MSN, CNM, FACNM, founder of CenteringPregnancy and the Centering Healthcare Institute (CHI), Nancy Bardacke, CNM, MA, founder of MBCP and the director of the MBCP program at the University of California, San Francisco (UCSF) Osher Center for Integrative Medicine, and Larissa Duncan, PhD, formerly associate professor of Family and Community Medicine at UCSF until 2015 and now the Elizabeth C. Davies chair in Child and Family Well-Being in the School of Human Ecology at the University of Wisconsin–Madison. Through funding support from the Mt. Zion Health Fund administered by UCSF and a career award from the National Institutes of Health/National Center for Complementary and Integrative Health (NIH/NCCIH; Duncan K01 AT005270), the team embarked on a series of systematic studies to develop, pilot, refine, and begin to test the impact of an enhanced version of CenteringPregnancy incorporating essential elements of MBCP, including foundational practices in mindfulness meditation, preparation for coping with childbirth pain and fear using mindfulness, and preparation for bringing mindful parenting into mother–infant interactions in the early postpartum period. A description of the development of the CPMS curriculum is presented in the following pages.

Step 1: Provider Survey

Our first step was to survey an array of Centering providers who were members of the Bay Area CenteringPregnancy Consortium. Providers from 17 sites in the greater San Francisco Bay Area were invited to enroll two participants per site in a research study in which they were asked to respond to an online survey designed to gauge their experiences of providing CenteringPregnancy, and in particular, their views of the sources of stress faced by the women they served and their views regarding the stress management elements of the CenteringPregnancy curriculum. Among 24 participants (including certified nurse-midwives [CNMs], family physicians, family nurse practitioners, and social workers) from 13 sites, there was strong agreement that more could be done to bolster skills for working with stress for Centering participants than was in the current Centering Pregnancy model; however, some of the Centering-Pregnancy providers were concerned that there was limited time to add additional content within the already quite full CenteringPregnancy curriculum. Providers identified pregnancy-related concerns, including mental health and medical challenges, as the most common area of focus in their discussions with participants about stress (with 16 of 24 providers highlighting this topic). We also learned of the many varied sources of life stress faced by CenteringPregnancy participants, such as immigration-related concerns, experiences of domestic violence, the challenges of caring for other children while pregnant, and working low-wage jobs with unpredictable shifts (Taub, Burns, Castro-Smyth, & Duncan, 2010).

This study provided valuable background for understanding the potential benefits of incorporating mindfulness skills into both provider training and the CenteringPregnancy group experience to address stress, as well as the challenges of fusing the two models. MBCP is a promising approach for alleviating pregnancy-related anxiety, as well as for supporting mindfulness as a coping strategy for dealing with a variety of sources of life stress (Duncan & Bardacke, 2010). Yet, creating additional stress for CenteringPregnancy providers as they worked to cover a wide range of topics and meet group participants with whatever might be arising for them in the moment would have been counterproductive.

Step 2: Cross-Training of Providers

To facilitate the integration of the two models, the MBCP developer (Bardacke) attended a CenteringPregnancy group as a participant-observer. The CenteringPregnancy group was led by a CHI faculty member (Deena Mallareddy, CNM) and was made up of a heterogeneous group of expectant women and their partners with diverse socioeconomic backgrounds and race/ethnicity. During this same timeframe, the CHI faculty member attended a MBCP course as a participant-observer

Step 3: Reviewing the CenteringPregnancy Curriculum Through the MBCP Lens

A curriculum workgroup was formed (composed of Duncan, Bardacke, Rising, Mallareddy, another CHI faculty member, Margaret "Margy" Hutchison, CNM, and Lisabeth Castro-Smyth) to review the CenteringPregnancy curriculum session by session and the facilitator's guide, the mothers' notebooks, and the self-assessment sheets. This review was done to ascertain how mindfulness concepts and practices from MBCP and mindful parenting elements from Duncan's other mindful parenting work (Duncan, Coatsworth, & Greenberg, 2009) might be interwoven into each CenteringPregnancy session. The workgroup took into account the results of the provider survey, Bardacke's experience as a participant-observer in CenteringPregnancy, and Mallareddy's experience as a participant-observer in MBCP and produced an initial outline of the CPMS curriculum.

Step 4: Curriculum Development Pilot Study

Using the first draft of the CPMS curriculum, the MBCP developer (Bardacke) participated in a second CenteringPregnancy group, this time as a group co-facilitator in which she led mindfulness practices drawn from MBCP, meeting regularly with Duncan between sessions to refine the approach session-by-session. The curriculum workgroup met again to process the results of this pilot and to further refine the session-by-session outline of the integrated curriculum based on their own experiences and their observations of the pregnant participants' experiences in the session.

Step 5: Provider Training Pilot and Curriculum Refinement

In preparation for a small clinical trial of the CPMS enhanced model, the curriculum workgroup was expanded to include an additional CHI faculty member (Laurie Jurkiewicz, CNM). Both Hutchison and Jurkiewicz attended a MBCP course as participants-observers and met bimonthly with Duncan and Bardacke to review the CPMS curriculum and to refine the integration of mindfulness skills in CenteringPregnancy. Hutchison and Jurkiewicz offered their suggestions based on their experiences of delivering CenteringPregnancy with the low-income patient population served by the Outpatient Midwifery Service of San Francisco General Hospital (SFGH) in partnership with the Homeless Prenatal Program in San Francisco. An additional step in the curriculum refinement for the CPMS clinical trial involved Bardacke creating and recording guided audio meditations that were somewhat shorter than those used in the MBCP program in order to encourage home practice among CPMS participants. In addition, Duncan, Bardacke, and their UCSF staff revised handouts from the MBCP program for delivery in CPMS.

Step 6: Adaptation of CPMS for Delivery in Spanish

Duncan led a staff team, including two bilingual research assistants (Castro-Smyth and Trilce Santana) in the translation and adaptation of the English-language version of the CPMS curriculum into Spanish, including the scripts of the guided audio materials developed by Bardacke for CPMS. Adjustments included verbatim translation of some elements, as well as careful adjustment of deeper, structural elements of the curriculum to ensure cultural relevance for the Latina population of the San Francisco Bay Area, including many recent immigrants to the United States. Audio recordings were made in Spanish by a native Spanish speaker contracted for this purpose.

CPMS: Curriculum

A small clinical trial (see Preliminary Results of the CPMS Clinical Trial section) was conducted to test the CPMS curriculum. Modifications to this version of the CPMS curriculum will be made based on review of the study results. Several aspects of the curriculum are worth noting.

A foundational decision was made that mindfulness practice would be introduced as a health-promoting life skill for reducing stress and that it would be practiced in the very first session. Participants learned that the skill of being in the present moment could be beneficial for decreasing stress now during pregnancy, helpful for managing pain and fear during labor, and would provide some coping tools for managing parenting and stress after the baby is born. Mindfulness was offered as a skill cultivated through meditation practice, and that like any skill, it takes practice, and so opportunities to meditate would be offered in each CenteringPregnancy session. Depending on the particular culture and background of each CPMS participant, the meaning of "meditation" could vary greatly. It is in the skill of a well-trained CPMS facilitator who can draw on her/his own meditation experience and practice that this way of training the mind can be demystified, normalized, and universalized.

Participants were also told that they would be given CDs/mp3s containing guided mindfulness meditation practices to listen to at home if they chose to do so and that they would be given suggestions and handouts for other ways they might begin to bring more present moment awareness into their lives.

It was important that the facilitators kept in mind that the women and support people attending the CenteringPregnancy group were primarily there for prenatal care, not to learn how to meditate. Great care was taken that the attitude in which the facilitators offered the meditation practices was one of invitation. Being clear that each person had a choice about whether to participate in the formal meditation practices or not was essential.

Preliminary Results of the CPMS Clinical Trial

To begin to investigate the potential benefits of incorporating mindfulness into CenteringPregnancy, we embarked on a small, quasiexperimental clinical trial of CPMS in comparison to CenteringPregnancy without the mindfulness enhancements. This research, conducted from 2010 to 2015, was funded by the NIH/NCCIH through grant number K01 AT005270. Low-income women receiving Medicaid-covered prenatal care at SFGH, an urban, public safety net hospital, were invited to participate in the study after enrolling in CenteringPregnancy. Study participation was not a requirement for receiving CenteringPregnancy, and participants were blinded to which version of the curriculum they received.

The majority of participants were members of racial/ethnic minority groups (e.g., 48.5% Latina), and both CPMS and CenteringPregnancy groups were conducted in English and in Spanish. Using a mixed methods approach, women participated in in-depth qualitative interviews (in their chosen language) about their experiences of pregnancy, prenatal care, labor and delivery, and early parenting, as well as psychological stress and coping strategies they used, and any adversity they faced in their lives. To examine physiological stress processes in addition to psychological stress, participants were invited to contribute blood samples (for assay of neuroendocrine hormones previously shown to be linked with preterm birth, i.e., adrenocorticotropic hormone and corticotropin-releasing hormone), home collection of saliva samples (for diurnal cortisol assay), and blood pressure assessments. They also responded to an array of quantitative survey measures that were administered verbally by bilingual study staff (to alleviate any literacy burdens) and were asked for consent for review of their medical records.

Medical record collection was completed in late 2015 and data analysis began in early 2016. Preliminary results indicate that women in CPMS experienced a significant reduction in pregnancy-related anxiety from early to late pregnancy, and lower trait anxiety in late pregnancy compared to the standard CenteringPregnancy condition (Duncan et al., 2016), suggesting that CPMS was having the intended effect of bolstering the stress reduction aspects of the CenteringPregnancy program. Furthermore, participants in CPMS commonly reported elements drawn from the MBCP curriculum as most helpful, demonstrating strong receptivity to the MBCP training elements and associated demands. For example, when asked "What was the most helpful thing you learned for having a healthy pregnancy?" participants offered responses such as: "How to reduce my stress with the breathing and how to not let little things get me" "How to manage stress and pain" and "Being present in my mind and my body" [translated from Spanish]. When asked "What was the most useful thing you learned about taking care of a new baby?" participants responded with reports such as "The baby's signals that you can tell from their face" [mindfulness of baby's facial expressions/emotions from session 7] and "How to stay calm when I can't stop the baby from crying."

Our intention is to examine the biological and psychological pathways by which the mindfulness enhancement of CenteringPregnancy may demonstrate its effect. We have also collected data on provider experiences of delivering the CPMS curriculum. Implementation and dissemination research is needed to understand how best to provide the necessary training to take this approach to scale. In addition, we have identified an area for improvement in ensuring the cultural relevance of mindfulness approaches when delivered to people of color (Watson, Black, & Hunter, 2016), an area of ongoing work for our group in collaboration with organizations with expertise in this area such as Mindfulness for the People founded by Angela Rose Black, PhD.

Extension of a Mindfulness Approach Into CenteringParenting

Our vision includes offering a continuum of developmentally appropriate mindfulness and mindful parenting courses across the life span. For example, following MBCP, participants would continue in a mindful parenting course over the first year of life, just as CenteringParenting well-family care is available in the first year of life following CenteringPregnancy. Our aim is to integrate mindful parenting skills training into CenteringParenting and to test the benefits of such an approach. In this way, groups who stay together from the prenatal through the postpartum period can support one another in continuing to develop a daily practice of mindful parenting, the seeds of which were planted during pregnancy in CPMS.

Next Steps for the Broader Implementation of CPMS

Currently, a key focus in mindfulness work globally is on how to address the challenge of training providers to offer mindfulness in professional settings where time, attention, and resources are limited. Some evidence suggests that mindfulness can facilitate provider presence in ways that are meaningful to the recipients of care, and we expect mindfulness training of CenteringPregnancy providers to be supportive of the facilitative leadership style so central to the power of Centering. Mindfulness training is also likely to be effective at reducing provider burnout and improving provider empathy (Krasner et al., 2009). For those settings most interested in bringing this enhanced version of CenteringPregnancy to their providers and clients, our recommendation is to begin with provider training in MBSR. MBSR is a well-tested and well-established way of developing one's own mindfulness practice and serves as the foundation for MBCP and CPMS. Advanced training in CPMS and MBCP is in development, and we hope it will soon be offered regularly in North America and beyond.

Conclusion: The Process of Transformation

CenteringPregnancy is a profoundly empowering, useful, and caring way to bring structural change into a health care system sorely in need of one. The experience of participating in the original CenteringPregnancy model already brings great benefit to both participants and care providers. By carefully infusing it with systematic training in mindfulness meditation as taught in the MBCP program, CPMS may be a way to deepen the impact of this systems change approach, providing skills for change for both participants and care providers from the inside out. While CPMS provider training, adjustments to the CPMS curriculum as presented here, and research on a larger scale are needed, the elements that have been birthed in the CPMS program seem to be sound and hold great promise for additional benefits to women and families during pregnancy, childbirth, and beyond.

References

Bardacke, N. (2012). *Mindful birthing: Training the mind, body, and heart for childbirth and beyond*. New York, NY: HarperCollins.

Duncan, L. G., & Bardacke, N. (2010). Mindfulness-based childbirth and parenting education: Promoting family mindfulness during the perinatal period. *Journal of Child and Family Studies, 19*(2), 190–202.

Duncan, L. G., Coatsworth, J. D., & Greenberg, M. T. (2009). A model of mindful parenting: Implications for parent–child relationships and prevention research. *Clinical Child and Family Psychology Review, 12*(3), 255–270.

Duncan, L. G., Cook, J. G., Santana, T., Castro-Smyth, L., Hutchison, M., Jurkiewicz, L., . . . Bardacke, N. (2016). *Prenatal mindfulness training as primary prevention of maternal anxiety: Reaching underserved pregnant women through CenteringPregnancy with Mindfulness Skills group medical visits*. Paper presented at the 24th annual meeting of the Society for Prevention Research, San Francisco, CA.

Heifetz, R. (2009). *The practice of adaptive leadership*. Boston, MA: Harvard Business Press.

Ickovics, J., Kershaw, T., Westdahl, C., Magriples, U., Massey, Z., Reynolds, H., & Rising, S. S. (2007). Group prenatal care and perinatal outcomes: A randomized controlled trial. *Obstetrics & Gynecology, 11,* 330–339.

Kabat-Zinn, J. (2005). *Coming to our senses: Healing ourselves and the world through mindfulness.* London, United Kingdom: Hachette.

Kabat-Zinn, J. (2013). *Full catastrophe living, revised edition: How to cope with stress, pain and illness using mindfulness meditation.* London, United Kingdom: Hachette.

Krasner, M. S., Epstein, R. M., Beckman, H., Suchman, A. L., Chapman, B., Mooney, C. J., & Quill, T. E. (2009). Association of an educational program in mindful communication with burnout, empathy, and attitudes among primary care physicians. *The Journal of the American Medical Association, 302*(12), 1284–1293.

Nugent, K. (2011). *Your baby is speaking to you: A visual guide to the amazing behaviors of your newborn and growing baby.* New York, NY: Houghton Mifflin Harcourt.

Segal, Z. V., Williams, J. M. G., & Teasdale, J. D. (2012). *Mindfulness-based cognitive therapy for depression.* New York, NY: Guilford Press.

Taub, R., Burns, A., Castro-Smyth, L., & Duncan, L. G. (2010). *Reducing health disparities through group prenatal care: Providers' perspectives on stress reduction.* Poster presented at 4th Annual Health Disparities Research Symposium at the University of California, San Franciso, San Francisco, CA.

Warriner, S., Hunter, L., & Dymond, M. (2016). Mindfulness in maternity: Evaluation of a course for midwives. *British Journal of Midwifery, 24*(3), 188–195.

Watson, N. N., Black, A. R., & Hunter, C. D. (2016). African American women's perceptions of mindfulness meditation training and gendered race-related stress. *Mindfulness, 7*(5), 1034–1043.

Part B: Centering Health and Oral Health: Moving Toward Healthy Women and Healthy Families

Sally H. Adams, PhD, and Lisa Chung, PhD

sally.adams@ucsf.edu and lisa.chung@ucsf.edu

To address unmet needs in oral health and mental health, some health care systems, where the traditional focus is on physical health concerns, are now broadening their content of care to include screening and treatment services in oral and mental health. The CPOP study is one example of such broadening of service.

Background

CenteringPregnancy's clinicians in the San Francisco Bay Area voiced the concern that many women in the Centering groups were experiencing oral health problems. This concern prompted the medical director of the Maternal, Child, & Adolescent Health Section within the San Francisco Department of Public Health to propose the integration of oral health into CenteringPregnancy. The director suggested oral health integration as a project for a postgraduate resident in Dental Public Health at University of California, San Francisco (UCSF).

Soon the idea evolved into a plan to submit a grant application to the National Institutes of Health/National Institute of Dental and Craniofacial Research Division (NIH/NIDCR). And core research team co-led by the principal investigator (PI), a behavioral scientist and the dental resident (now a faculty member in the School of Dentistry), was formed to develop a research proposal.

This new team began an assessment of the existing CenteringPregnancy model and curriculum and of potential partnerships with local sites engaged in the model. While the topic of oral health was found in some sections of the standard CenteringPregnancy curriculum, it was not consistently addressed. The assessment team included in their review CenteringPregnancySmiles (Kovarik et al., 2009; Skelton et al., 2009), which was developed by researchers at the University of Kentucky. The Smiles program is an oral health curriculum providing enriched oral health content in each of the 10 sessions. In the program, a dental hygienist often participates in the educational component and also conducts screenings and treatment of gingival disease of the women.

The review determined that the Smiles program, while comprehensive, was at the same time too resource dependent to be feasibly implemented broadly across all CenteringPregnancy sites. The team's conclusion highlighted the need for some kind of simple, brief, low-cost intervention dealing with oral health in the Bay Area CenteringPregnancy groups, with the ultimate goal of wide adoption beyond the San Francisco Bay Area.

To further assess the need for a more formal partnership with the local CenteringPregnancy groups, it was important to engage the leadership of Bay Area CenteringPregnancy Collaborative. The project lead invited the UCSF researchers to one of the regular gatherings of representatives from most of the CenteringPregnancy groups in the San Francisco Bay Area. The research team surveyed the CenteringPregnancy facilitators with results indicating that oral health was a common problem raised by CenteringPregnancy women in their groups. In addition, the facilitators expressed interest in developing more formal oral health content. These findings confirmed the prevalence of oral health need among Bay Area CenteringPregnancy women and provided a favorable setting for creating a community–academic partnership to develop a grant proposal.

The CenteringPregnancy founder, Sharon Schindler Rising, and the Bay Area CenteringPregnancy Consortium leader, Margie Hutchison, joined the San Francisco research team as co-investigators, lending their guidance and expertise on prenatal care and CenteringPregnancy to the team. The UCSF oral health team learned about the Centering model of prenatal care, its core components and essential elements, and overall style of facilitation. They attended CenteringPregnancy facilitator training workshops, worked closely with the CenteringPregnancy co-investigators, and met with local CenteringPregnancy-site lead facilitators and co-facilitators to continue building partnerships and gain a better understanding of what an oral health program would look like and how it could be integrated into CenteringPregnancy.

An overall vision for the project began to take shape with the following guiding principles: the project would be low-cost, brief, sustainable, facilitator-led, skills-building, and in line with the CenteringPregnancy model of interactive care. The research team developed a roadmap to guide a pilot study, under the NIH R21 Developmental Research Grant mechanism, in two phases: (a) development of an oral health promotion curriculum (later known as CPOP); and (b) pilot test of the CPOP curriculum. The goal of the pilot study was to develop and test an interactive educational and behavioral intervention to promote maternal and infant oral health for low-income underserved women receiving prenatal care through CenteringPregnancy.

Phase I: The CPOP Study

■ Developing the CPOP Curriculum and Research Study Instruments

Researchers used a community-engaged process to develop the curriculum, drawing upon several perspectives and areas of expertise. The team included CenteringPregnancy leaders, CenteringPregnancy facilitators, and women receiving CenteringPregnancy care, as well as dental clinicians/researchers and a social and behavioral scientist. An important factor was that all study procedures were developed to integrate smoothly into the clinic flows and practices. To achieve that goal, we involved clinic staff from the start of the project for their feedback, minimizing the impact of study activities on clinic operations.

■ Recruiting Sites and Facilitators

Our process began with identifying potential CenteringPregnancy program sites/locations as partners in development and implementation of the intervention. We planned to recruit facilitators from sites that would be participating as our intervention sites. We worked closely with the Bay Area CenteringPregnancy leadership to identify programs that were site approved, had experienced CenteringPregnancy facilitators, adequate staff support, and where enough women were enrolled in CenteringPregnancy to meet the sample size needs of the study. The study design required and recruited two intervention and two control locations, with one English- and one Spanish-language group each. Two or three facilitators at each intervention site were recruited to serve on the development and implementation team. Facilitators from the two control sites were not involved in the development of the intervention to prevent information crossover between sites.

■ Developing the Intervention

The intervention is based on a theoretical model for behavioral change—Social Cognitive Theory (Bandura, 1997)—that describes the reciprocal influences of personal factors, environmental factors, and behaviors. For this project, the team focused on personal factors of self-efficacy (the sense of confidence in ability) and knowledge; environmental factors of the CenteringPregnancy culture encouraging and emphasizing oral health; and the behavioral factors of improving behavioral skills in oral health. These three components were consistent with the CenteringPregnancy model emphasizing health assessments and care, health education, and community building.

In designing the intervention, we worked in an iterative process. We began with a basic list of curricular learning objectives drawn from federal, national, and state guideline recommendations for oral health care and supervision within prenatal care (American College of Obstetricians and Gynecologists Women's Health Care Physicians; Committee on Health Care for Underserved Women, 2013; California Dental Association Foundation; American College of Obstetricians and Gynecologists, District IX, 2010; Kumar & Samelson, 2009). The facilitators suggested activities consistent with the CenteringPregnancy model that could be used to deliver the curriculum. Two 15-minute modules resulted—one on maternal oral health and one on infant oral health suitable for presenting in two separate CenteringPregnancy sessions: the maternal module to be included in session 3 or 4 and the infant module in session 7 or 8. A one-page reference guide of the learning objectives and key points for each module was designed to help the facilitators cover all of the objectives and the associated activities.

Once a basic outline of the intervention was approved, we conducted four focus groups of women receiving their prenatal care in CenteringPregnancy. We explored their responses and suggestions related to the intervention materials. We had two focus group topics, and for each topic we conducted one group for Spanish speakers and one for English speakers. One focus group covered the curriculum and the second covered the assessments needed to evaluate the intervention. We asked the women to suggest any additional curriculum topics that they would like to see included in the modules. In the second focus group, we asked the women to provide feedback and suggestions, with a particular focus on our plan to conduct clinical dental exams. We were concerned that the women might be hesitant to have exams while pregnant because of possible safety issues for their unborn babies. Through this process, we learned that the women were very interested in oral health care and supervision, were eager to have the intervention modules become part of CenteringPregnancy, and were comfortable with the idea of having dental exams.

Once the design of the intervention was finalized, we conducted the training in a group setting, co-led by the UCSF dental researcher/project director and the CenteringPregnancy Bay Area lead. Training began with facilitators learning the scientific rationale and current evidence base for the intervention content and activities. Following this, a live demonstration by the CenteringPregnancy lead showed how the intervention modules would be conducted and delivered. At a later date, each facilitator conducted her own practice session with one of the CenteringPregnancy groups that was currently in session. These sessions were evaluated for fidelity with feedback provided.

Phase II: Pilot Test of the CPOP Curriculum

When we were ready to pilot test the interventions in CenteringPregnancy groups, we visited during their second session and described the study to them explaining the aims and activities. Interested women either stayed after the group for a few minutes to get more information or gave us contact information for a phone call at a later time. Women in the study signed informed consent forms that were available in English and Spanish, as were all assessments and materials. Almost every woman in the six intervention CenteringPregnancy groups agreed to participate in the study (total $n = 49$, 93% agreement), and 75% of the women recruited in the eight control groups also agreed (total $n = 52$), making for a total of 101 women. Each CenteringPregnancy group included 6 to 10 women.

Our goal was to make participation as convenient as possible for the clinics, facilitators, and CenteringPregnancy women. The effects of the interventions—change in women's knowledge, attitudes, behaviors, and oral health outcomes—were evaluated by having the women complete questionnaires and dental exams before and after the maternal module interventions were presented in the sessions. Both the intervention and control group study participants completed the questionnaires and dental exams. The women could complete the questionnaires (a) by phone or in person before or after their CenteringPregnancy care session, (b) through an interview if there were literacy issues, or (c) on their own with paper and pencil. The pre- and post-intervention dental exams were conducted by the study dental examiner in a separate space in the same building as their CenteringPregnancy group sessions. Most women preferred to complete the questionnaires by themselves at the same time as they came in for their dental exams.

■ Intervention Modules

The intervention modules were conducted as part of the CenteringPregnancy group sessions, and each module took about 15 minutes. For the maternal module, groups discussed common oral health problems that many of them were having, the importance of oral health, and the importance of receiving dental care during pregnancy, with an emphasis that getting dental care during pregnancy was safe (Michalowicz et al., 2008) and important for their and their infant's health. The women were asked to discuss whether they thought dental care during pregnancy was safe or whether they had concerns. These discussions provided the opportunity for women to talk about their oral health experiences and led into the second part of the module: proper oral hygiene practices.

Researchers provided each woman with a toolkit that included a toothbrush, fluoride toothpaste, floss, and a 2-minute timer. They learned about and practiced proper tooth brushing. Women learned a self-assessment referred to as the "toothpick test" (Caton & Polson, 1985), an activity to assess gum health. Illustrated instructions on flossing teeth were given to participants as part of the intervention. Although the women had wanted a hands-on session on proper flossing, we were unable to fit that content into the time frame allotted for the session. At subsequent CenteringPregnancy sessions, the women conducted the toothpick test at the same time as their self-assessments of their blood pressures and weights.

The infant module addressed oral hygiene practices for infants, healthy feeding practices, and the importance of avoiding sharing of saliva which is the primary way that infants and children acquire the bacteria that cause dental cavities (caries) from caregivers (Berkowitz, Turner, & Green, 1981; Li & Caufield, 1995) The importance of a dental visit at 1 year of age also was among topics discussed. Infant toolkits provided to each woman included soft cloths for cleaning the inside of the baby's mouth after feedings, infant tooth brushes, and fluoride toothpaste. Each intervention was audiotaped and the fidelity of the intervention delivery evaluated for completeness. The results of this evaluation showed that the facilitators delivered the interventions well—women received an average of 98% on the learning objectives from both modules. This assured us that the facilitators had mastery of the intervention content and delivered it well, which led to high intervention module fidelity.

Study Findings

Facilitators completed questionnaires at the end of the study to rate their experience of participating in the study. Overall, they expressed a high level of satisfaction with: (a) the time required to participate in the CPOP activities for the Intervention groups, (b) the interest and benefits to the women in their groups, and (c) the idea to conduct this study in a larger clinical trial. The facilitators agreed that the trainings should be conducted in a similar manner for future studies, but also thought that online trainings might be a possibility. Given the time constraints and challenge of getting facilitators together for group training, and considering possible broader adoption nationwide in the future, online trainings, though challenging to design, might be a good option.

The CenteringPregnancy study participants reported high levels of satisfaction with the study procedures, particularly the intervention modules and the hands-on tooth-brushing activity in the maternal module. Fewer than 18% reported any dissatisfaction with the dental exams. The times required to complete questionnaires and exams were satisfactory to the large majority.

Based on the results of the dental exams, we found that women in the intervention group had significant improvements in their oral health, compared to the control women. These included improvements in plaque levels (measure of oral hygiene), in percentages of sites that bled when probed (measure of gingival inflammation), and in levels of probing depths (measure of current or former gingival disease). We did not find that intervention mothers had higher levels of knowledge, attitudes, or oral health behaviors when compared to the control mothers. Specific findings of the maternal intervention are currently under review for publication. Through additional funding given to the investigators by the NIDCR, we were able to conduct a follow-up of some of the mother–infant dyads at 6 and 12 months postpartum. Preliminary findings suggest that, at 12 months postpartum, infants whose mothers had participated in the intervention were less likely to have acquired one of the main bacteria responsible for dental caries (*Streptococcus mutans*) when compared to mothers who had not received the intervention.

Having shown that the intervention had a positive effect on oral health for mothers and infants, we received funding from the NIDCR to develop a clinical trial application. While it is tempting to consider the results of the pilot study as evidence enough to implement the interventions widely without further full testing, it is important to test the intervention in a larger study in which facilitators and CenteringPregnancy participants are randomly assigned to either the intervention or the control group. Only through the randomization of patients and CenteringPregnancy facilitators to either the intervention or control groups can we be sure that the differences found in the study are due to the intervention and not due to particular characteristics of the patients or the facilitators that might influence them to choose the intervention group or the control group if they had the opportunity to do so. During this grant-planning period, we have established our CenteringPregnancy partner sites for the clinical trial, refined our study procedures, and have updated our assessments and other documents needed for the application process.

Lessons Learned

In our work with our CenteringPregnancy partners, we learned that the CenteringPregnancy leaders and facilitators are dedicated to providing the finest state-of-the art, evidence-based care to their families. We also learned that the leaders and facilitators are tireless managers, stretching every possible resource to maximize their effectiveness. We understand that taking the time to participate in this research is both a great opportunity for CenteringPregnancy providers, staff, and participants and an added burden on their system. The CPOP project would not have succeeded to this point without the full support of the leadership at CHI and the support of the San Francisco CenteringPregnancy organizations that have partnered with us for years.

Experience has taught us that CenteringPregnancy moms are eager to learn more about their health and their family's health and want to do what is best for all of them. Their interest in family and personal health contributed to their willingness to participate in the study. It reduced the burden for the women when the dental exams were scheduled to coincide with their group sessions.

Finally, we learned that trained CenteringPregnancy facilitators, that is, nondental providers, are capable of delivering effective oral health supervision, education, and anticipatory guidance. This combination of facilitators bringing oral health skills into clinical care can result in significant improvements in women's oral health and perhaps health of their families. In addition, health care systems benefit from brief, low-cost behavioral interventions that are capable of having a significant impact on oral health outcomes. If the results of the CPOP pilot study are validated in a randomized clinical trial, the resulting confidence in the model will be a major contribution to public health.

References

American College of Obstetricians and Gynecologists Women's Health Care Physicians; Committee on Health Care for Underserved Women. (2013). Committee opinion no. 569: Oral health care during pregnancy and through the lifespan. *Obstetrics & Gynecology, 122*(2, Pt. 1), 417–422.

Bandura, A. (1997). *Self-efficacy: The exercise of control.* New York, NY: W. H. Freeman.

Berkowitz, R. J., Turner, J., & Green, P. (1981). Maternal salivary levels of *Streptococcus mutans* and primary oral infection of infants. *Archives of Oral Biology, 26*(2), 147–149.

California Dental Association Foundation; American College of Obstetricians and Gynecologists, District IX. (2010). Oral health during pregnancy and early childhood: Evidence-based guidelines for health professionals. *Journal of the California Dental Association, 38*(6), 391–403, 405–440.

Caton, J. G., & Polson, A. M. (1985). The interdental bleeding index: A simplified procedure for monitoring gingival health. *Compendium of Continuing Education in Dentistry, 6*(2), 88, 90–92.

Kovarik, R., Skelton, J., Mullins, M. R., Langston, L., Womack, S., Morris, J., Martin, D., Brooks, R., & Ebersole, J. (2009). CenteringPregnancy Smiles: A community engagement to develop and implement a new oral health and prenatal care model in rural Kentucky. *Journal of Higher Education and Engagement, 13*(3), 101–112.

Kumar, J., & Samelson, R. (2009). Oral health care during pregnancy recommendations for oral health professionals. *The New York State Dental Journal, 75*(6), 29–33.

Li, Y., & Caufield, P. W. (1995). The fidelity of initial acquisition of mutans streptococci by infants from their mothers. *Journal of Dental Research, 74*(2), 681–685.

Michalowicz, B. S., DiAngelis, A. J., Novak, M. J., Buchanan, W., Papapanou, P. N., Mitchell, D. A., . . . Rogers, T. B. (2008). Examining the safety of dental treatment in pregnant women. *Journal of the American Dental Association, 139*(6), 685–695.

Skelton, J., Mullins, R., Langston, L. T., Womack, S., Ebersole, J. L., Rising, S. S., & Kovarik, R. (2009). CenteringPregnancySmiles: Implementation of a small group prenatal care model with oral health. *Journal of Health Care for the Poor and Underserved, 20*(2), 545–553.

Part C: Does CenteringPregnancy Promote Maternal Health Literacy?

Sandra A. Smith, PhD, MPH

sandras@u.washington.edu

Pregnancy and early parenting present mothers with a series of challenges to protect and promote personal and child health and manage health care for the dyad. How well a mother meets those challenges depends on her maternal health literacy. This section describes the ongoing CenteringPregnancy Health Literacy Promotion Trial. The project aims to assess changes in maternal health literacy among participants in two CenteringPregnancy sites and the impact of supplemental health educational materials on those changes. An overview of maternal health literacy and why it matters is followed by a discussion of what is known about improving maternal health literacy and what led researchers to hypothesize that group care is an ideal environment for health literacy promotion. The section closes with a brief description of the project and its implications.

Promoting Health Literacy: National and International Priority

Promoting maternal health literacy is a cross-cutting national priority to improve maternal–child health and transform the quality of health care. The United Nations Economic and Social Council (2010) calls on all countries to improve parents' health literacy and empower women as a global strategy to reduce the burdens of chronic disease and related disparities. These policies rise from increased understanding of the developmental origins of health and disease (Silveira, Portella, Goldani, & Barbieri, 2007) and of the influence of mothers' health behaviors, self-care, and health care practices during pregnancy and early parenting on her child's health and quality of life as an adult.

Health Literacy: One of Multiple Literacies

According to the theory of multiple literacies (Hull, Mikulecky, Clair, & Kerka, 2003), everyone reading this page has, at any one time, many literacies at different levels of proficiency. Functional literacy is the basic skill set that enables you to recognize and pronounce these words. Computer literacy enables you to send e-mail or produce a spreadsheet. Financial literacy enables you to maintain a good credit rating. Spanish literacy opens to you a whole range of information, options, and opportunities not available to those who have not developed that literacy.

Health Literacy Skills Enable You to Manage Heath and Health Care

Health literacy enables you to manage heath and health care for yourself, your family, and your community. You may have multiple health literacies that overlap and develop with need, opportunity, and support: mental health literacy, health insurance literacy, oral health literacy, maternal health literacy. Your proficiency might be high or nonexistent depending on the circumstance and your experience with the context and the media. More proficient health literacy brings more options and opportunities for health.

Maternal Health Literacy Defined

Maternal health literacy is defined as *the cognitive and social skills and motivations that determine a mother's ability to obtain, understand and use information [and services] in ways that enhance her health and that of her child* (Renkert & Nutbeam, 2001). A health literate mother is empowered for health. She has the skill and confidence to express her needs, make health-related choices, and transform those choices into her desired actions and outcomes (World Bank, 2005).

Literacy scholars describe three categories of literacy skills: functional, interactive, and critical skill sets. Functional skills are the "three Rs": reading, 'riting, and 'rithmatic, used to decode words and numbers. Some scholars argue that functional literacy is a necessary antecedent of health literacy. However, recent studies support adult learning theories that suggest skills in one category can compensate for the absence of skills in another; family or community members can supply missing skills; and skills beget skills. That is how individual health literacy develops and becomes a collective family and community asset. In one study, among 36 factors in mothers' progress toward optimal functioning during pregnancy and early parenting, reading ability was the least influential (Smith & Carroll, 2015).

For health empowerment, interactive and critical thinking skills seem to matter more than reading. Mothers, and the rest of us, use these social and cognitive skills together to make meaning from information and apply it in context. We personalize information by thinking and talking it through to interpret its relevance and usefulness in a specific real-life situation. It is through this process of interaction and reflection that health literacy is empowering.

What Improves Maternal Health Literacy?

The science around improving health literacy is in its infancy. Intervention studies remain rare, especially intervention geared to diverse, low-literacy populations and interventions in child health. In the United States, groundbreaking efforts to improve maternal health literacy through home visitation have demonstrated success. Home visiting is a preventive intervention that supports families and healthy development of children. Visitors are paraprofessionals, social workers, or public health nurses. Programs affiliated with health departments, school districts, and private organizations serve about 500,000 disadvantaged families annually.

Five recent studies (Carroll, Smith, & Thomson, 2014; Haynes et al., 2015; Mobley et al., 2014; Smith, 2009; Smith & Moore, 2012) report on four implementations of an intervention to promote maternal health literacy. The intervention integrated into home visitors' usual activities an empowerment approach to developing interactive and critical thinking skills, particularly reflection. The primary teaching and empowerment strategy was reflective questioning. Visitors were trained not to deliver standard content and not to answer questions, but rather to lead reflective conversations that require mothers to think critically. Reflective questions lead mothers to prioritize challenges, obtain information, marshal resources, plan actions, and progress toward their goals with increasing autonomy and confidence. The visitors used data from formal and informal assessments, observations, interviews, and, in some cases, medical records to formulate reflective questions and tailor standard content to individual families. To aid recall, encourage further learning, and direct them to vetted Internet resources, mothers were provided printed health education materials designed for low-skilled learners.

"I Talk Less; Parents Think More"

Home visitors participating in these studies built on their capacity to establish trusting relationships and to provide intervention of sufficient intensity to support lifestyle change. The use of reflective questioning, instead of traditional information-giving or educating, precipitated an essential change in practice. Visitors shifted out of their accustomed roles as health care or education professionals to take on roles as change agents akin to peer supporters, offering emotional support and help to make sense of complicated information and reflect on how to use it. Their health education intent shifted from thorough information-giving and knowledge gain to empowerment for health demonstrated by changes in health- and health care–related practices and behaviors. By leading reflective conversations, they shifted the focus of their visits from content to process, so that learning became mother-directed, problem-based, and collaborative. Visitors reported it took about 10 visits to feel comfortable with the new approach. One visitor summed up her experience of this shift saying, "Parents have their own answers. We just need to ask questions to get them thinking."

The aforementioned studies consistently found that, overall, mothers improved their maternal health literacy scores in home visitation by improving their use of health information and services, risk behaviors, and self/baby care. Mothers who were lower functioning at baseline made greater gains than their higher functioning counterparts, reducing disparities related to age, literacy, and mental health.

Does Centering Improve Maternal Health Literacy and Empower Mothers?

Home visiting is expanding because time constraints prevent delivery of the health promotion content of prenatal care (U.S. Department of Health and Human Services; Public Health Service, 1989) during traditional individual visits. The promising results of integrating maternal health literacy promotion into the usual activities of home visiting led researchers at the Center for Health Literacy Promotion to reason that CenteringPregnancy, with its emphasis on facilitated group interaction, purposeful self-reflection, and intent to empower mothers, might promote maternal health literacy through the group process. Interaction and reflection with a group of other pregnant women and their supporters might be even more effective as a catalyst to health literacy improvement than one-to-one reflective conversations with a home visitor. The group provides more opportunities for interaction with multiple peers currently facing similar challenges, as well as with medical and nonmedical health care professionals who present themselves as collaborating equals.

Home visitors aim to provide social support and to aid mothers in developing social networks. In Centering, the group provides rich social support for learning and behavioral change, with some groups continuing to meet after their Centering group ends. Home visitors rely on data to plan the reflective process and tailor intervention; in Centering, the group tailors the process to themselves. Home visiting services are not coordinated with prenatal care, and so mothers rarely see their records or have opportunity to discuss routinely recorded health indicators. Centering participants may increase their health literacy as they measure and record their own blood pressure and weight at each session. They may gain understanding of the measures, their progress, the use and ownership of medical records, along with confidence to ask questions.

How Much Information Is Enough?

How much information is enough to support adoption of healthy pregnancy behaviors and build mothers' confidence as protectors and managers of family health? The question led researchers to wonder whether supplementing the information in the CenteringPregnancy Notebook would increase behavioral change and confidence. It may be that the Notebook satisfies mothers' information needs or that access to digital information is approaching a point that makes more than minimal printed materials unnecessary, even in low-income populations with limited computer access. It may be that mothers place high value on the supplemental information as an easily accessed and shared reference.

Study Overview

The CenteringPregnancy Health Literacy Promotion Trial aims to assess the capacity of CenteringPregnancy to promote maternal health literacy and health empowerment. Participating mothers are Medicaid eligible and obtaining care at an academic medical center. Since studies indicate Medicaid recipients, on average, read at a fifth-grade level, and since for many women pregnancy brings their first significant encounter with the health care system, as a population, study participants are likely to have low functional literacy and lower baseline health literacy.

Two Centering sites were randomized as the intervention and comparison sites. All participants at both sites will complete the Maternal Health Literacy Self-Assessment at their second (pretest) and eighth or ninth sessions (posttest) and receive a small cash incentive for completing each assessment. The self-assessment of change in knowledge, health behaviors, and health care utilization is in keeping with the Centering process and focus on autonomy. Survey questions reflect the health promotion content of prenatal care as defined by the U.S. Public Health Service (U.S. Department of Health and Human Services; Public Health Service, 1989), the basis of the Centering curriculum, and of the supplemental materials. The assessments themselves increase awareness of key health behavior messages. They may generate discussion, and influence behavior. These impacts are equally likely in both groups. Beyond the self-assessment of literacy, the comparison group receives usual care.

In addition to the self-assessment, the intervention site will use *Beginnings Pregnancy Guide* (Smith, 1989–2014) along with the CenteringPregnancy Notebook. Each participant will receive supplemental information referenced by gestational age at the intake appointment and at each session. Participants will receive a copy of *Beginnings Parents Guide* at their final session. Facilitators and the groups together will determine when and to what degree the supplemental information is discussed. The trial will continue until 120 women at each site have completed prenatal care and the two assessments. Qualitative data from interviews with participating facilitators will inform findings. The project includes validity testing of the instrument.

The CenteringPregnancy Health Literacy Trial asks:

1. Is it feasible to integrate maternal health literacy promotion in CenteringPregnancy?
2. Is it beneficial to supplement CenteringPregnancy with *Beginnings Pregnancy Guide?*
3. Can the Maternal Health Literacy Self-Assessment be used as a meaningful measure of maternal health literacy?

4. Does CenteringPregnancy + self-assessment of health literacy promote maternal health literacy?
5. Does Centering + self-assessment + *Beginnings Guides* promote maternal health literacy more?
6. Do Centering participants and facilitators report *Beginnings Pregnancy Guide* adds value to their Centering experience?

Preliminary Results

At this writing, the intervention group is still collecting data. We can say no facilitator or participant has reported any difficulty or objection to incorporating the health literacy self-assessments. It seems feasible to integrate maternal health literacy promotion into CenteringPregnancy. One striking preliminary finding from the comparison group is that participating mothers are seeking additional information, primarily using smartphones.

The research team anticipates that mothers do improve their maternal health literacy in CenteringPregnancy. Positive findings will add weight to emerging evidence that facilitated interaction and reflection are the active ingredients in health literacy promotion. Further, positive results will add to the growing evidence of CenteringPregnancy as an essential element of a quality health care system, a means to reduce disparities and future burdens of chronic disease by promoting maternal health literacy at the very foundation of personal and public health.

Note

Mental health literacy should be differentiated from health-related literacy in mothers. A burgeoning body of literature from U.S. academic medical centers defines health literacy as functional literacy in a clinical setting. Reading tests using medical terms and documents suggest that most Americans, including one in three parents, have low health-related literacy, that is, they perform poorly on health-related tasks such as pronouncing medical terms, interpreting medication labels, and completing insurance forms. This line of research has aimed to link patients' health-related literacy to clinical outcomes. However, results have been mixed and sometimes contradictory so that the pathway from parents' reading skills to child health outcomes is far from clear.

References

Carroll, L., Smith, S. A., & Thomson, N. (2014). Parents as teachers health literacy demonstration project: Integrating an empowerment model of health literacy promotion into home-based parent education. *Health Promotion Practice, 16*(2), 282–290.

DeWalt, D. A., & Hink, A. (2009). Health literacy and child health outcomes: A systematic review of the literature. *Pediatrics, 124*(Suppl.), S265–S274. doi:10.1542/peds.2009-1162b

Haynes, G., Neuman, D., Hook, C., Haynes, D., Steeley, J., Kelly, M., . . . Paine, M. (2015). Comparing child and family outcomes between two home visitation programs. *Family and Consumer Sciences Research Journal, 43*(3), 209–228.

Hull, G. A., Mikulecky, L., St. Clair, R., & Kerka, S. (2003). *Multiple literacies: A compilation for adult educators.* Columbus: College of Education, The Ohio State University. Retrieved from www.calpro-online.org/eric/docs/compilation -literacies.pdf

Mobley, S. C., Thomas, S. D., Sutherland, D. E., Hudgins, J., Ange, B. L., & Johnson, M. H. (2014). Maternal health literacy progression among rural perinatal women. *Maternal and Child Health Journal, 18,* 1881–1892.

Renkert, S., & Nutbeam, D. (2001). Opportunities to improve maternal health literacy through ante-natal education: An exploratory study. *Health Promotion International, 16,* 381–388.

Silveira, P. P., Portella, A. K., Goldani, M. Z., & Barbieri, M. A. (2007). Developmental Origins of Health and Disease (DOHaD). *Jornal de Pediatria, 83*(6), 494–504.

Smith, S. (Ed.). (1989–2014). *Beginnings pregnancy guide.* Seattle, WA: Practice Development. Retrieved from www.BeginningsGuides.com

Smith, S. A., & Moore, E. (2012). Health literacy and depression in the context of home visitation. *Maternal and Child Health Journal, 16,* 1500–1508.

Smith, S. A. (2009). *Promoting health literacy: Concept, measurement, intervention* (Doctoral dissertation, Cincinnati, Union Institute & University, Publication No. AAT 3375168).

Smith, S. A., & Carroll, L. N. (2015, November). *Promoting maternal health literacy: Data guides intervention.* Presented by invitation to the Health Literacy Annual Research Conference, Bethesda, MD.

United Nations Economic and Social Council. (2010). Health literacy and the millennium development goals: United Nations economic and social council (ECOSOC) regional meeting background paper [Abstract]. *Journal of Health Communication, 15*(Suppl. 2), 211–223. doi:10.1080/10810730.2010.499996

U.S. Department of Health and Human Services; Public Health Service. (1989). *Caring for our future: The content of prenatal care. A report of the Public Health Service Expert Panel on the Content of Prenatal Care.* (NIH Publication No. 90-3182). Washington, DC: National Institutes of Health.

World Bank. (2005). *What is empowerment?* Washington, DC: Author. Retrieved from http://go.worldbank.org/V45HD4P100

12 Adapting CenteringPregnancy®-Based Group Antenatal Care Globally

Kathleen F. Norr and Crystal L. Patil

*There is no tool for development more effective than
the empowerment of women. —Kofi Annan*

Reflecting the global need for innovative strategies to improve the quality of health care, the Centering Healthcare™ model has generated widespread interest outside the United States. The primary focus has been adapting CenteringPregnancy, which has the longest implementation track record and strong evidence base for positive impacts. In this chapter, we describe how CenteringPregnancy can address quality of antenatal care (ANC) globally and review previous efforts to implement a CenteringPregnancy-based group care model outside the United States. Then, a comparison of the implementation process and outcomes to date identifies commonalities and unique features for three CenteringPregnancy-based group ANC initiatives in three very different contexts: the Netherlands (Rijnders, van der Pal, & Aalhuizen, 2012), a high-resource European country; Nepal (Maru, Harsha, & Nirola, 2015), a low-resource Asian country with especially challenging terrain; and the low-resource countries of Malawi and Tanzania (Patil et al., 2013) in sub-Saharan Africa. We focus on balancing adaptation to the specific context and retaining core components of CenteringPregnancy that are essential for its effectiveness; evaluation is integrated to build evidence for innovative group care models. Our conclusion focuses on the promise of CenteringPregnancy-based group ANC, implementation challenges and complexities associated with adaptation, and strategies to support global expansion of this innovative health care delivery model.

TABLE 12.1   Illustrating Global Health Inequities

Life expectancy: • 36-year gap in life expectancy comparing Malawi to Japan
Globally, out of every 100,000 women giving birth: • In low-resource countries, 230 women die • In high-resource countries, only 16 women die
In Afghanistan, Somalia, and Chad, the maternal mortality ratio is over 1,000 (out of 100,000 live births), while the same average figure for the WHO European Region is 21. Women in the richest 20% of the global population are up to 20 times more likely to have a birth attended to by a skilled health worker than a poor woman.
Every single day, 21,000 children die before their fifth birthday of pneumonia, malaria, diarrhea, and other diseases. Infants are even more vulnerable. Out of 1,000 infants born alive: • In low-resource countries, 47 will die before their first birthday • In high-resource countries, only 6 will die before their first birthday
Within-country gaps: • In the United States, infants born to African American women are 1.5–3 times more likely to die than infants born to other races/ethnicities • Children from the poorest 20% of households are nearly twice as likely to die before their fifth birthday as children in the richest 20%

WHO, World Health Organization.
Source: Creanga et al., 2012.

Improving maternal and child health requires reducing the distressingly high disparities in mortality rates that continue to persist between high- and low-resource countries. Disparities also exist in low-resource pockets within both high- and low-resource countries wherever women are disadvantaged by poverty, race/ethnicity, religion, or geographic barriers to care (Table 12.1) (Creanga et al., 2012; World Health Organization, 2011). ANC, as part of a continuum of care package, fails to maximize its potential contribution advancing health for women and children during pregnancy and beyond. Numerous missed opportunities occur due to poor quality of care, poor provider–client interactions, and because many women do not start ANC early or complete all visits, reflecting their perspectives on the value of ANC as delivered (Kerber, 2007; Roberts et al., 2015).

While the nature and root causes of the quality gap are somewhat different in low-resource and high-resource countries, short one-on-one visits of 15 minutes or less, after a somewhat longer first visit, prevail in both contexts. In many low-resource countries, high birth rates create high demand for ANC services, while acute shortages of health workers and severely underfunded health systems make providing these services exceptionally challenging. Observations in low-income countries document that women have long waits for service and that their ANC visits are brief with almost no health promotion, with a longer first visit and subsequent visits averaging only 11 minutes in one study in Tanzania (Conrad, De Allegri, Moses, et al., 2012; Conrad, Schmid, Tientrebeogo, et al., 2012; Magoma et al., 2011; Sarker et al., 2010; von Both, Flessa, Makuwani, Mpembeni, & Jahn, 2006). In most middle- to high-income countries, while there are sufficient health providers and adequate funding overall, pressures for efficiency and cost reductions have created powerful incentives for short ANC visits with minimal provider–client interactions or health promotion. In the United States, after a longer first visit, most clinics schedule a visit every 10 to 15 minutes (S. Rising, personal communication, 2016).

Achieving optimal health for childbearing women and their infants requires a seamless continuum of care across the lifecourse, from preconception through postbirth (The Partnership for Maternal, Newborn & Child Health [PMNCH], 2006, 2015). Because preconception care is woefully underdeveloped, ANC becomes the entry point to this childbearing care continuum for most women. Pregnancy is a time when women are eager to promote health for themselves and their babies. High-quality ANC can be the beginning of a positive health-promoting cascade that engages women and builds their trust in the health care system. With trust, women are more likely to come for services and accept health promotion advice during pregnancy, at delivery, and beyond.

Past experience shows that intensive efforts can achieve substantial reductions in mortality. For example, the unprecedented global Millennium Development Goals (MDGs) initiative reduced maternal mortality by nearly half and under-five mortality by more than half in just 15 years. The Sustainable Development Goals (Sachs, 2012) and universal application of existing evidence-based and low-cost interventions could push the global community to meet new targets (Darmstadt, 2008; Howson, Kinney, & Lawn, 2012). A focus on increasing quality of care at ANC and the overall health care experience for all women will make another substantial contribution in the global push to improve maternal and infant health outcomes (Tunçalp et al., 2015).

Efforts to improve quality of care (QOC) have included evidence-based practices, continuous quality improvement (CQI), and patient-centered care (Bhutta, Salam, Lassi, Austin, & Langer, 2014; Institute for Healthcare Improvement, 2003; Meyers, Durlak, & Wandersman, 2012; Robinson, Callister, Berry, & Dearing, 2008; Stewart et al., 2000). The evidence-based practices movement focuses on integrating proven strategies into care more quickly and systematically. CQI, modeled after industrial best practices, aims to improve QOC within a health facility using the classic Deming model of plan, do, study, act to rapidly introduce best practices (Deming, 1986). Patient-centered care is an effort to improve quality of care by tailoring health services to the specific needs of the client, collaborative provider–patient health decision making, and patient empowerment (Austin et al., 2014; Bhutta et al., 2014). Patient-centered care is widely endorsed and has been associated with better adherence; implementing genuine patient-centered care has proved challenging, especially in the context of short ANC visits. However, none of these approaches have been able to address the primary drivers of the quality gap in ANC because they have not reenvisioned the basic ANC model.

This model of 10 or more one-on-one visits with a provider has remained unchanged since its inception in the early 20th century (Bergsjø & Villar, 1997; Oakley, 1981).The only major modification to the original model has been reduction of the number of visits. On the basis of several large randomized trials that found no difference in outcomes with reduced visits, the World Health Organization (WHO) endorsed a four-visit model, called Focused Antenatal Care (FANC) (Villar et al., 2001). The assumption was that resources saved on fewer visits would be dedicated to the cost of higher quality visits. In low-resource settings, the expectation was that FANC would result in longer and patient-centered visits. Unfortunately, no mechanisms were put in place to ensure this would happen; so after the research ended, the reality of implementing FANC in low-resource settings with severe provider shortages was that patient-centered care could not be fully achieved. Women continued to receive brief, low-quality ANC visits—but substantially fewer of them (Conrad, Schmid, Tientrebeogo, et al., 2012; Magoma, Requejo, Campbell, Cousens, & Filippi, 2010; Nyamtema, Jong, Urassa, Hagen, & van Roosmalen, 2012; Tetui et al., 2012). A recent reanalysis of the same clinical trial data identified slightly higher perinatal mortality with the reduced visit model (Dowswell et al., 2010).

CenteringPregnancy Has the Potential to Improve ANC Quality of Care and Outcomes

CenteringPregnancy is the first truly innovative model that fundamentally alters the nature of ANC. A detailed description of a typical Centering-Pregnancy session is provided in Chapter 3. CenteringPregnancy's three core components (care within group space, interactive learning, and community-building) harness the well-established power of self-care, interactive learning, and the benefits of positive group dynamics. *The synergistic intertwining in time and space of these three components creates a holistic woman-centered model of ANC that empowers pregnant women and meets their needs for in-depth information and support.*

This book provides substantial reference that CenteringPregnancy improves outcomes for women and infants across the continuum of care. Satisfaction with care increases for both women and their providers (Andersson, Christensson, & Hildingsson, 2014; Klima, 2003; Liu, Chao, Jostad-Laswell, & Duncan, 2016; Massey, Rising, & Ickovics, 2006; McNeil et al., 2013; Tandon, Colon, Vega, Murphy, & Alonso, 2012). For women, increased satisfaction ties them into the health care system and is part of building trust, which is expected to lead to greater uptake of services along the entire cascade of care, including increased attendance at ANC, facility birth, and follow-up for self (postnatal and beyond) and infant (well-baby care) (Bakken et al., 2004; Schneider, Kaplan, Greenfield, Li, & Wilson, 2004). For health workers, the extended interaction through continuity of care establishes relationships and creates a more satisfying and less stressful encounter that enables providers to better understand the women they serve and provide the respectful high-quality care they were trained to offer (McNeil et al., 2013; Patil et al., 2013). Collectively, this can reduce job-related stress and burnout. A growing body of evidence documents that CenteringPregnancy has positive impacts on health outcomes, including greater prenatal and postnatal care attendance and satisfaction, better prenatal mental and physical health during pregnancy, babies being heavier and/or less likely to be premature, more births with a skilled birth attendant, more breastfeeding, and more family planning uptake, which will increase birth intervals (Ickovics et al., 2007; Ickovics et al., 2011; Ickovics et al., 2016; Kennedy et al., 2011).

CenteringPregnancy also offers distinct advantages to the health system overall and clinics. By providing care to a group of women at the same stage of pregnancy with similar concerns, CenteringPregnancy overcomes a fundamental weakness of individual care. Instead of repeating brief health promotion messages over and over, providers can provide in-depth information to a group of women simultaneously. This richer, more effective health promotion experience makes efficient use of provider time. A single provider plus a lower level assistant can serve eight to 12 women in a 2-hour session, equivalent to 10 minutes of provider time per woman for groups of 12 or 15 minutes per woman for groups of eight. Visits of 11 to 15 minutes are quite comparable with average visit times in both low-resource and high-resource countries (von Both et al., 2006). Thus, the CenteringPregnancy model has the potential to offer more care to each woman despite the constraints of provider shortages and/or cost-containment pressures common across many countries. CenteringPregnancy also provides other efficiencies for overall clinic flow. After the first visit, women come directly to the Centering-Pregnancy group space, eliminating repeated registration at subsequent visits and reducing the overall burden of registration and crowding in the registration and waiting area, a major contributor to stress for both women and workers. Eliminating waiting time also makes the length of an ANC visit more predictable and shows respect for women's time. This approach also uses provider time efficiently because they can start seeing early arrivals immediately.

Implementing CenteringPregnancy-Based Group ANC Globally: Challenges and Lessons Learned

Given all the advantages of the CenteringPregnancy group care model for women, providers, and health systems, it is not surprising that there is high enthusiasm for bringing this care innovation to the millions of pregnant women throughout the world who can benefit from CenteringPregnancy. Numerous efforts to do so have been initiated globally. Published work from initiatives working with the Centering Healthcare Institute (CHI) directly is available: Australia (Teate, Leap, Rising, & Homer, 2011), Canada (McNeil et al., 2012; McNeil et al., 2013; McDonald, Sword, Eryuzlu, & Biri, 2014), Ireland (McNeill & Reiger, 2014), Malawi and Tanzania (Patil et al., 2013), Nepal (Maru et al., 2015), Netherlands (Rijnders et al., 2012), Sweden (Andersson, 2014; Andersson, Christensson, & Hildingsson, 2012;

Andersson, Christensson, & Hildingsson, 2013; Andersson et al., 2014), and the UK (Gaudion, 2010; Gaudion et al., 2011). Other initiatives are just underway in Brazil, Colombia, Chile, China, Iceland, and Norway. Still other researchers exploring group care are from Iran (Jafari, Eftekhar, Fotouhi, Mohammad, & Hantoushzadeh, 2012), Ghana (Lori, Munro, & Chuey, 2016), Egypt (Ghani, 2015), Kenya, Mexico, Nigeria, and Rwanda. We note the model used and the current status of each initiative based on both published and unpublished information from Sharon Rising, who has spearheaded CHI collaboration with global initiatives. At least one initiative has been started in every WHO region of the world. In nearly all cases, pregnant women, providers, and health system administrators are excited about the potential of group care generally and CenteringPregnancy-based group ANC in particular. However, few of these initiatives have been able to be sustained or become a widespread alternative choice for ANC. Despite ambitious plans and hard work, only a few of these efforts have resulted in a well-documented, systematically evaluated, and potentially sustainable CenteringPregnancy-based group care program.

These collective experiences highlight how challenging it is to introduce and sustain this innovative model of care. CenteringPregnancy re-envisions the model of ANC, and health systems, clinics, individual providers, and administrators are likely to find such a major departure from their prior training and experiences especially challenging. Such implementation challenges are not unique to CenteringPregnancy. Despite the movement to institute evidence-based practice, a major scientific gap in health sciences is the lag between developing new evidence-based practices and achieving their widespread implementation (Barker, Reid, & Schall, 2016; Gitlin, 2013; Glasgow et al., 2012).

The characteristics of the innovation affect the ease of implementation, as identified by Rogers more than 40 years ago (Rogers, 1976). Simple innovations that can be tried out with low investment and "trialability" are easier to implement than more complex innovations. Centering-Pregnancy is a complex innovation that requires a certain minimum investment. The minimum would be one CenteringPregnancy group at one clinic, but because CenteringPregnancy training, like Centering-Pregnancy itself, uses interactive learning in a small group, it is usually more practical to train at least six to 12 providers at one time and to launch a minimum of one group per month for at least 6 months, since it takes at least 6 months to complete the first groups and evaluate the process and outcomes. Thus, bringing CenteringPregnancy to a different country requires a sizeable initial commitment and investment of human and other resources.

However, CenteringPregnancy offers several strategic advantages for implementation in new contexts. Although CenteringPregnancy has been tested with a randomized clinical trial in only one country, the United States, CenteringPregnancy has been implemented across widely different health care settings, including public health clinics, small private practices, and large care networks, and for diverse groups of pregnant women from different racial and ethnic groups with different language needs, ranging from rich to poor and from adolescents to adults. Positive outcomes have been identified in each of these populations, including public health settings serving impoverished, vulnerable, and/or non-English-speaking pregnant women. Moreover, the model's core components necessary for fidelity are well defined, and process evaluation has linked the core component of interactive learning to more positive outcomes (Novick et al., 2013). This broad success indicates that the CenteringPregnancy model is robust and has high potential for adaptation globally, including low-resource countries with multiple constraints and poor maternal and infant outcomes.

As the CenteringPregnancy model expands to new settings outside of the United States, different adaptations will be needed for successful implementation because the context of each setting is unique. Implementation science models have identified a common process, involving distinct stages of preparing, piloting, and expanding (Barker et al., 2016; Bergh & Pattinson, 2003; Damschroder et al., 2009; World Health Organization, 2010; World Health Organization, 2011). At each stage, adaptation of the innovation to the context is important for success because better contextual fit enhances feasibility, acceptability, and sustainability. However, the adaptation must retain fidelity to CenteringPregnancy's core components or the benefits of this health care innovation may be lost.

The context includes every aspect of the environment from the type of health care system to the clinic's room sizes as well as shared cultural norms and values affecting ANC such as gender discrimination and the role of mothers. The broad scope of potential factors can be daunting. Drawing on ideas from many implementation models, we present a simplified approach to adaptation that focuses on the specific contextual features that directly affect implementation of CenteringPregnancy (Figure 12.1). The site in which CenteringPregnancy is offered is within a specific clinic or care setting; therefore, characteristics of the clinic and staff that may facilitate or hinder implementation are the first set of contextual factors to consider. This proximate environment includes patient volume; number,

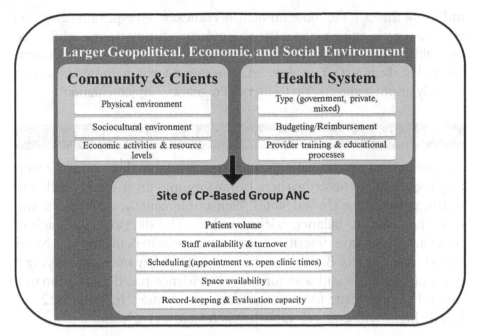

FIGURE 12.1 A simplified model of contextual factors affecting the adaptation of CenteringPregnancy.
ANC, antenatal care; CP, CenteringPregnancy.

qualifications, and turnover of personnel, including administrators, providers, and support staff; physical space availability; registration system; record-keeping; and evaluation processes and capacities.

Two other sets of factors that also affect implementation are the clients and communities served by the clinic and the larger health care system in which the clinic is embedded. Community and client factors that commonly affect ANC services can include a number of client characteristics: age, parity, education, and environment, especially the degree of difficulty accessing care related to the terrain and transportation networks. The sociocultural environment can include: prevailing family structures, familial and community supports for childbearing women, cultural values around gender inequalities, and women's roles. Economic activities and resources including the level of income, women's work at home and outside the home, and family separation due to migration for jobs are important to understand.

Health system factors include the type of system (national health care, private or mixed), the reimbursement system especially as it relates to ANC delivery and clinic sites' level of control over resources for care at that clinic, and the training and continuing education system for administrators, providers, and lower level workers. All of these specific factors are embedded in the larger society, but this broad context typically affects CenteringPregnancy indirectly, through the more immediate context (e.g., type of religion and religious organizations may relate to gender inequality norms, while type of health care system and reimbursement is tied into the overall economic and political context). Therefore, adaptation can focus on those factors that actually impinge directly on CenteringPregnancy implementation.

Three Initiatives: Implementing CenteringPregnancy Globally

To explore the common lessons learned when implementing CenteringPregnancy, we describe three promising initiatives in very different settings outside the United States, their implementation processes, and how they tried to balance fidelity and fit. The developers of each of these initiatives have described their experiences in detail in Field Notes found in Appendix B. Each of these initiatives began by identifying a particular problem and searching for an evidence-based innovation that might be appropriate for their problem and context. In Table 12.2, we briefly highlight some relevant details related to each site.

Preparation

Introducing CenteringPregnancy into a new context requires engaging stakeholders and obtaining all necessary permissions as well as modifying CenteringPregnancy to fit the context and preparing the health care setting. All three initiatives obtained buy-in and support from key stakeholders. Stakeholders in all three countries had immediate positive responses to the group model (Figure 12.2). They recognized that group ANC overcomes major inefficiencies in the existing ANC model and opens up the possibly of improving quality of care by redirecting the resources already present. Although they started on a small scale, both the Netherlands and Malawi and Tanzania initiatives had a vision of nationwide scale-up from the start. Therefore, they sought buy-in at the national level from the Ministry of Health and national experts and at the local level from the administrators and providers at sites. In the Netherlands, the midwifery professional organization, nursing education, and health research leaders were also engaged. The Malawi and Tanzania initiative had team members engaged in nursing education and research and active members in their professional organizations.

These international efforts all engaged stakeholders at higher levels initially than is usual in expansion of CenteringPregnancy to new clinics

TABLE 12.2 Basic Setting Details for the Three Initiatives

Country	Netherlands	Nepal	Malawi and Tanzania
Resources	High	Low	Low
Context	Affluent country with sufficient numbers of well-trained providers and a well-developed health care system	A district in a very remote and impoverished district of the low-resource country of Nepal with an underfunded national health system	Low-resource country, underfunded health care system and extreme provider shortage
Problem	Highest perinatal mortality in Europe	Low health facility delivery rate contributing to high maternal mortality	High maternal and infant mortality, low quality of care, provider shortages, insufficient completion ANC and postnatal visits
Implementation Team	Independent practice midwives, representatives from midwifery professional associations, educational facility, and research institute	Nongovernmental organization that has collaborative agreement to run the district hospital and its 12 clinics, and district administrators	Doctorally prepared midwives and researchers from Malawi, Tanzania, and United States
Justification of Centering-Pregnancy	Woman-centered, evidence-based approach would empower women and potentially have favorable impacts on perinatal outcomes	Supportive environment to increase self-efficacy and help women obtain male relative approval and plan for a health facility birth	Woman-centered, evidence-based approach would improve ANC quality of care, satisfaction, and perinatal outcomes
Expansion Goals	Nationwide	District	District and national

ANC, antenatal care.

Netherlands

With its mixed health care system, small independent midwifery practices provided an ideal setting because of their autonomy and flexibility. The researchers spread their ideas and identified three practices ready to innovate. A small research grant supported efforts.

Malawi & Tanzania

Sits were identified in rural Malawi and urban Dar es Salaam to maximize diversity in clinic size and context. Small research grants were obtained to provide the resources necessary to pilot the program.

Nepal

To meet their more focused goal of district-wide implementation, they enlisted the support of the district health officer (DHO) of each of the mid-level practitioners who run and administer the village-level clinics. They did not obtain additional funding but funded the project from the regular hospital and clinics budget.

FIGURE 12.2 Preparation varied by funding and planned scale of implementation.

in the United States. Most other countries have a more centralized health care system, usually a national program with oversight from the Ministry of Health or a mixed public–private system with centralized standards of care and reimbursement. Also, in comparison, the introduction of CenteringPregnancy in the United States is most often initiated by a few providers at a single clinic without plans for expansion. Recently, wider efforts are underway to expand CenteringPregnancy in health networks and in public health systems.

The next part of preparation is examining the fit between CenteringPregnancy as offered in the United States and the new health care system and clients and community and then modifying CenteringPregnancy and/or the health care setting as needed. Both the Malawi and Tanzania and Nepal initiatives were in countries where FANC was the nationally approved model of ANC care, so both had to adapt from the 10 CenteringPregnancy sessions in the United States to a number closer to the four-visit FANC model. Independently, both initiatives decided on six visits.

Whether in the United States or a new country, introducing CenteringPregnancy also requires adaptations to the clinic administration. Many of these issues are similar to issues faced when introducing

CenteringPregnancy to a new setting in the United States, discussed in Chapter 7, but contextual differences in other countries make these adaptations (Figure 12.3) more challenging and more varied.

- *Space:* A room or space for group meetings needs to be identified. In many clinics designed for individual care, space where CenteringPregnancy group sessions can occur is often less than ideal, although committed initiators usually manage to work out space issues.
- *Scheduling*: Clinics also need to make plans to recruit women into group care and to schedule group sessions.
  - *Recruiting for Group ANC Appointments*: This was especially challenging in the Malawi and Tanzania and Nepal initiatives, where no appointment system is in place and women receive care on a first-come, first-served basis.
  - *Volume*: The degree to which a clinic can be successful in recruiting is also dependent upon volume. The smallest rural clinic in Malawi struggled to recruit enough women at the same gestational age for a group, while there were no problems forming groups in the large urban clinic in Tanzania. Some of the smaller midwifery practices in the Netherlands also struggled to fill groups.
  - *Entry Into ANC*: The problem of filling groups is exacerbated when women come for their first ANC visit at widely differing stages of pregnancy and determination of gestational age is limited. The universal use of ultrasounds to determine the number of weeks pregnant is not feasible; this problem can be at least partially addressed by working with clients and the community. For example, if women do not come to ANC early enough to be incorporated into CenteringPregnancy groups, community campaigns can heighten awareness of the benefits of early ANC.
- *Record Keeping and Evaluation*: Antenatal records that can be linked to birth outcomes are important for assessing whether the innovation is in fact improving outcomes. In the Netherlands, a record review made a relatively low-cost initial outcomes evaluation feasible. In Malawi and Tanzania, the lack of electronic records and separate clinic and delivery records kept by date of service (rather than patient) make this nearly impossible. This gap forced both the countries to conduct their own repeated surveys, adding greatly to costs and requiring research funding.

Netherlands

Relatively few modifications were made. As a high-resource country with an ANC model of up to 10 visits, the practice of individual ANC is similar to individual practice in the United States. However, low-risk ANC in the Netherlands is provided almost entirely by midwives in either small independent clinics or hospital-based clinics, so that individual ANC is less interventionist and more women-centered than in the United States. The manual was translated and a few content changes were made to fit better with the cultural norms.

Malawi & Tanzania

Adapted to fit the FANC model. Five visits were antenatal, and the last group visit occurred at the 6-week postpartum visit and focused on the post-birth issues. Because HIV is a major health issue,content had to be added regarding HIV prevention,couples HIV testing,and the prevention of mother-to-child transmission (PMTCT).

Nepal

Adapted to fit the FANC model. All six visits were antenatal visits. The initiative integrated another intervention into their adapted Centering Pregnancy model: women's talking circles *(see Appendix B)*. These circles have been effective in Nepal and other countries in helping women develop appropriate solutions to local problems affecting women's health, and they hoped that this addition would help women address the need to plan for facility births and obtain male permission to do so.

FIGURE 12.3 Sustainable adaptation requires that the program fit into the current system and has enough flexibility to change over time.
ANC, antenatal care; FANC, Focused Antenatal Care.

■ Pilot

All three initiatives recognized the importance of a small-scale pilot to identify and resolve implementation challenges. Collaborations with CHI and the training of providers was a critical first step. Initially the Netherlands and the Malawi and Tanzania initiatives sent a small number of key people to a CHI training in the United States (Figure 12.4). They then worked within their own country setting to begin the preparation for implementation. These three countries had training conducted by experienced trainers affiliated with CHI (along with a translator). The Netherlands initiative consulted with CHI as they translated and adapted materials. The Malawi and Tanzania initiative included an experienced CenteringPregnancy trainer and provider (see profile for Dr. Carrie

Netherlands

Centering Pregnancy started in three independent midwifery practices with a built-in planning for sustainability by establishing a coordinating committee, training and certification program, regular support meetings, representation from midwifery education, professional organization, and researchers and wide publicity to spread the concepts to policy makers.

Malawi & Tanzania

Pretested by session, then conducted full-scale pilots at two rural sites in Malawi and a large urban site in Tanzania.

Nepal

Multisite pilot for a shortened duration, first 6 months. Process evaluation reviewed afterwards required several modifications to the model before going forward.

FIGURE 12.4 Pilot data are necessary to make sure that the program fits well within the current system and provides an opportunity to make adjustments before implementing at a larger scale.

Klima in Chapter 8) who was heavily involved in session adaptations. The Nepal initiative had conversations with CHI but no formal collaboration and their training was conducted by Dr. Maru, who had a major role in the initiation and its evaluation but no prior experience offering CenteringPregnancy-based group ANC.

All three sites evaluated the pilot. All found that both women and providers enthusiastically embraced the group ANC model, as illustrated by sample quotes from mothers and providers in all three countries (Figure 12.5).

The Nepal initiative conducted only a process evaluation and addressed problems in the expansion stage. One change included reducing the scope of the "talking circles" to just creating plans for facility birth. Their most challenging problem was the lack of congruence between group visits and a program that encouraged ANC attendance with incentive to both women and clinics when women attended ANC at the designated week's gestation. The common group meeting for 12 women was often outside the designated range. After failed negotiation, the Nepal program moved to group ANC on designated days, allowing women to attend the group that met the requirements to receive their incentives. They recognize that this violates one of the essential elements of CenteringPregnancy, that group membership is stable over time. Future evaluation will consider the impact of this change on outcomes. Another substantive change was

Netherlands

[Centering is] the first of all the trainings I received in 20 years of midwifery that really makes me happy... it will make a difference.

–Midwife

Tell me and I forget, teach me and I remember, involve me and I learn.

–Ancient proverb, true for pregnant women

Malawi & Tanzania

[Nurses] know Centering is a better way than what we are usually doing here now...It has an advantage too, because on the days that I do Centering, I don't tire like I do other days. You see, I don't tire because other days, we will measure nearly 40 mothers. Truly, you will tire. For this reason, it is a better way to mothers.

–Midwife, Tanzania

Now that you've given us care this way, you can't take it away!

–Pregnant woman, Malawi

Nepal

When we counsel a women individually, time is not managed very well. We have to keep repeating the same thing to each woman individually and sometimes it is not done so well. In group, it is easier since everyone listens to the session together. They can discuss their concerns and problems with each other. Women who hide their problems and concerns also benefit from these sessions by listening to the discussions. During individual sessions, women might feel uncomfortable to share their problems, but here they are discussed openly.

–Provider

Before, no matter how educated do uneducated we were, we used to feel uncomfortable and shy to talk with people or in front of people. Now, after coming to these sessions and participating in discussions, we have learned to talk as well. Above all, we have learned to talk, and feel comfortable expressing ourselves now.

–Pregnant woman

FIGURE 12.5 Perspectives on experiencing CenteringPregnancy-based group antenatal care.

focusing the "talking circles" solely on creating plans for a facility birth. Other changes included more intensive facilitative leadership training, resulting in higher fidelity to the model.

The Netherlands and the Malawi and Tanzania initiatives both also conducted pilot outcome evaluations. In the Netherlands, a record review of 579 women in CenteringPregnancy, compared to all others in the

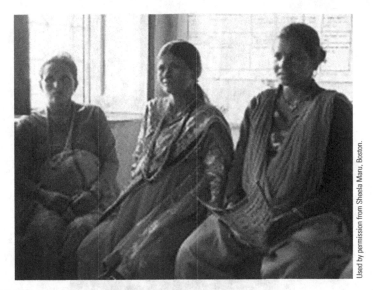

FIGURE 12.6 Woman participating in group session in Nepal.

Used by permission from Sheela Maru, Boston.

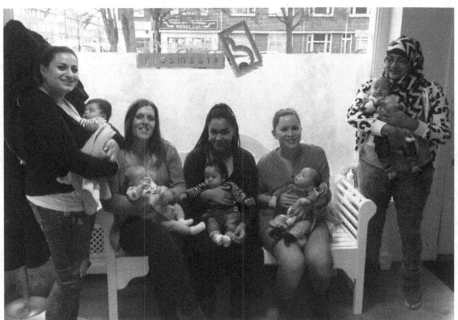

FIGURE 12.7 Netherlands: Women with their new babies.

Used by permission from Marlies Rijnders, Amsterdam.

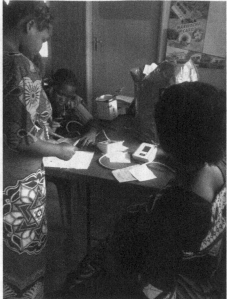

Used with permission from Crystal L. Patil, Chicago.

FIGURE 12.8 Malawi: Pregnant women helping one another conduct self-assessment measures.

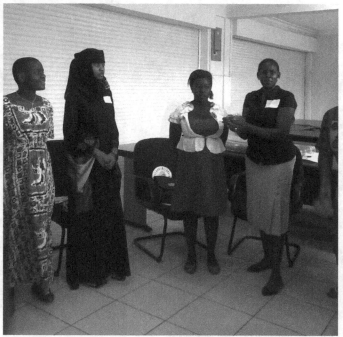

Used with permission from Crystal L. Patil, Chicago.

FIGURE 12.9 Tanzania: Pregnant women participating in a group activity.

same practices, had less augmentation and use of pharmaceutical pain relief among nulliparous women and more breastfeeding. The Malawi and Tanzania pilot was a small randomized clinical trial of 192 women; more favorable outcomes for women in CenteringPregnancy included more ANC and postpartum visit attendance, more HIV and prevention of maternal-to-child transmission (PMTCT) knowledge, less mental distress (depression/anxiety/somatization), and greater pregnancy-related empowerment. Neither pilot found significant differences in adverse maternal and perinatal outcomes. Both found significantly much higher satisfaction among women who received CenteringPregnancy compared to those in standard care.

Expansion

The three initiatives are at very different stages regarding expansion. The Netherlands initiative has experienced substantial expansion in just 3 years; today, almost 47 midwifery practices and five hospitals offer CenteringPregnancy. Three sites also introduced CenteringParenting®, a group care model for mothers and infants. Several developments along the way supported expansion. The coordinating committee has established a process of initial certification and ongoing practice and continuing training to maintain certification. A CenteringPregnancy internship for midwifery students was introduced that both provided very appropriate student co-facilitators at no cost to the practice and engaged students in this innovative model of ANC while they were still learning what "standard practice" is. The major barrier to long-term sustainability is that CenteringPregnancy was and still is not being reimbursed by health insurances or funded in any other way. To justify more adequate reimbursement, the initiative is now examining CenteringPregnancy costs for training and materials, effects, and cost savings due to more optimal outcomes. Funding is needed to cover some of the costs associated with CenteringPregnancy such as training, supervision, and materials. Efforts to obtain standardized payments are underway, along with research on health outcomes and costs and cost savings from averted adverse outcomes.

The Malawi and Tanzania initiative is now publishing pilot results and seeking funding for a large randomized controlled trial that will be powered to identify any significant differences in adverse effects. The urban municipality where the pilot occurred has agreed to host the trial and to later play a leading role in working for national expansion. In Nepal, the initiative has achieved its goal of district-wide expansion. They are engaged in an outcomes evaluation using a prospective nonrandomized controlled trial and continue to use detailed process evaluation to monitor fidelity and quality.

Lessons Learned About Adapting CenteringPregnancy Outside the United States

Initiatives to introduce CenteringPregnancy outside of the United States confirm that this innovative model is robust and adaptable in a variety of contexts. All three settings found ways to accommodate a CenteringPregnancy-based group ANC within the health system. These adapted CenteringPregnancy-based group ANC models were enthusiastically supported by stakeholders. Women and providers strongly agreed that this innovation provided substantial improvement in the quality of care provided to pregnant women. Providers felt more satisfied with their work, and women gained confidence in the health care system and their providers.

Three stages of the implementation process—preparation, pilot, and expansion—were described for each initiative (Barker, Reid, & Schall, 2016; Bergh & Pattinson, 2003; Wandersman, Imm, Chinman, & Kaftarian, 2000). Clearly, envisioning implementation as a process with these distinct stages can be used to guide new global expansion efforts. The preparation stage included engaging stakeholders, adapting CenteringPregnancy sessions to the context, and preparing the setting for implementation. A pilot, limited in scope and/or time, is an opportunity to work out initial difficulties. Process and outcome evaluation during the pilot is critical to provide early evidence of benefits that build enthusiasm for this innovative model. While the expansion stage is more varied, two of the three initiatives can be considered well-established in their new contexts, while the third is actively seeking funding to conduct a definitive study of feasibility and impact of CenteringPregnancy on a larger scale.

As has been found in prior efforts to implement an innovative care model, each of these initiatives had to make adaptations to better fit the unique context. Importantly, they also needed to prepare the clinical setting for the administrative changes needed to support the CenteringPregnancy model. A feature common to each initiative was the close collaboration between practicing providers and researchers, with regular involvement of local and higher level health system administrators and policy persons. Only in Nepal did a major impediment emerge that required compromising one aspect of fidelity: Their group membership was not stable throughout pregnancy, and this was done to make the model feasible and acceptable given the government reimbursement issues that would arise with timing of each visit for individual women. They plan to evaluate the potential for less positive outcomes due to this change. This relatively smooth progress was facilitated by a systematic approach to implementation, with careful attention to balancing fit and fidelity and engaging relevant stakeholders.

These initiatives also provide support for the WHO call to "consider the end at the beginning" (World Health Organization, 2010). The Netherlands initiative especially provides a model for others in developing a supportive infrastructure for long-term sustainability of a health innovation. Their attention to certification and lifelong learning, multisectoral involvement, and disseminating accomplishments are all examples of what Barker, Reid, and Schall (2016) identify as creating a supportive infrastructure.

Evaluation is critical to provide evidence for expanding an innovative ANC model in countries outside the United States. All three initiatives devoted a substantial part of their resources to evaluation of the implementation process and the impacts of CenteringPregnancy-based group ANC. All the initiatives recognized the importance of evaluation to provide justification for expansion. All incorporated extensive evaluation, especially considering the relatively small scope during piloting. In addition to positive acceptance from midwives and women, there were positive health outcomes in both the Netherlands and the Malawi and Tanzania sites. Extensive evaluation in these global examples was possible because of the link between researchers and practitioners throughout the implementation process.

In comparing these three initiatives, the level of country-wide resources did not appear to present a major barrier to implementation. In all three cases, there was widespread receptiveness at policy levels to innovative model of ANC. In the low-resource countries, the challenges of making major improvements to high mortality rates within the existing model were clear to all stakeholders. Awareness of quality gaps in the current system meant that stakeholders were open to innovation and more willing to take chances. CenteringPregnancy-based group ANC was intuitively appealing to those in health care because of its potential to enhance quality of care despite resource limitations. In the Netherlands, readiness to try innovative approaches was galvanized by a national report identifying a performance gap in the existing health system, reflected in higher perinatal mortality than other European countries. The major difference we observed related to resources was that the more developed professional organization in the Netherlands had continuing education programs and established perinatal research efforts. These established organizational structures were important resources that facilitated more rapid implementation and sustainability.

Potential Health System Impacts of Introducing an Innovative Group Care Model

The benefits of introducing CenteringPregnancy-based group ANC go beyond its immediate impacts on ANC and the health of women and children. CenteringPregnancy-based group ANC establishes new provider–client relationships based on collaborative responsibility for health and mutual respect. Experience in this model of care, whether direct or indirect, builds the capacities for reflective practice of all health workers, including administrators, providers, and the lower level workers. Building capacity is especially important for lower level workers. Recent task-shifting initiatives have given lower level workers many new responsibilities. However, training for lower level workers has generally been task-oriented and has not always provide adequate preparation in leadership and vision for these expanded roles (Campbell, Sochas, Cometto, & Matthews, 2016).

Regardless of resource availability, a CenteringPregnancy-based group ANC model has major implications for the movement to enhance quality of care and strengthen health care systems. In low-resource countries, ANC is a substantial portion of all outpatient services, especially where there are high birth rates; therefore, innovations in ANC have the potential to "spill over" to all outpatient services. Women bring their expectations for quality of care from ANC to delivery and postbirth care, and ANC providers often also provide in-patient intrapartum and postpartum care.

Besides the direct impact of group ANC on quality of care, implementing and evaluating a new care model builds the clinic and health system's capacity for health care innovations in all areas of health care. Such an effort is an investment in evidence-based practice to improve quality of care. Innovation provides experiential learning regarding the potential of innovations to improve quality of health care delivery and client outcomes.

Building a Global Community to Support CenteringPregnancy-Based Group ANC

These three initiatives and the many others in early development suggest that the time is right for expanding CenteringPregnancy-based group ANC. Interconnections among various groups attempting to achieve similar goals will foster sharing of lessons learned, facilitating more rapid and less difficult expansion. Ongoing dialogue is needed to identify the best organizational structure to support these efforts. At a minimum, a place like a secure website where implementers can share their experiences and stories has much to offer. Such a platform could also allow sharing of materials like session guides and training workshops and perhaps a set of common evaluation measures that would facilitate cross-national comparisons. An archive of published research articles and presentations would also help advance expansion of the model. There is also a need to develop a network of experienced trainers with international experience. CHI has developed a legal entity, Centering Healthcare Institute International, to provide consultation and training to international sites interested in implementing Centering Healthcare.

It is also important to work with regional and international professional organizations or build on global meeting such as the International Congress of Midwives and/or regional meetings of international groups organizing conferences. These conferences could provide a sponsored workshop, special programs, or other mechanisms to support a group ANC interest group and planned sessions focused on new research. There could also be pre- or postconference workshops that would offer support and guidance for initiatives in the preparation stage regarding engaging stakeholders and adaptation of sessions and regarding evaluation and research for those in the later stages of pilot and expansion.

The successes described in this chapter suggest that CenteringPregnancy-based group ANC is robust and readily transferrable. Reenvisioning of ANC is appropriate in many settings and addresses the persistent QOC issues in ANC. The emphasis on collaborative provider–client relationships based on mutual respect, interactive learning that is more effective, and building on the clients' individual and collective wisdom are all strategies that are relevant for quality improvement efforts across the health care system.

References

Andersson, E. (2014). Group based antenatal care—Expectations, attitudes and experiences from parents' and midwives' perspective. Retrieved from https://openarchive.ki.se/xmlui/bitstream/handle/10616/42005/Thesis_English_Ewa_Andersson.pdf?sequence=5

Andersson, E., Christensson, K., & Hildingsson, I. (2012). Parents' experiences and perceptions of group-based antenatal care in four clinics in Sweden. *Midwifery, 28*(4), 502–508. doi:10.1016/j.midw.2011.07.006

Andersson, E., Christensson, K., & Hildingsson. I. (2013). Mothers' satisfaction with group antenatal care versus individual antenatal care: A clinical trial. *Sexual & Reproductive HealthCare, 4*(3) 113–120. doi:10.1016/j.srhc.2013.08.002

Andersson, E., Christensson, K., & Hildingsson, I. (2014). Swedish midwives' perspectives of antenatal care focusing on group-based antenatal care. *International Journal of Childbirth, 4*(4), 240–249. doi:10.1891/2156-5287.4.4.240

Austin, A., Langer, A., Salam, R. A., Lassi, Z. S., Das, J. K., & Bhutta, Z. A. (2014). Approaches to improve the quality of maternal and newborn health care: An overview of the evidence. *Reproductive Health, 11*(2), 1–9. doi:10.1186/1742-4755-11-S2-S1

Bakken, S., Holzemer, W. L., Brown, M. A., Powell-Cope, G. M., Turner, J. G., Inouye, J., . . . Corless, I. B. (2004). Relationships between perception of engagement with health care provider and demographic characteristics, health status, and adherence to therapeutic regimen in persons with HIV/AIDS. *AIDS Patient Care STDs, 14*(4), 189–197. doi:10.1089/108729100317795

Barker, P. M., Reid, A., & Schall, M. W. (2016). A framework for scaling up health interventions: Lessons from large-scale improvement initiatives in Africa. *Implementation Science, 11*, 1–12. doi:10.1186/s13012-016-0374-x

Bergh, A., & Pattinson, R. C. (2003). Development of a conceptual tool for the implementation of kangaroo mother care. *Acta Paediatrica, 92*(6), 709–714. doi:10.1080/08035250310002399

Bergsjø, P., & Villar, J. (1997). Scientific basis for the content of routine antenatal care. *Acta obstetricia et gynecologica Scandinavica, 76*(1), 15–25. doi:10.3109/00016349709047779

Bhutta, Z. A., Salam, R. A., Lassi, Z. S., Austin, A., & Langer, A. (2014). Approaches to improve quality of care (QoC) for women and newborns: Conclusions, evidence gaps and research priorities. *Reproductive Health, 11*(Suppl. 2), S5. doi:10.1186/1742-4755-11-S2-S5

Campbell, J., Sochas, L., Cometto, G., & Matthews, Z. (2016). Evidence for action on improving the maternal and newborn health workforce: The basis for quality care. *International Journal of Gynecology & Obstetrics, 132*(1), 126–129. doi:10.1016/j.ijgo.2015.11.003

Centering Healthcare Institute. (2016). Centering. Retrieved from http://centeringhealthcare.org

Conrad, P., De Allegri, M., Moses, A., Larsson, E. C., Neuhann, F., Müller, O., & Sarker, M. (2012). Antenatal care services in rural Uganda: Missed opportunities for good-quality care. *Qualitative Health Research, 22*(5), 619–629. doi:10.1177/1049732311431897

Conrad, P., Schmid, G., Tientrebeogo, J., Moses, A., Kirenga, S., Neuhann, F., . . . Sarker, M. (2012). Compliance with focused antenatal care services: Do health workers in rural Burkina Faso, Uganda and Tanzania perform all ANC procedures? *Tropical Medicine & International Health, 17*(3), 300–307. doi:10.1111/j.1365-3156.2011.02923.x

Creanga, A. A., Berg, C. J., Syverson, C., Seed, K., Bruce, F. C., & Callaghan, W. M. (2012). Race, ethnicity, and nativity differentials in pregnancy-related mortality in the United States: 1993–2006. *Obstetrics & Gynecology, 120*(2, Pt. 1), 261–268. Retrieved from http://journals.lww.com/greenjournal/Fulltext/2012/08000/Race,_Ethnicity,_and_Nativity_Differentials_in.11.aspx

Damschroder, L. J., Aron, D. C., Keith, R. E., Kirsh, S. R., Alexander, J. A., & Lowery, J. C. (2009). Fostering implementation of health services research findings into practice: A consolidated framework for advancing implementation science. *Implementation Science, 4*(1), 50. doi:10.1186/1748-5908-4-50

Darmstadt, G. L., Walker, N., Lawn, J. E., Bhutta, Z. A., Haws, R. A., & Cousens, S. (2008). Saving newborn lives in Asia and Africa: Cost and impact of phased scale-up of interventions within the continuum of care. *Health Policy Plan, 23*(2), 101–117. doi:10.1093/heapol/czn001

Deming, W. (1986). *Out of crisis.* Cambridge: Massachusettes Institute of Technology.

Dowswell, T., Carroli, G., Duley, L., Gates, S., Gülmezoglu, A. M., Khan-Neelofur, D., & Piaggio, G. G. (2010). Alternative versus standard packages of antenatal care for low-risk pregnancy. *Cochrane Database of Systematic Reviews, 10*, CD000934.

Gaudion, A. (2010). *The CenteringPregnancy model of group antenatal care: A feasibility study in S E London.* London, England: NHS Foundation Trust. Retrieved from http://fnp.nhs.uk/sites/default/files/contentuploads/cp_kings_gaudion_2010.pdf

Gaudion, A., Bick, D., Menka, Y., Demilew, J., Walton, C., Uiannouzis, K., . . . Rising, S. S. (2011). Adapting the CenteringPregnancy model for a UK feasibility study. *British Journal of Midwifery, 19*(7), 433–438. doi:10.12968/bjom.2011.19.7.433

Ghani, R. M. A. (2015). Perception toward conducting the CenteringPregnancy model in the Egyptian teaching hospitals: A step to improve the quality of antenatal care. *European Journal of Biology and Medical Science Research, 3*(1), 9–18.

Gitlin, L. N. (2013). Introducing a new intervention: An overview of research phases and common challenges. *American Journal of Occupational Therapy, 67*, 177–184. doi:10.5014/ajot.2013.006742

Glasgow, R. E., Vinson, C., Chambers, D., Khoury, M. J., Kaplan, R. M., & Hunter, C. (2012). National Institutes of Health approaches to dissemination and implementation science: Current and future directions. *American Journal of Public Health, 102*(7), 1274–1281. doi:10.2105/AJPH.2012.300755

Howson, C. P., Kinney, M. P., & Lawn, J. E. (2012). *Born too soon: The global action report on preterm birth.* Geneva, Switzerland: March of Dimes, PMNCH, Save the Children, WHO. Retrieved from www.who.int/pmnch/media/news/2012/201204_borntoosoon-report.pdf

Ickovics, J. R., Earnshaw, V., Lewis, J. B., Kershaw, T. S., Magriples, U., Stasko, E., . . . Tobin, J. N. (2016). Cluster randomized controlled trial of group prenatal care: Perinatal outcomes among adolescents in New York City health centers. *American Journal of Public Health, 106*(2), 359–365. doi:10.2105/AJPH.2015.302960

Ickovics, J. R., Kershaw, T. S., Westdahl, C., Magriples, U., Massey, Z., Reynolds, H., & Rising, S. S. (2007). Group prenatal care and perinatal outcomes: A randomized controlled trial. *Obstetrics & Gynecology, 110*(2, Pt. 1), 330–339.

Ickovics, J. R., Reed, E., Magriples, U., Westdahl, C., Rising, S. S, & Kershaw, T. S. (2011). Effects of group prenatal care on psychosocial risk in pregnancy: Results from a randomised controlled trial. *Psychology Health, 26*(2), 235–250. doi: 10.1080/08870446.2011.531577

Institute for Healthcare Improvement. (2003). The breakthrough series: IHI's collaborative model for achieving breakthrough improvement. Retrieved from www .ihi.org/resources/Pages/IHIWhitePapers/TheBreakthroughSeriesIHIsCollaborative ModelforAchievingBreakthroughImprovement.aspx

Jafari, F., Eftekhar, H., Fotouhi, A., Mohammad, K., & Hantoushzadeh, S. (2012). Comparison of maternal and neonatal outcomes of group versus individual prenatal care: A new experience in Iran. *Health Care for Women International, 31*(7), 571–584. doi:10.1080/07399331003646323

Kennedy, H. P., Farrell, T., Paden, R., Hill, S., Jolivet, R. R., Cooper, B. A., & Rising, S. S. (2011). A randomized clinical trial of group prenatal care in two military settings. *Military Medicine, 176*(10), 1169–1177.

Kerber, K. J., de Graft-Johnson, J. E., Bhutta, Z. A., Okong, P., Starrs, A., & Lawn, J. E. (2007). Continuum of care for maternal, newborn, and child health: From slogan to service delivery. *The Lancet, 370*(9595), 1358–1369. doi:10.1016/ S0140-6736(07)61578-5

Klima, C. S. (2003). CenteringPregnancy: A model for pregnant adolescents. *Journal of Midwifery & Women's Health, 48*(3), 220–225. doi:10.1016/ S1526-9523(03)00062-X

Liu, R., Chao, M. T., Jostad-Laswell, A., & Duncan, L. G. (2016, March). Does CenteringPregnancy group prenatal care affect the birth experience of underserved women? A mixed methods analysis. *Journal of Immigrant and Minority Health.* Advance online publication. doi:10.1007/s10903-016-0371-9

Lori, J. R., Munro, M. L., & Chuey, M. R. (2016). Use of a facilitated discussion model for antenatal care to improve communication. *International Journal of Nursing Studies, 54*, 84–94. doi:10.1016/j.ijnurstu.2015.03.018

Magoma, M., Requejo, J., Campbell, O., Cousens, S., & Filippi, V. (2010). High ANC coverage and low skilled attendance in a rural Tanzanian district: A case for implementing a birth plan intervention. *BMC Pregnancy and Childbirth, 10*(1), 13. Retrieved from www.biomedcentral.com/1471-2393/10/13

Magoma, M., Requejo, J., Merialdi, M., Campbell, O., Cousens, S., & Filippi, V. (2011). How much time is available for antenatal care consultations? Assessment of the quality of care in rural Tanzania. *BMC Pregnancy and Childbirth, 11*(1), 64. Retrieved from www.biomedcentral.com/1471-2393/11/640

Maru, S., Harsha, A., & Nirola, I. (2015). Group antenatal care: The power of peers for increasing institutional birth in Achham, Nepal. Retrieved from www .mhtf.org/document/group-antenatal-care-the-power-of-peers-for-increasing -institutional-birth-in-achham-nepal

Massey, Z., Rising, S. S., & Ickovics, J. (2006). CenteringPregnancy group prenatal care: Promoting relationship-centered care. *Journal of Obstetric, Gynecologic, and Neonatal Nursing, 35*(2), 286–294. doi:10.1111/j.1552-6909.2006.00040.x

McDonald, S. D., Sword, W., Eryuzlu, L. E., & Biri, A. B. (2014). A qualitative descriptive study of the group prenatal care experience: Perceptions of women with low-risk pregnancies and their midwives. *BMC Pregnancy and Childbirth, 14,* 334. doi:10.1186/1471-2393-14-334

McNeil, D. A., Vekved, M., Dolan, S. M., Siever, J., Horn, S., & Tough, S. C. (2012). Getting more than they realized they needed: A qualitative study of women's experience of group prenatal care. *BMC Pregnancy and Childbirth, 12*(1), 17. doi:10.1186/1471-2393-12-17

McNeil, D. A., Vekved, M., Dolan, S. M., Sieve, J., Horn, S., & Tough, S. (2013). A qualitative study of the experience of CenteringPregnancy group prenatal care for physicians. *BMC Pregnancy and Childbirth, 13*(Suppl. 1), S6. doi:10.1186/1471-2393-13-S1-S6

McNeill, J. A., & Reiger, K. M. (2014, March). Rethinking prenatal care within a social model of health: An exploratory study in Northern Ireland. *Health Care for Women International, 36*(1), 5–25. Retrieved from www.tandfonline.com/doi/ abs/10.1080/07399332.2014.900061#.VfBZZxFVhBc

Meyers, D. C., Durlak, J. A., & Wandersman, A. (2012). The quality implementation framework: A synthesis of critical steps in the implementation process. *American Journal of Community Psychology, 50*(3/4), 462–480. doi:10.1007/ s10464-012-9522-x

Novick, G., Reid, A. E., Lewis, J., Kershaw, T. S., Ickovics, J. R., & Rising, S. S. (2013). Group prenatal care: Model fidelity and outcomes. *American Journal of Obstetrics & Gynecology, 209*(2), 112.e1–112e6. Retrieved from http://linkinghub.elsevier.com/ retrieve/pii/S0002937813003001

Nyamtema, A., Jong, A., Urassa, D., Hagen, J., & van Roosmalen, J. (2012). The quality of antenatal care in rural Tanzania: What is behind the number of visits? *BMC Pregnancy and Childbirth, 12*(1), 70. doi:10.1186/1471-2393-12-70

Oakley, A. (1981). The origins and development of antenatal care. In M. Enkin & L. Chalmers (Eds.), *Effectiveness and satisfaction in antenatal care* (pp. 1–21). Philadelphia, PA: Lippincott.

The Partnership for Maternal, Newborn & Child Health. (2006). Opportunities for Africa's newborns: Practical data, policy and programmatic support for newborn care in Africa. Retrieved from www.who.int/pmnch/media/publications/ africanewborns/en

The Partnership for Maternal, Newborn & Child Health. (2015). *PMNCH progress report 2015.* Retrieved from www.who.int/pmnch/knowledge/publications/ pmnch_2015_report/en

Patil, C. L., Abrams, E. T., Klima, C., Kaponda, C., Leshabari, S. C., Vonderheid, S. C., . . . Norr, K. F. (2013). CenteringPregnancy-Africa: A pilot of group antenatal care to address Millennium Development Goals. *Midwifery, 29*(10), 1190–1198. doi:10.1016/j.midw.2013.05.008

Rijnders, M., van der Pal, K., & Aalhuizen, I. (2012). CenteringPregnancy® offers pregnant women a central position in Dutch prenatal care [CenteringPregnancy® biedt zwangere centrale rol in Nederlandse verloskundige zorg]. *Tijdschr voor Gezondheidswetenschappen, 90*(8), 513–516.

Roberts, J., Sealy, D., Marshak, H. H., Manda-Taylor, L., Gleason, P., & Mataya, R. (2015). The patient-provider relationship and antenatal care uptake at two referral hospitals in Malawi: A qualitative study. *Malawi Medical Journal, 27*(4), 145–150. doi:10.4314/mmj.v27i4.6

Robinson, J. H., Callister, L. C., Berry, J. A., & Dearing, K. A. (2008). Patient-centered care and adherence: Definitions and applications to improve outcomes. *Journal of the American Academy of Nurse Practitioners, 20*(12), 600–607. doi:10.1111/j.1745-7599.2008.00360.x

Rogers, E. M. (1976). New product adoption and diffusion. *Journal of Consumer Research, 2*(4), 290–301. Retrieved from www.jstor.org/stable/2488658

Sachs, J. D. (2012). From millennium development goals to sustainable development goals. *Lancet, 379*(9832), 2206–2211. doi:10.1016/S0140-6736(12)60685-0

Sarker, M., Schmid, G., Larsson, E., Kirenga, S., De Allegri, M., Neuhann, F., . . . Müller, O. (2010). Quality of antenatal care in rural southern Tanzania: A reality check. *BMC Research Notes, 3*(1), 209. Retrieved from www.biomedcentral.com/1756-0500/3/209

Schneider, J., Kaplan, S. H., Greenfield, S., Li, W., & Wilson, I. B. (2004). Better physician-patient relationships are associated with higher reported adherence to antiretroviral therapy in patients with HIV infection. *Journal of General Internal Medicine, 19*(11), 1096–1103. doi:10.1111/j.1525-1497.2004.30418.x

Stewart, M., Brown, J. B., Donner, A., McWhinney, I. R., Oates, J., Weston, W., & Jordan, J. (2000). The impact of patient-centered care on outcomes. *The Journal of Family Practice, 49*(9), 796–804. Retrieved from www.ncbi.nlm.nih.gov/pubmed/11032203

Tandon, S. D., Colon, L., Vega, P., Murphy, J., & Alonso, A. (2012). Birth outcomes associated with receipt of group prenatal care among low-income Hispanic women. *Journal of Midwifery & Women's Health, 57*(5), 476–481. doi:10.1111/j.1542-2011.2012.00184.x

Teate, A., Leap, N., Rising, S. S., & Homer C. S. E. (2011). Women's experiences of group antenatal care in Australia: The CenteringPregnancy pilot study. *Midwifery, 27*(2), 138–145. Retrieved from www.sciencedirect.com/science/article/pii/S026661380900028X

Tetui, M., Ekirapa, E. K., Bua, J., Mutebi, A., Tweheyo, R., & Waiswa, P. (2012). Quality of antenatal care services in eastern Uganda: Implications for interventions. *The Pan African Medical Journal, 13*, 27. Retrieved from www.pubmedcentral.nih.gov/articlerender.fcgi?artid=3527020&tool=pmcentrez&rendertype=abstract

Tunçalp, Ö., Were, W. M., MacLennan, C, Oladapo, O. T., Gülmezoglu, A. M., Bahl, R., . . . Bustreo, F. (2015). Quality of care for pregnant women and newborns: The WHO vision. *BJOG: An International Journal of Obstetrics & Gynaecology, 122*(8), 1045–1049. doi:10.1111/1471-0528.13451

Villar, J., Ba'aqeel, H., Piaggio, G., Lumbiganon, P., Miguel Belizán, J., Farnot, U., Al-Mazrou, Y., . . . Garcia, J. (2001). WHO antenatal care randomised trial for the evaluation of a new model of routine antenatal care. *The Lancet, 357*(9268), 1551–1564. doi:10.1016/S0140-6736(00)04722-X

von Both, C., Flessa, S., Makuwani, A., Mpembeni, R., & Jahn, A. (2006). How much time do health services spend on antenatal care? Implications for the introduction of the focused antenatal care model in Tanzania. *BMC Pregnancy and Childbirth, 6*, 22. Retrieved from http://ukpmc.ac.uk/abstract/MED/16796749

Wandersman, A., Imm, P., Chinman, M., & Kaftarian, S. (2000). Getting to outcomes: A results-based approach to accountability. *Evaluation and Program Planning, 23*(3), 389–395. doi:10.1016/S0149-7189(00)00028-8

World Health Organization. (2010). Nine steps for developing a scaling-up strategy. Retrieved from www.who.int/reproductivehealth/publications/strategic_approach/9789241500319/en

World Health Organization. (2011a). Beginning with the end in mind: Planning pilot projects and other programmatic research for successful scaling up. Retrieved from www.who.int/reproductivehealth/publications/strategic_approach/9789241502320/en

World Health Organization. (2011b). Fact file on health inequities. Retrieved from www.who.int/sdhconference/background/news/facts/en

13 Moving Forward Into the Mainstream

The small group is the bridge between our own individual existence and the larger community—(Block, 2008, p. 95)

As human beings, we are meant to be in conversation with one another. In circles, we share our stories, surface solutions to our challenges, and form bonds of strength that guide us as we continue our lives.

In this book, we explore a model of care that is revolutionary because it is counterintuitive to the accepted individual care model found in almost all of today's health settings. The journey has involved over 20 years of experience with CenteringPregnancy® sites in almost every state with growing international activity. Affirmations for giving and receiving care through Centering circles continue to be expressed by most everyone exposed to this powerful model. So, how do we move what is widely recognized as a viable alternative model of group care into the mainstream so as to become the "this is the way we do care" model?

This final chapter explores issues raised in previous chapters from the perspective of how to integrate Centering Healthcare™ into the dialogue of health care reform.

In their book, *Unraveled: Prescriptions to Repair a Broken Health Care System*, Weeks and Weinstein declare:

> We have incredible technology and have made major strides in applying that technology. Providing high quality care is so much more . . . understanding the whole patient, his or her values, environment, wants and needs. (2016, p. 4)

Weeks and Weinstein go on to urge a consumer-oriented health system calling on providers and consumers to drive an "industrial revolution" in health care.

As we begin our discussion in this chapter, we urge readers to move from the frozen spot of *now* firmly engrained in us, to focus on what is about to emerge. To unfreeze our perception of what is and what is to come, we need to slow down and open up to new thoughts and insights that may be there, ready for our acknowledgment. In *Theory U*, which explores processes of organizational change, this level of paying attention is called *presencing,* where there is heightened awareness and connection (Scharmer & Kaufer, 2013).

You might consider asking yourself: What do you think will happen with health care over the next 10 to 20 years? What can you do right now to make a difference that may lead to a new emerging future for you and your community? Our hope is that the model described in this book will help to shape that emerging future.

The New 10 Rules for Redesign

We have referenced, in this book, the seminal Institute of Medicine work, *Crossing the Quality Chasm*, published in 2001, which outlined both aims and rules for system redesign. In that document, one of the six aims is the core need for health care to be patient centered, which is defined as "providing care that is respectful and responsive to individual patient preferences, needs, and values, and ensuring that patient values guide all clinical decisions" (Institute of Medicine, 2013). In traditional short visits, the aim of customizing care is to ensure that the patient's values guide all clinical decisions, which seems like an impossible task. CenteringPregnancy provides a setting that encourages discussion of these individual needs within an atmosphere of respect for differences. This nurturing environment surfaces opportunities for relationship-centered care leading to growth for both the clinicians and the women.

In 2016, the Institute of Healthcare Improvement (IHI) published an update, *10 New Rules to Accelerate Healthcare Redesign,* recognizing that it has been well over 10 years since the first rules were published and still there is need for health care redesign. As the 2016 publication says, "The 10 new rules provide ambitious leaders in healthcare with much needed fuel to take a leap. After all, you can't cross a chasm with a few small steps" (Loehrer, Feeley, & Berwick, 2015).

In Table 13.1, we have taken these 10 new rules and matched them to some of the basic elements of the Centering model.

TABLE 13.1   10 New Rules to Accelerate Health Care Redesign and Centering Care Model Design

10 New Rules	Centering Model Design
Change the balance of power	✓ Patients and clinicians are centered in relationship ✓ Skilled facilitation supports the process
Standardize what makes sense	✓ Educational content allows emphasis to vary with group needs ✓ Care, interactive learning, and community building all happen in the group space
Customize to the individual	✓ Educational content allows emphasis to vary with group needs ✓ Facilitative leadership encourages exploration of cultural values
Promote well-being	✓ Participants share their own knowledge and experience ✓ Participants are involved in self-care activities
Create joy in work	✓ Clinician satisfaction documented to bring joy ✓ Participant satisfaction is contagious
Make it easy	✓ Group process promotes trust and openness ✓ Making group care the standard of care maximizes routines
Move knowledge, not people	✓ Participants have access to and track their own health information ✓ Services needed are brought to the group space
Collaborate and cooperate	✓ Interdisciplinary collaboration is fostered ✓ Steering committee guides internal and external processes

(continued)

TABLE 13.1   10 New Rules to Accelerate Health Care Redesign and Centering Care Model Design (*continued*)

10 New Rules	Centering Model Design
Assume abundance	✓ Health assessment occurs in the group space ✓ Group process promotes trust and openness ✓ Patients share resources with other group members
Return the money	✓ Evaluation of outcomes reinforces multi-level savings for reinvestment in community health care

From Loehrer, Feeley, and Berwick (2015). Centering elements contributed by Sharon Schindler Rising.

Table 13.1, showing the 10 new rules and supporting elements of the Centering Healthcare model, provides clinicians and leaders with assurance that the Centering group model is in alignment with broader efforts to redesign care. Following are some specific ways that four of these rules are applied in the Centering Healthcare model:

- *Change the balance of power:* Providers intent on change should be at the table in board rooms, design rooms, and financial planning boards; they need to talk to funders, researchers, and auxiliary groups. They need to be in any arena where decisions are made about space, funding materials, advertising programs, or social network platforms. If we believe that change is essential, we owe this commitment to be present to change the balance of power to ourselves and to those for whom we care. Maternal and child health advocates have politely waited in line to accept whatever crumbs are left; such waiting is no longer acceptable.

  In Centering Healthcare groups, the power balance is shared by the clinician/facilitator and the persons in each group cohort. Facilitation skills demand attentive listening and remembering that: It doesn't matter what we don't talk about; we are talking about what matters to the group.

- *Promote well-being:* This book offers examples of creative approaches to well-being such as teen mothers eating more nutritious foods, acknowledging they have learned to love spinach; a young woman and a grandfather struggling with their diagnoses of diabetes, but learning in a group that they are not alone and, like others, that they can learn to manage. We have included compelling stories of families and providers who lived and worked with painful diagnoses about their infants and leaned on each other for support in ways that opened their hearts and helped them grow through these tragedies.

- *Create joy in work:* In these pages, we relate stories of how eager new health professionals are ready and wanting to provide quality care, but how quickly their frustrations rise. Several professionals tell about the pain, shock, and disappointment of having no time to hear patients' stories; they tell of working with providers who minimize the trauma inherent in their roles as clinicians, or deny them of opportunity to express the difficulty of the lessons they are learning. When one resident says, "I love this model. The problem is that it's the opposite of what I am being taught," she is expressing frustration over the disconnect she feels. Some clinicians who have worked hard to master the knowledge base are reluctant to relinquish their domain to listen to the women's stories. Yet these same providers face hours of seeing patients when they don't have time to do more than the "belly check and fetal heart tones" and end their workdays tired, frustrated, and disillusioned. They deserve the opportunity to explore new options, receive quality training in the Centering model, and have exposure to colleagues who *have* rekindled their joy at work.

We have talked about the triple aim of better health, better care, and lower cost that has been widely adopted as a way to set and review metrics focused on improvement. We also are encouraged by the work of Bodenheimer and Sinsky on a fourth aim focused on improving the work life of clinicians and staff. The very real burnout experienced by care providers is likely to increase partly due to expectations for availability of the primary care workforce. The joy found by clinicians and staff in their Centering group work relates directly to this aim (Bodenheimer & Sinsky, 2014).

Joy is evident when Centering patients eagerly share their appreciation for not having to wait in crowded waiting rooms and instead, have opportunity to make new friends and have creative learning experiences. *We came at the same time and left at the same time and something happened the whole time we were there.* When partners are included, they also express gratitude for being in Centering groups at this important time of their lives.

- *Assume abundance:* We, as midwives, family nurses and medical practitioners, pediatricians and obstetricians, administrators, and policy makers must learn to question the term "abundance" and how it and other resources are distributed in health care. We have learned that mothers and babies are seldom the priority for funding and space allocation in our high-tech health care institutions. Most often, our requests are the last to be heard. We need adequate space to provide care in a group as opposed to requests for expensive machines and technologies. In fact, we don't need much technology at all to provide Centering Healthcare. We need to remember that we are the advocates for our nation's precious resource: mothers and children.

"For many years, Americans have been dying at younger ages than people in almost all other high-income countries. This disadvantage has been getting worse for three decades, especially among women" (Institute of Medicine, 2013). We have expensive drugs, the latest in technology and equipment, the best trained scientists in the world, the most expensive care, and yet, and yet.

In the past two decades, money and energy have been poured into increasing access for prenatal care, yet better outcomes have not necessarily been the result. Missing in these developments has been a broader view of the needs of women for health care that addresses a continuum of issues that impact women from pre-conceptional care, obesity, chronic depression, education, and referral when needed for contraception and prevention of disease (Handler & Johnson, 2016).

We need a sense of abundance that comes from stretching our hearts. We need to walk in the shoes of the women we serve who have no money to pay the next rent, who have no food security, whose situation is complicated by not having grocery stores in their neighborhood, and who, if lucky enough, are working two part-time jobs to make ends meet. We need to act first and worry later. We need to bring ourselves to speak at every meeting in every venue. *We need to stop valuing high volume and start valuing better relationships.*

What does abundance mean in health care today and who brings it to the table? Our mothers in group bring their extra clothes and baby items to share, they sponsor baby showers for themselves, and they bring food to group and proudly share cultural recipes. They provide rides and childcare for one another and grieve with the mother and family experiencing loss. What abundance! "What made for change was communities that believed they had capacities, skills, abilities and could create power when they came together in a community—that is how change happens" (Block & McKnight, 2009). *Let our patients remind us of abundance and show us ways to tap into that energy.*

These new rules for the acceleration of health care design should give us the courage to be strong advocates for a disruptive design for giving and receiving health care, precisely what is found in the Centering Healthcare model.

Life Course

In an editorial titled "Toward a National Strategy on Infant Mortality," Lu and Johnson remind the health community, "each stage of life is influenced by all the life stages that precede it, and it, in turn, influences all the life stages that follow it" (2014, p. S13).

The potential for empowerment and growth found in CenteringPregnancy raises these important questions: Would our outcomes be different/better if we used life course theory to ground our practice, research, and relationships within and outside of the health care setting? What would happen if the majority of our care in life happened in groups?

Imagine more settings like the Mama Cares groups at Children's Hospital of Philadelphia (CHOP) where women carrying babies with major defects talk together and families are welcome to be present, including at the time of birth. Such a program exemplifies caring for an entire family in ways that could have profound effects on the psychological life course of the adults and the children. The Healing Circle for staff at CHOP provides an extraordinary opportunity for all of the staff to share together deeply about their own experience with providing this amount of caring day after day. The Centering-like circle is a unique time for intimate reflection. This group sharing could make the difference in the ability of each person to continue the intense, personal work with grieving families, again affecting the life course of everyone involved. (See Chapter 8 for more details.)

Some years ago Rising developed Lifecycle Components of Women's Health Care, a model for exploring components across the life cycle affecting women from their time as young girls to old age. The components included sexuality, exercise, nutrition, substance abuse, safety, self-esteem, mental health, and interpersonal relations.

Each of these components is present throughout women's lives but may manifest differently at different times. For example, young girls work

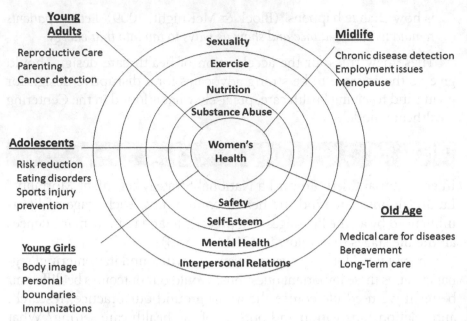

FIGURE 13.1 Lifecycle Components of Women's Health Care model.
Source: Sharon Schindler Rising.

on personal boundaries, adolescents on risk reduction, young women on reproductive issues, midlife "travelers" on menopause, and older age on physical challenges or bereavement. Time spent in Centering circles, 20 to 40 years before some of these important life components, can yield tremendous benefits for group members as life goes on—the benefit of listening and responding in wisdom and empathy to one's children, family members, and oneself or each other as life unfolds.

Misae Vela Brohl, a nurse practitioner in Denver, tells of her experiences with her CenteringParenting® groups, some of which still are meeting yearly for their care and that of their growing children now 8 and 9 years old. Referencing one group, she says, "They have become a community . . . they are friends and their children are friends. They look forward to getting together . . . this is their support group." It is possible to imagine the positive effect this long-term group experience is having on both the mothers' and children's ability to navigate the societal challenges concerning parents today.

Healthy People 2020, in addressing the social determinants of health (SDOH), has set a goal to "create social and physical environments that promote good health for all" (Office of Disease Prevention and Health

Promotion, 2016). The five key areas/determinants are: (a) economic stability, (b) education, (c) social and community context, (d) health and health care, and (e) neighborhood and environment. Screening for these SDOH during the prenatal period will surface individual needs and more broadly, those of the agency's population. By working to establish policies that positively influence these conditions, including those that encourage changes in individual behavior, it is possible to improve health for large numbers of people. These changes can be sustained over time leading to a healthier community for living, learning, working, and playing.

A powerful movement referenced by Thurow's *The First 1,000 Days*, is working worldwide to provide enhanced nutrition to women, babies, and children during this critical time of development. "What happens in those 1,000 days through pregnancy to the second birthday determines to a large extent the course of a child's life—his or her ability to grow, learn, work, and succeed" (2016, p. 7). The impact of poor nutrition early in life has lasting effects that can transcend generations. Women who grow up malnourished often birth girls who are low birth weight and who may grow up to be malnourished mothers. Many of these babies are born preterm or have low birth weight and become one of every four children in the world who is stunted. Strategies include a strong effort to increase breastfeeding and to enrich agricultural products with micronutrients. Evidence shows that with this focus on nutrition, more than 1 million lives can be saved and that individuals, communities, and countries can all be helped to rise out of poverty. This work is a fit for CenteringPregnancy and Parenting groups worldwide as they emphasize good nutrition, group support, and behavioral change.

Making successful, sustainable change requires that all members of the community look for ways to collaborate, and for most this will mean outside of the usual work areas. Perhaps one way to say this is that all members of the community need to be "present" to the issues affecting the population, looking for ways to bring personal and professional assets to the table. In one inspired implementation project, in an inner-city school in Washington, DC, the principal, David Palank, introduced Dialogue Circles, "Conversations in which participants make a conscious attempt to suspend their assumptions . . . and focus on individual and group learning" (Plank, 2015). As principal, he used the dialogue circle method and found it was a powerful tool for increasing generosity, trust, social connection, and cooperation among students

Circles and Listening

Across the country, our children are experiencing toxic stress and increased family neglect, leading to poor educational and social outcomes. More and more children are in state custody. In Vermont, the rate for custodial care for the youngest and most vulnerable children, ages 0 to 5, more than doubled between 2014 and 2016 (Vermont Agency of Education & Human Services, 2016).

That means the social determinants for these families have been stressed to the breaking point. Decades of research support what we see: babies and young children who suffer early childhood traumas are more likely to be sick, to do poorly in school, and to develop behavioral problems in early grades. Unfortunately these children often are caught in interpersonal violence, drop out of school, and are incarcerated by the age of 17 (Centers for Disease Control and Prevention, 2016). The Centering models are designed to help young mothers learn skills, ask questions, and support decisions that begin to empower them to care for themselves and their children in positive and productive ways.

■ Benefits for Teens

The first evaluation study of a teen CenteringPregnancy model occurred at Barnes Jewish Hospital in St. Louis and was published in 2004. Outcomes included better attendance for prenatal and postpartum visits, improved health outcomes, and increased satisfaction of care when compared to teens in traditional care (Grady & Bloom, 2004). Trotman and other researchers in their study of adolescents also confirm better attendance, more appropriate weight gain, and increased commitment to breastfeeding. Of significance, there also was an increase in use of long-acting reversible contraception and decreased incidence of depression (Trotman et al., 2015).

What is also needed to protect the health and well-being of our young people is to provide food security, safe neighborhoods, excellent schools, gun safety, and restorative justice programs to prevent and reduce incarceration. In short, it means that now is the time for communities to be receiving the help they need. John Santelli, MD, chair of the Heilbrunn Department of Population and Family Health in the Columbia University Mailman School of Public Health, New York, New York, makes an eloquent case for this investment:

From a life course perspective, adolescents stand at the cross roads of the major challenges to global health: HIV/AIDS, intentional and unintentional injuries, sexual and reproductive health, and chronic disease. Investments in adolescent health have the potential to alter the future course of global health.

Why Do Centering Circles of Care Work?

We have opportunities to listen to stories in individual care, but the setting and time constraints make deep listening difficult.

More and more we are learning about the importance of stories, of listening and hearing and honoring the lives of those we care for. David Isay, the founder of Story Corps, tells us, "The soul is contained in the human voice" (2016). The act of being listened to can be revolutionary in people's lives. Structuring an environment where each person can be heard and find his or her own voice provides a safe space for exploring each life and learning from one other. Such experiences can show each person how to live a better, more empowered life. There is growing interest in listening to the stories patients tell, such as in the Narrative Medicine Program of Columbia University, developed by Rita Charon, MD (Narrative Medicine Master of Science, Columbia University School of Professional Studies, 2016). This program brings together people from multiple disciplines to learn how health care is perceived by those who receive it, with tellers of stories ranging from speakers on racial disparity to those dealing with death and dying.

From 2005 to 2009, the Collaborative for Development Action (CDA) conducted a Collaborative Learning Project to listen to the voices of people in the countries receiving international assistance. Conversations were conducted with a broad cross-section of people from local workers to government ministers. Many people commented on how thankful they were just to be listened to in a way that reinforced the value of their ideas and judgments. This act of listening brought about "a fundamental shift in the relationship between the aid providers with aid recipients" (Anderson, Brown, & Jean, 2012, p. 146).

Stories and narratives can provide more insights for clinicians and researchers to understand the context of the patients' lives and struggles. Woolf's investigators are working to develop guidelines for gathering stories and a methodology for determining the stories' importance in clinical decision making (Woolf, Zimmerman, Haley, & Krist, 2016). This nascent movement toward the integration of narrative bodes well for CenteringPregnancy, where the premise of each group session is the importance of hearing each woman's story as she shares it as part of the group process.

Providers are in need of the same kinds of sacred spaces—spaces where they might identify the ways their training obliterated or damaged their desire to heal themselves as they cared for others. Dr. Rachel Remen has developed a curriculum for medical students, "The Healers' Art, Because Medicine is an Act of Love," which is now offered at more than 70 medical schools (The Remen Institute for the Study of Health and Illness, Wright State University Boonshoft School of Medicine, 2016). The goal of Remen's and other programs is to give medical students the opportunity to explore how to keep themselves well as they care for others.

Patients mine narratives from family members, friends, and the media when making health decisions in exam rooms, hospital rooms, and living rooms. (Dohan et al., 2016, p. 720)

 "My friend called me and said that her clinician was encouraging her to have an induction of labor and she wasn't sure that was a good idea. So I asked her, 'What does your group say?' She responded, 'What group?'"

Human contact, such as smiling, making eye contact, and telling stories has, by these simple acts, the capacity to encourage people to work together. In *The Moral Molecule*, Paul J. Zak describes research which demonstrated that oxytocin, the hormone far more familiar as the agent responsible for the onset of labor or the release of milk in the nursing mother, can also be released by self-disclosure, an effect that is magnified by trust (2013a). This effect of oxytocin also makes the listener more inclined to trust. Zak's experiments indicated that when individuals viewed an emotional story, they released oxytocin, making them more likely to donate earnings they were receiving from the experiment itself. "What we know is that oxytocin makes us more sensitive to social cues around us. In many situations, social cues motivate us to engage to help others, particularly if the other person seems to need our help" (2013b). It begins to explain, then, the dynamic we have reported so frequently in this book: listening to another's stories moves members of the group to reach out with support and understanding.

> Researchers who are working to understand the importance of listening, hearing, quantifying the data from the narrative, have said it well, "Although numbers are powerful, stories trump numbers, and relationships trump stories."—(Elwyn, Frosch, Volandes, Edwards, & Montori, 2010, p. 706)

Achieving Sustainability

There is considerable discussion in this book about the challenges of implementing a new model that is totally disruptive to the established system justified by, "We have always done it this way." What is understood even less well is how to achieve sustainability, or the step after initiation, and the steps after that.

In the early days of watching and evaluating the effects of Centering on health outcomes and also the effect of Centering on systems, we suggested in our training workshops, "Just set this up as a pilot program." This was a fine way to start with a new care model that still needed data for us to understand the challenges as well as the health outcomes. As more and more data arrived, it was clear that the model did lead to more satisfied patients and clinicians and better health outcomes and that it would need system resources for support. So then we said, "Establishing Centering as a pilot is like a bubble on the top of the system. What happens to bubbles?" Quickly people understood that to be successful, Centering needed to get into the mainstream of health care delivery.

A book that speaks to the need for sustainability is Stephen Lundin's, *Fish! Sticks* (Lundin, Christensen, & Paul, 2003). Lundin wrote several books based on his experience with the innovation he witnessed at the Pike Street Fish Market in Seattle where a culture of fun and excitement pervaded the air, causing spontaneous energy to erupt. It is impossible to be passive when a big fish that you've ordered is being thrown to you! *Fish! Sticks* is focused on getting change infused into the fabric of the institution. It then becomes simply the way things are done.

The efforts for sustainability need to happen even before implementation of the model. There may be initial grant funding, but a line item needs to be established that will ensure funding after the grant period ends. The steering committee's oversight will help to encourage continued buy-in across the agency. Patient members of this committee will be helpful in assessing the success of marketing and suggesting new strategies to enhance patient enrollment in groups. A plan for periodic training in group facilitation for new staff and opportunities for seasoned facilitators to improve their skills will help to ensure sustainability and continued satisfaction of staff and patients with the model. Disrupting the current care model is hard work. Make sure your new model will last by planning ahead for sustainability.

Heading Into the Mainstream: What Do We Still Need To Know?

Investing in prenatal care research must be part of the comprehensive prenatal care agenda. (Handler & Johnson, 2016)

"We know that it works but we're not sure why it works" is frequently heard to describe our experience with providing care in Centering groups. Researchers, clinicians, and policy makers continue to look for answers; Centering sites are expected to collect at least a minimal data set. While it makes sense that providing care in Centering groups will lead to increased satisfaction of patients and staff, it doesn't make sense to many clinicians that sitting in a group and listening will lead to a reduction in preterm birth, even though there is evidence that it does!

As we head into the mainstream, it is clear that more support in terms of research and hard evidence is needed to show that providing health care in circles makes for better outcomes. There is a continuing need for proof that providing care in circles where participants are heavily involved in gathering their own health data, setting personal goals, and sharing with each other around important life issues will actually be more beneficial than the current, short, individual visits with additional monitoring of the mother and fetus. True randomized trials are difficult, especially when patient choice should be considered. As group care benefits become more widely acknowledged and people experiencing care in groups share the benefits with their friends, it will be harder and harder to truly randomize.

Data continue to support several outcomes: reduction in preterm birth, increased breastfeeding (both initiation and continuation), increased uptake and use of efficacious family planning methods, and longer spacing between pregnancies. In addition, there is a better attendance at group visits, and group members report stronger support networks and more success at reaching personal weight goals, and greater satisfaction with care. Data from cost studies also is showing promising reductions in cost for group care. We are curious about what makes groups work, why outcomes are better, and what we can learn to make this model even more effective with greater uptake. A recent article titled, "Group Prenatal Care: Has Its Time Come? asks many of the key questions (Picklesimer, Heberlein, & Covington-Kolb, 2015).

Future Research Questions

We have grouped a collection of research questions under several headings: community focused, characteristics of excellence, life course benefits, health outcomes, and institutional benefits. And we have followed this with a discussion of qualitative themes that have emerged from several of the publications on the Centering model.

Community Focused

- How does the community building that happens in groups affect the community? Are group participants more involved in issues in their community that affect wellness and the social determinants of health?
- How are community-based services such as Healthy Start, Head Start, home visiting, and legal aid articulating with Centering groups to strengthen impact?

Characteristics of Excellence

- How many Centering groups have members who continue contact after their group care involvement has ceased and are there measureable outcomes from those that continue?
- What are the major factors at the site level that indicate potential for successful implementation?
- What are the characteristics of Centering sites that have achieved model sustainability?
- What processes internationally are related to successful implementation of Centering or CenteringPregnancy-based ANC?

Life Course Benefits

- What are the long-term effects on family nutrition when mothers have been involved in Centering groups? Is there a reduction in obesity, especially in the children?
- What are the measureable mother/baby/family outcomes in a longitudinal study starting with CenteringPregnancy and following through at least 2 years of CenteringParenting?
- What cultural issues are most relevant to group facilitation and how does culturally sensitive care in groups affect the participants?
- How do Centering groups fit into the life course theory and efforts to address maternal child health disparities?

Health Outcomes

- What is the effect of participation in Centering groups on stress hormones and is there a relation to preterm birth?
- Does participation in Centering groups serve as a mediator for depression?
- In a large multisite study, does the preterm effect hold and are there other outcomes we have yet to study?
- What are the differences in outcomes when dads are involved in groups?

Institutional Benefits

- What are the benefits and challenges of mother–baby dyad care for the dyad, the system, and the clinicians, and are these challenges worth the benefits?
- Do staff involved with Centering groups experience more job satisfaction and longevity at the site? Is there a measureable effect on the workforce?
- Do students and residents exposed to providing care in Centering groups transfer that experience to individual care and to subsequent professional work?
- What is the cost benefit of Centering care to the site, the providers, the larger system, and the insurers?
- What are the longitudinal benefits, such as reduced chronic care issues and increased family stability, that might be measured?

Qualitative Data: Themes

Then there are themes that have surfaced from the qualitative studies looking at physicians, midwives, and women's responses to Centering care (Baldwin & Phillips, 2011; Herrman, Rogers, & Ehrenthal, 2012; McDonald, Sword, Eryuzlu, & Biringer, 2014; McNeil et al., 2012; McNeil, Vekved, Siever, Horn, & Tough, 2013; Novick, 2009). Some of these themes are:

- Knowledge is power: Women access information and use it with more confidence.
- Connecting and not feeling alone: Continuity with the clinician and with the same group leads to feelings of safety and support.
- Supporting each other: Women often reach out to others in the group and provide support through offering rides, sharing extra clothing or baby items, providing needed childcare, supporting another during labor, and so on.
- Respect: Women find they can share some of their most personal concerns with others who listen without bias and in an atmosphere of confidentiality.
- Reassurance: The comments, "I'm not the only one going through this" or "Someone would raise an issue that I had but was too embarrassed to ask," speak to the power of the circle.
- Taking ownership of care: Women understand their health data and ask for test results. The discussions focus on what matters to them and result in confidence in their decisions. They learn what they should worry about and make appropriate calls for help.
- Getting more in one place at one time, fun: Women and clinicians laugh together, hold hands, give each other affirmations. All the care components happen in the group space.
- "I'm a better mother . . . I'm a better clinician." All group participants seem to gain confidence, skills, and knowledge. These learnings become embedded in the behavior of the individuals and are seen in communication styles with family members or in interactions in individual care encounters.

While some might consider studies on these themes to be "softer" data, it is impossible to minimize the importance of these feelings of connection and empowerment to overall well-being, health, and joy at work. Many of these themes beg further study.

Most of the needed studies will require significant funding and co-operation among academic institutions, health care facilities, and other agencies. The requirement for indirect costs by each institution makes funding these studies costly and difficult. The military could be one excellent venue for a large group study that could more easily include randomization, possibly done by site rather than within sites and reduce concern about selection bias. Another avenue for collection of large data sets could come through the insurance industry and their claims data.

To maximize the impact of smaller studies, a decision to use particular validated and reliable surveys across studies could lead to confidence in the use of aggregate data. A recent review of group prenatal care studies compared to those from traditional care identified the lack of comparable tools for assessment of many outcomes among the studies to make conclusions difficult (Carter et al., 2016). A group of academic researchers could work with the Centering Healthcare Institute (CHI) to create a repository of suggested tools for use by a variety of researchers. A connection with government institutions such as the Agency for

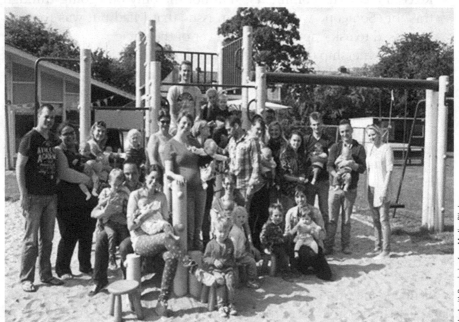

A Centering Group, the Netherlands.

Healthcare Research and Quality (AHRQ) or private groups such as Westat could facilitate the work on these data sets. The CenteringCounts data tool of CHI also could be expanded to collect research data from sites participating in these larger studies. One review of Centering publications concludes: "Building consistent study results across a number of studies is needed and is the essential next step in developing this body of knowledge" (Manant & Dodgson, 2011, p. 101).

Summary: A Call to Action

Our institutions can only offer service—not care. We cannot purchase care. Care is the freely given commitment from the heart of one to another. . . . And it is this care that is the basic power of a community of citizens. . . . Our way is made possible by the power to care. (Block & McKnight, 2009)

We know the downstream/upstream story. We continue to work hard to fix the problems, some that result from the social determinants of health and others that result from poor health choices. One article referenced the *I Love Lucy* episode where Lucy and Ethel have jobs in the candy factory, wrapping the candy. At first it is fun, but as the conveyer belt starts to accelerate they can't keep up. As Lucy starts eating the candy she soon winds up with, "a full mouth, full hands, and candy piling up." She runs out of options. This is much like the downstream story we can relate to in our sites and communities today (Rising, & Senterfitt, 2009).

The work of Rachel Remen and the model for medical student education shared by Amy MacDonald both give us hope. The need for new ways of learning for our interprofessional students is absolute. These models demonstrate hope for new "cracks" in the system that let new light in.

More than a decade ago, pioneering nurse-midwife Vera Keane asked:

Just what makes life "better?" Certainly, good physical health is the most basic component. Centering provides ample opportunities in its construct for participants to check on and learn about their own health status and how to improve it. Centering goes far beyond that. Its structure fosters the personality development and mental health of participants through its nurturing, supportive and confidence-building approach. It is in this arena that Centering is sowing seeds of a revolution that could, over time, help more people to think about and deal with one another in positive ways. (V. Keane, personal correspondence, 2003)

Listening to each other and working together in partnership to make the needed changes in care is essential to bringing forth better care, better health, and lower costs. Verbiest and others call for a "new social movement to create an agenda for women's reproductive health and economic justice that will usher in a new period of health, social, and financial development" (Verbiest, Malin, Drummonds, & Kotelchuck, 2015, p. 741). We can maximize the power of groups by encouraging a focus on racial justice and equity.

The challenges to reform health care are legion and complex. We believe that Centering Healthcare already is responding to this challenge. The process of writing this book brought us into contact with people all across the country: clinicians, patients, administrators. . . . Listening to their stories reinforced for us what we already knew: this is a powerful, renewing way to give and receive care.

What is the question? Centering is the answer.

References

Baldwin, K., & Phillips, G. (2011). Voices along the journey: Midwives' perceptions of implementing the CenteringPregnancy model of prenatal care. *The Journal of Perinatal Education, 20*(4), 210–217.

Block, P. (2008). *Community: The structure of belonging.* San Francisco, CA: Berrett-Koehler.

Block, P., & McKnight, J. (2009). *Community capacities and community necessities.* Opening remarks at the "From Clients to Citizens Forum," Coady International Institute, St. Francis Xavier University, Antigonish, Nova Scotia, Abundant Community. Retrieved from www.abundantcommunity.com/home/getting_started/community_capacities_and_community_neecessities.html

Bodenheimer, T., & Sinsky, C. (2014). From triple to quadruple aim: Care of the patient requires care of the provider. *Annals of Family Medicine, 12*(6), 573–576.

Carter, E., Temming, L., Akin, J., Fowler, S., Macones, G., Colditz, G., & Tuuli, M. (2016). Group prenatal care compared with traditional prenatal care: A systematic review and meta-analysis. *Obstetrics & Gynecology, 128*(3), 551–561.

Centers for Disease Control and Prevention. (2016). Association between aces and negative outcomes, about adverse childhood experiences. Retrieved from http://search.cdc.gov/search?query=Association+Between+ACEs+and+Negative+Outcomes%2C+About+Adverse+Childhood+Experiences.+&utf8=%E2%9C%93&affiliate=cdc-main

Dohan, D., Garrett, S. B., Rendle, K. A., Haley, M., & Abramson, C. (2016). The importance of integrating narrative into health care decision making. *Health Affairs, 35*(4), 720–725. Retrieved from http://content.healthaffairs.org doi10.1377/hitaff.2015.1373

Elwyn, G., Frosch, D., Volandes, A. E., Edwards, A., & Montori, V. M. (2010). Investing in deliberation: A definition and classification of decision support interventions for people facing difficult health decisions. *Medical Decision Making, 30*(6), 701–11.

Grady, M. A., & Bloom, K. C. (2004). Pregnancy outcomes of adolescents enrolled in a CenteringPregnancy program. *Journal of Midwifery & Women's Health, 49*(5), 412–420.

Handler, A., & Johnson, K. (2016). A call to revisit the prenatal period as a focus for action within the reproductive and perinatal care continuum. *Maternal Child Health Journal.* doi:10.1007/s10995-016-2187-6

Herrman, J., Rogers, S., & Ehrenthal, D. (2012). Women's perceptions of CenteringPregnancy: A focus group study. *MCN: The American Journal of Maternal/Child Nursing, 37*(1), 19–26.

Institute of Medicine. (2013, January). U.S. Health in international perspectives: Shorter lives, poorer health. Retrieved from http://nationalacademies.org/hmd/reports/2013/us-health-in-international-perspective-shorter-lives-poorer-health.aspx

Isay, D. (2016, May 12). "Listening as an Act of Love". Interview with Krista Tippett, *On Being.* Retrieved from www.onbeing.org/program/david-isay-listening-as-an-act-of-love/6268

Loehrer, S., Feeley, D., & Berwick, D. (2015). 10 new rules to accelerate healthcare redesign. *Healthcare Executive, 30*(6), 66–69.

Lu, M. C., & Johnson, K. A. (2014). Toward a national strategy on infant mortality. *American Journal of Public Health, 104*(Suppl. 1), S13–S16. doi:10.2105/ajph.2013.301855

Lundin, S., Christensen, J., & Paul, H. (2003). *Fish! Sticks: A remarkable way to adapt to changing times and keep your work.* New York, NY: Hyperion.

Manant, A., & Dodgson, J. (2011). CenteringPregnancy: An integrative literature review. *Journal of Midwifery & Women's Health, 56*(2), 94–102.

McDonald, S., Sword, W., Eryuzlu, L., & Biringer, A. (2014). A qualitative descriptive study of the group prenatal care experience: Perceptions of women with low-risk pregnancies and their midwives. *BMC Pregnancy and Childbirth, 14*(334), 2–12. Retrieved from www.biomedcentral.com/1471-2393/14/334

McNeil, D.A., Vekved, M., Dolan, S.M., Siever, J., Horn, S., & Tough, S. (2012). Getting more than they realized they needed: A qualitative study of women's experience of group prenatal care. *BMC Pregnancy and Childbirth, 12*(17), 1–10. Retrieved from www.biomedcentral.com/1471-2393/12/17

McNeil, D.A., Vekved, M., Dolan, S.A., Siever, J., Horn, S., & Tough, S. (2013). A qualitative study of the experience of CenteringPregnancy group prenatal care for physicians. *BMC Pregnancy and Childbirth, 13*(Suppl. 1), S6. Retrieved from www.biomedcentral.com/1471-2393/13/S1/S6

Narrative Medicine Master of Science, Columbia University School of Professional Studies. (2016). Retrieved from http://sps.columbia.edu/narrative-medicine

Novick, G. (2009). Women's experience of prenatal care care: An integrative review. *Journal of Midwifery & Women's Health, 54*(3), 226–237.

Office of Disease Prevention and Health Promotion. (2016). Healthy People 2020. Retrieved from www.healthypeople.gov/2020/topics-objectives/topic/social-determinants-of-health

Plank, D. (2015). How dialogue circles promote student growth. Retrieved from www.middleweb.com/21429/how-dialogue-circles-promote-student-growth

The Remen Institute for the Study of Health and Illness, Wright State University Boonshoft School of Medicine. (2016). Retrieved from www.rishiprograms.org/category/updates

Rising, S. S., & Senterfitt, C. (2009). Repairing health care: Building relationships through groups. *Creative Nursing, 15*(4), 178–183.

Scharmer, O., & Kaufer, K. (2013). *Leading from the emerging future: From ego-system to eco-system economies.* San Francisco, CA: Berrett-Koehler.

Thurow, R. (2016). *The first 1,000 days: A crucial time for mothers and children—And the world.* New York, NY: Public Affairs.

Trotman, G., Chhatre, G., Darolia, R., Tefera, E., Damle, L., & Gomez-Lobe, V. (2015). The effect of CenteringPregnancy versus traditional prenatal care models on improved adolescent health behaviors in the perinatal period. *Journal of Pediatric & Adolescent Gynecology, 28*(5), 395–401. doi:10.1016/j.jpag.2014.12.003

Verbiest, S., Malin, C., Drummonds, M., & Kotelchuck, M. (2015). Catalyzing a reproductive health and social justice movement. *Maternal and Child Health Journal, 20*(4), 741–748.

Vermont Agency of Education & Human Services. (2016, January). Report to senate committees on education and on health and welfare and the house committees on education and on human services, 6–9. Retrieved from http://education.vermont.gov

Weeks, W., & Weinstein, J. (2016). *Unraveled: Prescriptions to repair a broken health care system.* North Charleston, SC: CreateSpace Independent Publishing Platform.

Woolf, S., Zimmerman, E., Haley, A., & Krist, A. (2016). Authentic engagement of patients and communities can transform research, practice, and policy. *Health Affairs, 35*(4), 590–594. doi:10.1377/hlthaff.2015.1512

Zak, P. (2013a). How stories change the brain. Retrieved from http://greatergood.berkeley.edu/article/item/how_stories_change_brain

Zak, P. (2013b). *The moral molecule: How trust works.* New York, NY: Penguin Group.

Bibliography

Centering Healthcare Quantitative Research

Brumley, J., Cain, A., & Stern, L. J. (2016). Gestational weight gain and breastfeeding outcomes in group prenatal care. *Journal of Midwifery & Women's Health, 61*(5), 557–562.

Carter, E., Temming, L., Akin, J., Fowler, S., Macones, G., Colditz, G., & Tuuli, M. (2016). Group prenatal care compared with traditional prenatal care: A systematic review and meta-analysis. *Obstetrics & Gynecology, 128*(3), 551–561.

Cunnigham, S., Grilo, S., Lewis, J., Novick, G., Rising, S. S., Tobin, J., & Ickovics, J. (2016). Group prenatal care attendance: Determinants and relationship with care satisfaction. *Maternal Child Health Journal.* Advance online publication. doi:10.1007/s10995-016-2161-3

Earnshaw, V. A., Rosenthal, L., Cunningham, S. D., Kershaw, T., Lewis, J., Rising, S. S., Stasko, E., . . . & Ickovics, J. R. (2016). Exploring group composition among young, urban women of color in prenatal care: Implications for satisfaction, engagement, and group attendance. *Women's Health Issues, 26*(1), 110–115. doi:10.1016/j.whi.2015.09.011

Fausett, M., Gill, B., Esplin, M., Shields, A., & Staat, B. (2014). CenteringPregnancy is associated with fewer early, but not overall, preterm deliveries [Oral concurrent session 1]. *American Journal of Obstetrics & Gynecology, 210*(1), S9.

Fenick, A., Gilliam, W., Leventhal, J., Rising, S. S., Gilliam, A., & Rosenthal, M. (2011, April 30–May 3). *Health care utilization in infants receiving group pediatric care.* Abstract presented at Presidential Plenary at Pediatric Academic Society, Denver, CO.

Gareau, S., Lòpez-De Fede, A., Loudermilk, B., Cummings, T., Hardin, J., Picklesimer, A., . . . Covington-Kolb, S. (2016). *Maternal Child Health Journal.* doi:10.1007/s10995-016-1935-y

Gould Rothberg, B., Magriples, U., Kershaw, T., Rising, S., & Ickovics, J. (2011). Gestational weight gain and subsequent postpartum weight loss among young, low-income, ethnic minority women. *American Journal of Obstetrics & Gynecology, 52,* 1–11.

Grady, M. A., & Bloom, K. (2004). Pregnancy outcomes of adolescents enrolled in a CenteringPregnancy program. *Journal of Midwifery & Women's Health, 49*(5), 412–420.

Hackley, B., Applebaum, J., Wilcox, W., & Arevalo, S. (2009). Impact of two scheduling systems on early enrollment in a group prenatal care program. *Journal of Midwifery & Women's Health, 54*(3), 168–175.

Hale, N., Picklesimer, A., Billings, D., & Covington-Kolb, S. (2013). 96: The effect of CenteringPregnancy Group prenatal care on enrollment in the postpartum family planning Medicaid waiver program. *American Journal of Obstetrics & Gynecology, 208*(1), S55.

Hale, N., Picklesimer, A., Billings, D., & Covington-Kolb, S. (2014). The impact of CenteringPregnancy group prenatal care on postpartum family planning. *American Journal of Obstetrics & Gynecology, 210*, 50.e1–50.e7.

Heberlein, E., Frongillo, E., Picklesimer, A., & Covington-Kolb, S. (2016). Effects of group prenatal care on food insecurity during late pregnancy and early postpartum. *Maternal Child Health Journal, 20*(5), 1014–1024.

Heberlein, E., Picklesimer, A., Billings, D., Covington-Kolb, S., Farber, N., & Frongillo, E. (2015). The comparative effects of group prenatal care on psychosocial outcomes. *Archive of Women's Mental Health, 19*(2), 259–269. doi:10.1007/s00737-015-0564-6

Ickovics, J. R., Earnshaw, V., Lewis, J. B., Kershaw, T. S., Magriples, U., Stasko, E., . . . Tobin, J. N. (2015). Cluster randomized controlled trial of group prenatal care: Perinatal outcomes among adolescents in New York City health centers. *American Journal of Public Health*, e1–e7. doi:10.2105/AJPH.2015.302960

Ickovics, J. R., Kershaw, T., Westdahl, C., Magriples, U., Massey, Z., Reynolds, H., & Rising, S. (2007). Group prenatal care and perinatal outcomes: A randomized controlled trial. *Obstetrics & Gynecology, 110*(2, Pt. 1), 330–339.

Ickovics, J. R., Kershaw, T., Westdahl, C., Rising, S. S., Klima, C., Reynolds, H., & Magriples, U. (2003). Group prenatal care and preterm birth weight: Results from a matched cohort study at public clinics. *Obstetrics & Gynecology, 102*(5, Pt. 1), 1051–1057.

Ickovics, J. R., Reed, E., Magriples, U., Westdahl, C., Rising, S. S., & Kershaw, T. S. (2011). Effects of group prenatal care on psychosocial risk in pregnancy: Results from a randomized controlled trial. *Psychological Health, 26*(2), 235–250.

Kennedy, H. P., Farrell, T., Paden, R., Hill, S., Jolivet, R., Cooper, B., & Rising, S. S. (2011). A randomized clinical trial of group prenatal care in two military settings. *Military Medicine, 176*, 1169–1177.

Kershaw, T. S., Magriples, U., Westdahl, C., Rising, S. S., & Ickovics, J. (2009). Pregnancy as a window of opportunity for HIV prevention: Effects of an HIV intervention delivered within prenatal care. *American Journal of Public Health, 99*(11), 2079–2086.

Klima, C., Norr, K., Vonderheid, S., & Handler, A. (2009). Introduction of CenteringPregnancy in a public health clinic. *Journal of Midwifery & Women's Health, 54*(1), 27–34.

Machuca, H., Arevalo, S., Hackley, B., Applebaum, J., Mishkin, A., Heo, M., & Shapiro, A. (2016). Well baby group care: Evaluation of a promising intervention for primary obesity prevention in toddlers. *Childhood Obesity, 12*(3), 171–178. doi:10.1089/chi.2015.0212

Magriples, U., Boynton, M., Kershaw, T., Lewis, J., Rising, S. S., Tobin, J., . . . Ickovics, J. (2015). The impact of group prenatal care on pregnancy and postpartum weight trajectories. *American Journal of Obstetrics & Gynecology, 213,* 688.e1–688.e9.

Magriples, U., Kershaw, T. S., Rising, S. S., Massey, Z., & Ickovics, J. R. (2008). Prenatal health care beyond the obstetrics service: Utilization and predictors of unscheduled care. *American Journal of Obstetrics & Gynecology, 198*(1), 75.e1–75.e7.

Magriples, U., Kershaw, T. S., Rising, S. S., Westdahl, C., & Ickovics, J. R. (2009). The effects of obesity and weight gain in young women on obstetric outcomes. *American Journal of Perinatology, 26*(5), 365–371.

Milan, S., Kershaw, T., Lewis, J., Westdahl, C., Rising, S. S., Patrikios, M., & Ickovics, J. (2007). Caregiving history and prenatal depressive symptoms in low-income adolescents and young adult women: Moderating and mediating effects. *Psychology of Women Quarterly, 31,* 241–251.

Novick, G., Reid, A., Lewis, J., Kershaw, T., Rising, S. S., & Ickovics, J. (2013). Group prenatal care: Model fidelity and outcomes. *American Journal of Obstetrics & Gynecology, 209*(2), 112.e1–112.e6. doi:10.1016/j.ajog.2013.03.026

Picklesimer, A., Billings, D., Hale, J., Blackhurst, D., & Covington-Kolb, S. (2012). The effect of CenteringPregnancy group prenatal care on preterm birth in a low-income population. *American Journal of Obstetrics & Gynecology, 206,* 415.e1–415.e7.

Reid, J. (2007). CenteringPregnancy®: A model for group prenatal care. *Nursing for Women's Health, 11*(4), 384–388.

Schellinger, M. M., Abernathy, M. P., Amerman, B., May, C., Foxlow, L., Carter, A., . . . Haas, D. (2016). Improved outcomes for Hispanic women with gestational diabetes using the CenteringPregnancy® group prenatal care model. *Maternal and Child Health Journal.* Advance online publication. doi:10.1007/s10995-016-2114-x

Shah, N., Fenick, A., & Rosenthal, M. (2016). A healthy weight for toddlers? Two-year follow-up of a randomized controlled trial of group well-childcare. *Clinical Pediatrics.* Advance online publication. doi:10.1177/0009922815623230

Shakespear, K., Waite, P. J., & Gast, J. (2010). A comparison of health behaviors of women in CenteringPregnancy and traditional prenatal care. *Maternal and Child Health Journal, 14,* 202–206.

Skelton, J., Mullins, R., Langston, L. T., Womack, S., Ebersole, J. L., Rising, S. S., & Kovarik, R. (2009). CenteringPregnancy smiles: Implementation of a small group prenatal care model with oral health. *Journal of Health Care for the Poor and Underserved, 20*(2009), 545–553.

Tandon, S. D., Colon, L., Vega, P., Murphy, J., & Alonso, A. (2012). Birth outcomes associated with receipt of group prenatal care among low-income Hispanic women. *Journal of Midwifery & Women's Health, 57*(5), 476–481.

Tanner-Smith, E., Steinka-Fry, K., & Lipsey, M. (2013a). Effects of CenteringPreg-
    nancy group prenatal care on breastfeeding outcomes. *Journal of Midwifery &
    Women's Health, 58*(4), 389–395.
Tanner-Smith, E., Steinka-Fry, K., & Lipsey, M. (2013b). The effects of Centering-
    Pregnancy group prenatal care on gestational age, birth weight, and fetal demise.
    Modern Child Health Journal, 18(4), 801–809. doi:10.1007/s10995-013-1304-z
Tanner-Smith, E., Steinka-Fry, K., & Gesell, S. (2014). Comparative effectiveness
    of group and individual prenatal care on gestational weight gain. *Maternal and
    Child Health Journal, 18,* 1711–1720.
Tarney, C. M., Berry-Caban, C., Jain, R. B., Kelly, M., Sewell, M. F., & Wilson, K. L.
    (2015). Association of spouse deployment on pregnancy outcomes in a U.S.
    military population. *Obstetrics & Gynecology, 126*(3), 569–574. doi:10.1097/
    AOG.0000000000001003
Tilden, E. L., Emeis, C. L., Caughey, A. B., Weinstein, S. R., Futernick, S. B., & Lee,
    C. S. (2016). The influence of group versus individual prenatal care on phase
    of labor at hospital admission. *Journal of Midwifery & Women's Health, 61*(4),
    427–434. doi:10.1111/jmwh.12437
Trotman, G., Chhatre, G., Darolia, R., Tefera, E., Damle, L., & Gomez-Lobo, V.
    (2015). The effect of Centering Pregnancy versus traditional prenatal care
    models on improved adolescent health behaviors in the perinatal period. *Journal
    of Pediatric and Adolescent Gynecology, 28*(5), 395–401. doi:10.1016/j.jpag
    .2014.12.003
Walton, R. B., Shaffer, S., & Heaton, J. (2015). Group prenatal care outcomes in
    a military population: A retrospective cohort study. *Military Medicine, 180*(7),
    825–829. doi:10.7205/MILMED-D-14-00273
Westdahl, C., Milan, S., Magriples, U., Kershaw, T., Rising, S. S., & Ickovics, J. R.
    (2007). Social support and social conflict as predictors of prenatal depression.
    Obstetrics & Gynecology, 110(1), 134–140.
Yoshida, H., Fenick, A., & Rosenthal, M. (2014). Group well-childcare: An analysis
    of cost. *Clinical Pediatrics, 53,* 387–394. doi:10:1177/0009922813512418
Zielinski, R., Stork, L., Deibel, M., Kothari, C. L., & Searing, K. (2014). Improving
    infant and maternal health through CenteringPregnancy: A comparison of ma-
    ternal health indicators and infant outcomes between women receiving group
    versus traditional prenatal care. *Open Journal of Obstetrics & Gynecology, 4*(9),
    497–505. doi:10.4236/ojog.2014.49071

Centering Healthcare Qualitative Research

Baldwin, K. (2006). Comparison of selected outcomes of CenteringPregnancy versus
    traditional prenatal care. *Journal of Midwifery & Women's Health, 51*(4), 266–272.
Baldwin, K., & Phillips, G. (2011). Voices along the journey: Midwives' perceptions
    of implementing the CenteringPregnancy model of prenatal care. *Journal of Peri-
    natal Education, 20,* 4, 210–217.
Barr, W., Aslam, S., & Levin, M. (2011). Evaluation of a group prenatal care-based
    curriculum in a family medicine residency. *Family Medicine, 43*(10), 712–717.

Chao, M., Abercrombie, P., Santana, T., & Duncan, L. (2015). Applying the RE-AIM framework to evaluate integrative medicine group visits among diverse women with chronic pelvic pain. *Pain Management Nursing, 16,* 920–929.

Gareau, S., Fede, A., Loudermilk, B. L., Cummings, T., Hardin, J., Picklesimer, A., . . . Covington-Kolb, S. (2016). Group prenatal care results in Medicaid savings with better outcomes: A propensity score analysis of CenteringPregnancy participation in South Carolina. *Maternal and Child Health Journal, 20,* 1384–1393. doi:10.1007/s10995-016-1935-y

Heberlein, E. C., Picklesimer, A. H., Billings, D. L., Covington-Kolb, S., Farber, N., & Frongillo, E. A. (2016). Qualitative comparison of women's perspectives on the functions and benefits of group and individual prenatal care. *Journal of Midwifery & Women's Health, 61*(2), 224–234. doi:10.1111/jmwh.12379

Herrman, J., Rodgers, S., & Ehrenthal, D. (2012). Women's perceptions of CenteringPregnancy: A focus group study. *American Journal of Maternal/Child Health, 37*(1), 19–27.

Kennedy, H. P., Farrell, T., Paden, R., Hill, S., Jolivet, R., Willetts, J., & Rising, S. S. (2009). "I wasn't alone": A study of group prenatal care in the military. *Journal of Midwifery & Women's Health, 54*(3), 176–183.

Klima, C., Vonderheid, S., Norr, K., & Park, C. (2015). Development of the pregnancy-related empowerment scale. *Nursing and Health, 3*(5), 120–127. doi:10.13189/nh.2015.030503

Little, S., Motohara, S., Miyazaki, K., Arato, N., & Fetters, M. (2013). Prenatal group visit program for a population with limited English proficiency. *Journal of the American Board of Family Medicine, 26*(6), 728–737. doi:10.3122/jabfm.2013.06.130005

Liu, R., Chao, M. T., Jostad-Laswell, A., & Duncan, L. G. (2016). Does CenteringPregnancy group prenatal care affect the birth experience of underserved women? A mixed methods analysis. *Journal of Immigrant and Minority Health,* 1–8. doi:10.1007/s10903-016-0371-9

Mittal, P. (2011). CenteringParenting: Pilot implementation of a group model for teaching family medicine residents well-childcare. *The Permanente Journal, 15*(4), 40–41.

Mooney, S., Russell, M., Prairie, B., Savage, C., & Weeks, W. (2008). Group prenatal care: An analysis of cost. *Journal of Health Care Finance, 34*(4), 31–41.

Novick, G., Sadler, L., Kennedy, H. P., Cohen, S., Groce, N., & Knafl, K. (2010). Women's experience of group prenatal care. *Qualitative Health Research, 21*(1), 97–116.

Novick, G., Sadler, L. S., Knafl, K. A., Groce, N. E., & Kennedy, H. P. (2012). "In a hard spot": Providing group prenatal care in two urban clinics. *Midwifery, 29*(6), 690–697. doi:10.1016/j.midw2012.06.013

Novick, G., Sadler, L., Knafl, K., Groce, N., & Kennedy, H. P. (2012). The intersection of everyday life and group prenatal care for women in two urban clinics. *Journal of Health Care for the Poor and Underserved, 23,* 589–603.

Novick, G., Womack, J., Lewis, J., Stasko, E., Rising, S. S., Sadler, L., . . . Ickovics, J. (2015). Perceptions of barriers and facilitators during implementation of a complex model of group prenatal care in six urban sites. *Research in Nursing and Health, 38*(6), 462–474. doi:10.1002/nur.21681

Phillippi, J., & Myers, C. (2013). Reasons women in Appalachia decline Centering-Pregnancy care. *Journal of Midwifery & Women's Health, 58*(5), 516–522.

Robertson, B., Aycock, D. M., & Darnell, L. A. (2009). Comparison of Centering-Pregnancy to traditional care in Hispanic mothers. *Maternal and Child Health Journal, 13,* 407–414.

Rosenthal, J., Connor, K., & Fenick, A. (2014). Pediatric residents' perspectives on relationships with other professionals during well-childcare. *Journal of Interprofessional Care, 28*(5), 481–484. doi:10.3109/13561820.2014.909796

Tilden, E. L., Emeis, C. L., Caughey, A. B., Weinstein, S. R., Futernick, S. B., & Lee, C. S. (2016). The influence of group versus individual prenatal care on phase of labor at hospital admission. *Journal of Midwifery & Women's Health, 61*(4), 427–434. doi:10.1111/jmwh.12437

Trudnak, T. C., Arboleda, E., Kirby, R. S., & Perrin, K. (2013). Outcomes of Latina women in CenteringPregnancy group prenatal care compared with individual prenatal care. *Journal of Midwifery & Women's Health, 58*(4), 396–403.

Vonderheid, S., Klima, C., Norr, K., Grad, M. A., & Westdahl, C. (2013). Using focus groups and social marketing to strengthen promotion of group prenatal care. *Advances in Nursing Science, 36*(4), 320–325.

Xaverius, P., & Grady, M. A. (2014). CenteringPregnancy in Missouri: A system level analysis. *The Scientific World Journal, 2014*(2014), 1–10. doi:10.1155/2014/285386

General Centering Healthcare Publications

Alliman, J., Jolles, D., & Summers, L. (2015). The innovation imperative: Scaling freestanding birth centers, CenteringPregnancy, and midwifery-led maternity health homes. *Journal of Midwifery & Women's Health, 60*(3), 244–248.

Barger, M., Faucher, M. A., & Murphy, P. A. (2015). Part II: The CenteringPregnancy model of group prenatal care. *Journal of Midwifery & Women's Health, 60*(2), 211–213. doi:10.1111/jmwh.12307

Bloomfield, J., & Rising, S. S. (2013). CenteringParenting: An innovative dyad model for group mother–infant care. *Journal of Midwifery & Women's Health, 58*(6), 683–689.

Buzi, R. S., Smith, P. B., Kozinetz, C. A., Peskin, M. F., & Wiemann, C. M. (2015). A socioecological framework to assessing depression among pregnant teens. *Maternal and Child Health Journal, 19*(10), 2187–2194. doi:10.1007/s10995-015-1733-y

Buzi, R. S., Smith, P. B., Wiemann, C. M., Peskin, M. F., Chacko, M. R., & Kozinetz, A. (2014). Project passport: An integrated group-centered approach targeting pregnant teens and their partners. *Journal of Applied Research on Children: Informing Policy for Children at Risk, 5*(1), 6.

Carlson, N. S., & Lowe, N. (2006). CenteringPregnancy: A new approach in prenatal care. *The American Journal of Maternal/Child Nursing, 31*(4), 218–223.

Catling, C. J., Medley, N., Foureur, M., Ryan, C., Leap, N., Teate, A., & Homer, C. S. (2015). Group versus conventional antenatal care for women. *Cochrane Database of Systematic Reviews.* doi:10.1002/14651858.CD007622.pub3/abstract

Chao, M., Abercrombie, P., Santana, T., & Duncan, L. (2012). Centering as a model for group visits among women with chronic pelvic pain. *Journal of Obstetric, Gynecologic, & Neonatal Nursing, 41*(5), 703–710. doi:10.1111/j.1552-6909.2012.01406.x

DeCesare, J. Z., & Jackson, J. R. (2015). CenteringPregnancy: Practical tips for your practice. *Archives of Gynecology and Obstetrics, 291*(3), 499–507. doi:10.1007/s00404-014-3467-2

DeFrancesco, M., & Rising, S. S. (2010). A new way to be "patient-centered" and help your practice. *The Female Patient, 35,* 46–48.

Devitt, N. (2013). Does the CenteringPregnancy group prenatal care program reduce preterm birth? The conclusions are premature. *Birth, 40*(1), 67–69.

Foster, G., Alviar, A., Neumeier, R., & Wooten, A. (2012). A tri-service perspective on the implementation of a CenteringPregnancy model in the military. *Journal of Obstetric, Gynecologic, & Neonatal Nursing, 41*(2), 315–321.

Garretto, D., & Bernstein, P. S. (2014). CenteringPregnancy: An innovative approach to prenatal care delivery. *American Journal of Obstetrics & Gynecology, 210*(1), 14–15.

Hollowell, J., Oakley, L., Brocklehurst, P., & Gray, R. (2011). The effectiveness of antenatal care programmes to reduce infant mortality and preterm birth in socially disadvantaged and vulnerable women in high-income countries: A systematic review. *BMC Pregnancy and Childbirth, 11,* 13. Retrieved from www.biomedcentral.com/1471-2393/11/13

Karsnitz, D., & Holcomb, M. (2012). CenteringPregnancy: An evidence-based model of prenatal care. In B. Anderson & S. Stone (Eds.), *Best practices in midwifery: Using the evidence to implement change* (pp. 31–42). New York, NY: Springer Publishing.

Klima, C. (2003). CenteringPregnancy: A model for pregnant adolescents. *Journal of Midwifery & Women's Health, 48*(3), 220–225.

Klima, C., Vonderheid, S., Norr, K., & Park, C. (2015). Development of the pregnancy-related empowerment scale. *Nursing and Health, 3*(5), 120–127.

Kolb, K., Picklesimer, A., Covington-Kolb, S., & Hines, L. (2012). CenteringPregnancy electives: A case study in the shift toward student-centered learning in medical education. *Journal of the South Carolina Medical Association, 108*(4), 103–105.

Kovarik, R., Skelton, J., Mullins, M.R., Langston, L., Womack, S., Morris, J., . . . Ebersole, J. (2009). CenteringPregnancy Smiles: A community engagement to develop and implement a new oral health and prenatal care model in rural Kentucky. *Journal of Higher Education Outreach and Engagement, 13*(3), 101–112.

Lathrop, B. (2013). A systematic review comparing group prenatal care to traditional prenatal care. *Nursing for Women's Health, 17*(2), 118–130.

Manant, A., & Dodgson, J. E. (2011). CenteringPregnancy: An integrative literature review. *Journal of Midwifery & Women's Health, 56*(2), 94–102.

Massey, Z., Rising, S. S., & Ickovics, J. (2006). CenteringPregnancy Group Prenatal Care: Promoting relationship-centered care. *Journal of Obstetric, Gynecologic, and Neonatal Nursing, 35*(2), 286–294.

McKeever, A. (2013). Preterm Birth Prevention: Marrying CenteringPregnancy and community health workers. *Journal of Obstetric, Gynecologic,& Neonatal Nursing, 42*, S21.

Novarik, R., Skelton, J., Mullins, M. R., Langston, L., Womack, S., Morris, J., . . . Ebersole, J. (2009). CenteringPregnancy Smiles: A community engagement to develop and implement a new oral health and prenatal care model in rural Kentucky. *Journal of Higher Education Outreach and Engagement,13*(3), 101–112.

Novick, G. (2004). CenteringPregnancy and the current state of prenatal care. *Journal of Midwifery & Women's Health, 49*(5), 405–411.

Ohno, M., Rodriguez, M., Wiener. S., & Caughey, A. (2012). *CenteringPregnancy for the prevention of preterm birth: A cost effectiveness analysis.* Presented at the 34th Annual Meeting of the Society for Medical Decision Making, Phoenix, AZ. Retrieved from https://smdm.confex.com/smdm/2012az/webprogram/Paper6929.html

Picklesimer, A., Herberlein, E., & Covington-Kolb, S. (2015). Group Prenatal Care: Has its time come? *Clinical Obstetrics and Gynecology, 58*(2), 380–391.

Reid, J. (2007). CenteringPregnancy®: A model for group prenatal care. *Nursing for Women's Health, 11*(4), 382–388.

Rising, S. S. (1998). CenteringPregnancy: An interdisciplinary model of empowerment. *Journal of Nurse-Midwifery, 43*(1), 46–54.

Rising, S. S., & Jolivet, R. (2009). Circles of community: The CenteringPregnancy© group prenatal care model. In R. Davis-Floyd, L. Barclay, B. A. Daviss, & J. Tritten (Eds.), *Birth models that work* (pp. 365–384). Berkeley: University of California Press.

Rising, S. S., Kennedy, H. P., & Klima, C. (2004). Redesigning prenatal care through CenteringPregnancy. *Journal of Midwifery & Women's Health, 49*(5), 398–404.

Rising, S. S., & Senterfitt, C. (2009). Repairing health care: Building relationships through groups. *Creative Nursing, 15*(4), 178–183.

Rotundo, G. (2011–2012). CenteringPregnancy: The benefits of group prenatal care. *Nursing for Women's Health, 15*(6), 508–518.

Rowley, R. A., Phillips, L. E., O'Dell, L., Husseini, R. E., Carpino, S., & Hartman, S. (2015). Group prenatal care: A financial perspective. *Maternal and Child Health Journal, 20*, 1–10. doi:10.1007/s10995-015-1802-2

Schwarz, J., Froh, E., & Bitowski, B. (2015, November 7– 11). *Mama Care: An innovative care model for pregnant women with a prenatally diagnosed birth defect.* Presented at the 43rd Biennial Convention, STTI Las Vegas, NV. Retrieved from https://stti.confex.com/stti/bc43/webprogram/Paper77467.html

Sheeder, J., Weber Yorga, K., & Kabir-Greher, K. (2012). A review of prenatal group care literature: The need for a structured theoretical framework and systematic evaluation. *Maternal and Child Health Journal, 16*(1), 177–187.

Stemig, C. (2008). CenteringPregnancy: Group prenatal care. *Creative Nursing, 14*(4), 182–183.

Strickland, C., Merrell, S., & Kirk, J. (2016). CenteringPregnancy: Meeting the quadruple aim in prenatal care. *North Carolina Medical Journal, 77*(6), 394–397.

Tanner-Smith, E., Steinka-Fry, K., & Lipsey, M. (2012). *A multi-site evaluation of the CenteringPregnancy programs in Tennessee.* Final report presented to the Tennessee Department of Health, Peabody Research Institute, Vanderbilt University, Nashville, TN.

Thielen, K. (2012). Exploring the group prenatal care model: A critical review of the literature. *Journal of Perinatal Education, 21*(4), 209–218.

Tilden, E. L., Hersh, S. R., Emeis, C. L., Weinstein, S. R., & Caughey, A. B. (2014). Group prenatal care: Review of outcomes and recommendations for model implementation. *Obstetrical & Gynecological Survey, 69*(1), 46–55. doi:10.1097/OGX.0000000000000025

Trotter, K. (2013). The promise of group medical visits. *Nurse Practitioner, 38*(5), 48–53.

Walker, D., & Rising, S. S. (2004–2005). Revolutionizing prenatal care: New evidence-based prenatal care delivery models. *Journal of New York State Nurses Association, 35*(2), 18–21.

Walker, D., & Worrell, R. (2008). Promoting healthy pregnancies through perinatal groups: A comparison of CenteringPregnancy® group prenatal care and childbirth education classes. *The Journal of Perinatal Education, 17*(1), 27.

International Centering Healthcare Articles

Allen, J., Kildea, S., & Stapleton, H. (2015). How does group antenatal care function within a caseload midwifery model? A critical ethnographic analysis. *Midwifery, 31*(5), 489–497. doi:10.1016/j.midw.2015.01.009

Andersson, E., Christensson, K., & Hildingsson, I. (2012). Parents' experiences and perceptions of group-based antenatal care in four clinics in Sweden. *Midwifery, 28*(2012), 502–508. doi:10.1016/j.midw.2011.07.006

Andersson, E., Chjristensson, K., & Hildingsson, I. (2013). Mothers' satisfaction with group antenatal care versus individual antenatal care: A clinical trial. *Sexual & Reproductive Healthcare, 4*(2013), 113–120. doi:10.1016/j.srhc.2013.08.002

Benediktsson, I., McDonald, S., Vekved, M., McNeil, D., Dolan, S., & Tough, S. (2013). Comparing CenteringPregnancy® to standard prenatal care plus prenatal education. *BMC Pregnancy and Childbirth, 13*(Suppl. 1), S5.

Craswell, A., Kearney, L., & Reed, R. (2016). Expecting and connecting: Group pregnancy care: Evaluation of a collaborative clinic. *Women and Birth.* Advance online publication. doi:10.1016/j.wombi.2016.03.002

Gaudion, A., Bick, D., Menka, Y., Demilew, J., Walton, C., Yiannouzis, K., . . . Rising, S. S. (2011). Adapting the CenteringPregnancy® model for a UK feasibility study. *British Journal of Midwifery, 19*(7), 433–438.

Gaudion, A., & Menka, Y. (2010). No decision about me without me: CenteringPregnancy. *The Practising Midwife, 13*(10), 15–18.

Gaudion, A., Menka, Y., Demilew, J., Walton, C., Yiannouzis, K., Robbins, J., & Bick, D. (2011). Findings from a UK feasibility study of the CenteringPregnancy® model. *British Journal of Midwifery, 19*(12), 796–802.

Gaudion, A., & Yiannouzis, K. (2011). 12 bumps are better than one. *Midwives: The Official Magazine of the Royal College of Midwives, 3*, 34–35.

Ghani, R. M. A. (2015). Perception toward conducting the CenteringPregnancy model in the Egyptian teaching hospitals: A step to improve the quality of antenatal care. *European Journal of Biology and Medical Science Research, 3*(1), 9–18.

Homer, C., Ryan, C., Leap, N., Foureur, M., Teate, A., & Catling-Paull, C. J. (2012). Group versus conventional antenatal care for pregnant women. *Cochrane Database of Systematic Reviews, 11*, CD007622.

Jafarim, F., Eftekhar, H., Fotouhi, A., Mohammad, K., & Hantoushzadeh, S. (2010). Comparison of maternal and neonatal outcomes of group versus individual prenatal care: A new experience in Iran. *Health Care for Women International, 31*(7), 571–584. doi:10.1080/07399331003646323

Kearns, A. D., Caglia, J. M., ten Hoope-Bender, P., & Langer, A. (2015). Antenatal and postnatal care: A review of innovative models for improving availability, accessibility, acceptability and quality of services in low-resource settings. *BJOG: An International Journal of Obstetrics & Gynaecology, 123*(4), 540–548. doi:10.1111/1471-0528.13818

Klima, C., Patil, C., Norr, K., Leshabari, S., Kaponda, C., & Rising, S. (2016). Exporting CenteringPregnancy may contribute to improving antenatal care and improving maternal and child health in Sub-Saharan Africa. *Journal of Midwifery & Women's Health, 61*(5), 660.

Kweekel, L., Gerrits, T., Rijnders, M., & Brown, P. (2016). The role of trust in CenteringPregnancy: Building interpersonal trust relationship in group-based prenatal care in the Netherlands. *Birth.* doi:10.1111/birth.12260

Maier, B. J. (2013). Antenatal group care in a Midwifery Group Practice: A midwife's perspective. *Women and Birth, 26*(1), 87–89.

Maru, S., Harsha, A., & Nirola, I. (2015). Group antenatal care: The power of peers for increasing institutional birth in Achham, Nepal. Retrieved from www.mhtf.org/document/group-antenatal-care-the-power-of-peers-for-increasing-institutional-birth-in-achham-nepal

McDonald, S. D., Sword, W., Eryuzlu, L. E., & Biringer, A. B. (2014). A qualitative descriptive study of the group prenatal care experience: Perceptions of women with low-risk pregnancies and their midwives. *BMC Pregnancy and Childbirth, 14*(1), 334. doi:10.1186/1471-2393-14-334

McDonald, S. D., Sword, W., Eryuzlu, L., Neupane, B., Beyene, J., & Biringer, A. (2016). Why are half of women interested in participating in group prenatal care? *Maternal and Child Health Journal, 20*(1), 97–105. doi:10.1007/s10995-015-1807-x

McNeil, D. A., Vekved, M., Dolan, S. M., Siever, J., Horn, S., & Tough, S. C. (2012). Getting more than they realized they needed: A qualitative study of women's experience of group prenatal care. *BMC Pregnancy and Childbirth, 12*, 17.

McNeil, D. A., Vekved, M., Dolan, S. M., Siever, J., Horn, S., & Tough, S. C. (2013). A qualitative study of the experience of CenteringPregnancy group prenatal care for physicians. *BMC Pregnancy and Childbirth, 13*(Suppl. 1), S6.

McNeill, J. A., & Reiger, K. M. (2015). Rethinking prenatal care within a social model of health: An exploratory study in Northern Ireland. *Health Care for Women International, 36*(1), 5–25. doi:10.1080/07399332.2014.900061

Patil, C. L., Abrams, E. T., Klima, C., Kaponda, C. P., Leshabari, S. C., Vonderheid, S. C., . . . Norr, K. F. (2013). CenteringPregnancy-Africa: A pilot of group antenatal care to address millennium development goals. *Midwifery, 10*, 1190–1198.

Rijnders, M., van der Pal, K., & Aalhuizen, I. (2012). CenteringPregnancy® offers pregnant women a central position in Dutch prenatal care [CenteringPregnancy® biedt zwangere centrale rol in Nederlandse verloskundige zorg]. *Tijdschr voor gezondheidswetenschappen, 90*(8), 513–516.

Ruiz-Mirazo, E., Lopez-Yarto, M., & McDonald, S. D. (2012). Group prenatal care versus individual prenatal care: A systematic review and meta-analysis. *Journal of Obstetrics Gynaecology Canada, 34*(3), 223–229.

Teate, A., Leap, N., & Homer, C. (2012). Midwives' experiences of becoming CenteringPregnancy facilitators: A pilot study in Sydney, Australia. *Women and Birth, 25*, 3. doi:10.1016/j.wombi.2012.08.002

Teate, A., Leap, N., Rising, S. S., & Homer, C. S. (2011). Women's experiences of group antenatal care in Australia: The CenteringPregnancy pilot study. *Midwifery, 27*(2), 138–145.

A

Pilot Study of CenteringParenting® in Two Public Health Clinics: Calgary, Alberta

A research group in Calgary, Alberta, has worked for several years on piloting a redesign of their public health well-baby model which includes childhood vaccinations, health assessment, and education. Public health nurses have provided care in a traditional one-on-one model, but recent changes in the vaccine schedule, including numbers of vaccines, have created a time burden on the visit. This contributed to a decrease in the time for education at the visits. In addition, funding constraints had a negative impact on the number of and availability of parenting classes.

The research group completed their 2-year feasibility study in 2015 of a CenteringParenting model piloted in two Calgary clinics. Twenty-two families from four groups in two sites participated in the study. These families attended six sessions with three to seven other families throughout the first year of the child's life. Sessions were held at about the 1-, 2-, 4-, 6-, 9- and 12-month birthdays and included the administration of appropriate vaccines. The groups were facilitated by two public health nurses and focused on core topics with special attention to areas of interest to the group. All three components of the Centering model: health care, interactive learning, and community building, were included. The primary research question was: Does the CenteringParenting model meet the needs of parents, nurses, and decision makers?

All women in CenteringParenting self-reported that they felt welcomed, respected, listened to, and encouraged to apply new information. They also became more confident in their parenting skills and parenting roles, were better able to manage stress, and were confident that they knew where to get answers to any questions.

Sixteen mothers participated in focus groups or individual interviews, and several themes emerged that were consistent with other Centering programs. Women appreciated the instrumental support that they received from the facilitators and each other. They enjoyed the group time and felt they connected with other mothers in the group. They most appreciated the opportunity to share the challenges of new motherhood at a time when others not in their situation could not understand how they were feeling.

The team also conducted interviews with all five nurse facilitators. Although the nurses enjoyed facilitating the group and making connections with the mothers in a different way, several issues surfaced. They experienced some conflict in meeting practice standards particularly around immunization practices. They felt time constraints in meeting the mothers' support and information needs as well as doing the immunizing. Four decision makers also were interviewed. They felt that CenteringParenting stimulated a new way of thinking about their standards of practice and identified the need for more flexibility. They saw CenteringParenting as an important option, particularly for high-risk families. They also identified that changes in some structures and processes would be required to implement the program more widely.

The data supported the research question: CenteringParenting met the needs of parents, nurses, and decision makers. Mothers expressed high satisfaction with the model. Nurses had mixed feelings but generally enjoyed facilitating groups. Future work will focus on addressing the challenges surfaced by the pilot and also may include a randomized controlled trial to determine the effectiveness of CenteringParenting.

Content abstracted from "CenteringParenting Pilot in Two Calgary Public Health Clinics," 2015, and printed with permission of Deborah McNeil, PhD RN, and Cyne Johnston, PhD.

B

Field Notes From The Netherlands, Nepal, and Malawi/Tanzania

Field Notes: Introduction of Centering Healthcare in the Netherlands

Marlies Rijnders, PhD, RM

TNO Child Health, Leiden, The Netherlands

CenteringPregnancy® began in response to a Dutch Ministry of Health committee's call for more woman-centered care to help improve their relatively unfavorable perinatal outcomes and quality of care (Mohangoo et al., 2008; van der Velden, 2009). In 2011, a research proposal was drafted by a research midwife who reviewed research on empowerment of pregnant women and realized that CenteringPregnancy could be *the* model of woman-centered care that had the potential to not only empower women but also improve perinatal outcomes. Foundation funding was obtained to pilot CenteringPregnancy to determine whether CenteringPregnancy could be implemented in independent Dutch midwifery practices with different client populations.

Preparation

We expected that implementation would be more successful if embedded from the start in practice and in the professional and educational system and underpinned by research. The research midwife who wrote the proposal was from a national research institute for applied research (TNO). She recruited three midwifery practices based on the midwives' enthusiasm and their client diversity. The research midwife formed a team that included a staff member of the Royal Dutch Organization of Midwives (KNOV) and a lecturer at the Amsterdam Midwifery Academy

(VAA). The team then consulted with Sharon Rising, the chief executive officer of the Centering Healthcare Institute (CHI).

Pilot

The pilot began with a 2-day training in the Netherlands conducted by Margie Rickell, a CHI consultant. The first training included the multisectoral team plus additional practicing midwives and support personnel from the three pilot practices. The training was a great success. Immediately, a core group came together to coordinate CenteringPregnancy implementation. The core group included the multisectoral team that planned training plus a midwife from each practice. The group translated and adapted the manual and Mother's Notebook for the Dutch in consultation with CHI. CenteringPregnancy started within 2 months after training in these three midwifery practices. Every month, the core group and other available CenteringPregnancy-trained midwives met to prepare upcoming sessions and discuss their experiences. CenteringPregnancy was offered only during the first 2 years by midwifery practices or hospitals within a series of research projects that covered costs such as the training, supervision, and materials. Within these research projects, 26 midwifery practices and five hospitals participated.

Expansion

CenteringPregnancy has grown rapidly in the Netherlands, spreading in just 4 years from three midwifery practices to 47 plus five hospitals, and CenteringParenting® has started at three locations. As word spread, more and more midwifery practices wanted to offer CenteringPregnancy. Most did so even though they had no research grants or other funding. Some practices managed to receive limited local funding to cover the costs of the co-facilitator. Successful proposals for local funding were shared with other midwifery practices so they could seek funding. Getting funding was sometimes plain luck; as one midwife describes: "It really helped to have had the right pregnant civil servant in one of the groups."

Challenges to CenteringPregnancy

The most serious threat for sustainability is lack of reimbursement by health insurance plans or any other way to cover the (unpaid) time investment of care providers and costs for the cofacilitator, training, materials, and, sometimes, space. The Dutch Royal Organization of Midwives has begun procedures to provide reimbursement of CenteringPregnancy by health insurance companies as soon as results of a study of costs and effects of CenteringPregnancy become available in late 2016. In the meantime, the core group is preparing an overview of actual costs of CenteringPregnancy, possible financing options, and cost-savings strategies. This information will help organizations that currently offer CenteringPregnancy, or want to do so, make the right choices to sustain CenteringPregnancy.

Other factors that sometimes negatively influence the implementation of CenteringPregnancy include a lack of commitment of some providers within the organization, unwillingness to change professional behavior, and failure to integrate the CenteringPregnancy model within the current organization, often affecting the balance of work with private life and burnout for those midwives trying to sustain CenteringPregnancy. Three midwifery practices stopped offering CenteringPregnancy. One stopped because they considered it to be too expensive, although they valued CenteringPregnancy for their clients. Another stopped, despite a very enthusiastic midwife, full groups, and enthusiastic women because of lack of support of colleagues. The third stopped temporarily when two "frontier" midwives moved, resulting in the fatigue of the remaining midwives. Recently, one of the midwives returned, and so the practice will restart CenteringPregnancy soon because they highly value CenteringPregnancy for the women they serve. Two practices could not recruit enough women for groups. All practices that stopped or never started were offered intensive support, but this did not result in an adequate uptake of CenteringPregnancy.

When CenteringPregnancy expanded from independent midwifery practice into larger hospitals, the more complex hospital structure made implementation more complicated. Administrators and other personnel not directly involved in CenteringPregnancy were supportive of this innovative antenatal care (ANC) model, but their other administrative and clinical duties meant they could not focus as intensively on CenteringPregnancy implementation in the way that the independent midwifery practices could. High provider turnover also made implementation more difficult. CenteringPregnancy-trained midwives in hospitals now provide workshops for new providers to build enthusiasm for CenteringPregnancy. Sending their colleagues an e-mail with "anecdotal" information about their groups and thanking them for the recruitment of women also is working very well to sustain commitment.

The implementation of CenteringParenting in Youth Health Care still is a challenge. The provision and content of Youth Health Care in the Netherlands is mandated by law and provided under municipal responsibility by hierarchically organized institutions that are constantly under pressure to economize care. So far, CenteringParenting has been implemented in relatively small organizations that could act swiftly. However, even then implementation was still much more time-consuming, with many more barriers to deal with compared to the implementation of CenteringPregnancy in midwifery practices or even hospitals.

Factors Contributing to Sustainability of CenteringPregnancy

The rapid implementation and sustained success of CenteringPregnancy was facilitated by a favorable climate for care innovation, organizational factors in Dutch maternity care, and multiple strategies for long-term sustainability introduced by the core group. CenteringPregnancy was introduced at a time when there was growing awareness of the relatively high perinatal mortality seen in the Netherlands. This awareness created a favorable national climate for innovation congruent with the new emphasis on empowerment and responsibilities of patients. This climate helped to initiate and fund CenteringPregnancy implementation and research regarding its implementation and outcomes in the Netherlands.

Several factors in Dutch maternity care were very helpful for the rapid implementation of CenteringPregnancy. Midwives work independently in midwifery practices; so each small group could decide for themselves whether or not to start with CenteringPregnancy without needing to persuade a bureaucratic organization. Another enhancing factor for implementation was the incredible enthusiasm of the midwives. This was partly a result of eagerness to improve their own business. CenteringPregnancy also appealed to midwives because CenteringPregnancy seemed to be one of the few changes oriented toward "midwifery care." Some midwives described the CenteringPregnancy training as the "the first of all the trainings I received in 20 years of midwifery that really makes me happy because it will make a difference." Quite a few said they were tired or even burned out after years of fighting against unnecessary medicalization of birth. Participating in CenteringPregnancy increased midwives' job satisfaction. Through CenteringPregnancy, they experienced more of a partnership with the women and their partners. The women's positive responses to CenteringPregnancy sustained the midwives' enthusiasm, as when one group member said:

"It's reassuring to hear that other women also experience inconveniences. That satisfies me in a way. It's not just me; it's not something strange; it's just normal and part of the process. These thoughts make me feel calm and confident."

As these stories were shared with other midwives, it made them in turn enthusiastic for CenteringPregnancy.

Perhaps the most important factor in the success of this initiative is the support provided by a fantastic core group of midwives who, from the very beginning, developed strategies to enhance sustainability. They dedicated lots of time to the implementation of CenteringPregnancy. They worked very well together, contributed a variety of expertise and networks, and had strong support from their colleagues and their employing organizations in terms of released time, finances, and assistance.

First, the core group established a program of certification, lifelong learning, and ongoing support to ensure fidelity to the CenteringPregnancy model and high quality. The program includes: a planning visit at any new sites, a 2-day initial training, initial certification after offering at least three groups and attending at least three supervision sessions, and ongoing recertification based on offering CenteringPregnancy groups and attending supervision sessions and an expert module. Supervision sessions offered monthly reemphasize the essential elements of CenteringPregnancy, share experiences, and create a network of experienced and less experienced CenteringPregnancy-trained professionals for mutual support. Expert modules provide more in-depth knowledge and skills training, such as a recent module on the effects of group dynamics on group cohesion.

Second, they integrated CenteringPregnancy into midwifery education by developing a clinical module for students. After attending a 3-hour workshop about CenteringPregnancy developed by the lecturer–midwife of the CenteringPregnancy core group, each student serves as a co-facilitator for all sessions in one group. This internship is very popular because, unlike other prenatal internships, the student gets to know a group of women through pregnancy. Midwifery practices benefit because a student co-facilitator is without cost, and students are more skillful than other co-facilitators during health assessment. This internship builds support to include CenteringPregnancy in the new curriculum of midwifery education and students' interest in becoming CenteringPregnancy providers.

Third, CenteringPregnancy-Netherlands engaged in extensive dissemination about the program to reach pregnant women, midwives, educators, researchers, and health policy leaders. Activities have included a website for professionals, a private Facebook page, an active Twitter account, a film about CenteringPregnancy in the Netherlands, and frequent interviews for professional and women's magazines and newspapers. To make CenteringPregnancy visible for all stakeholders in the Dutch maternity care, the core group provided many scholarly presentations at symposia, professional meetings, and midwifery academies, published five CenteringPregnancy articles for the *Dutch Journal of Midwives* in 2015 to 2016, (Aalhuizen & Rijnders, 2015a; 2015b; Kraan van der, Rijnders, Groessen, & Aalhuizen, 2015; Rijnders & Aalhuizen, 2016) and has a paper in English under review (Rijnders et al., 2015). In addition, another article on CenteringPregnancy has just been published in *Birth* (Kweekel et al., 2016).

Finally, an integral part of the implementation process of CenteringPregnancy in the Netherlands was evaluation to gain insight into the potential effects of CenteringPregnancy. The core group designed and carried out research that has grown in scope and rigor as the program expanded. Initially, 18 months after CenteringPregnancy was started, a retrospective cohort study used medical records to compare the 579 women who received CenteringPregnancy and all the other women who received individual ANC at the same clinics and had very similar demographic characteristics and obstetric histories. Significant findings included decreases of 8% in augmentation and 10% in use of pharmaceutical pain relief among nulliparous women in CenteringPregnancy and more breastfeeding for all women in CenteringPregnancy. There were no differences in adverse maternal and perinatal outcomes. A questionnaire also showed significantly better experiences with care among women who received CenteringPregnancy. However, because of the retrospective study design, we cannot say whether unmeasured factors like psychosocial characteristics account for the differences in outcomes. We have to wait until 2017 for more certainty, when the results of the prospective effectiveness study will be available, which include data on potential psychosocial differences between groups, perinatal outcomes, psychosocial outcomes, lifestyle, knowledge, and costs from 13 midwifery practices and two hospitals offering CenteringPregnancy. Future developments will be aimed at sustainability, reimbursement, and lifelong learning of CenteringPregnancy-trained professionals. New proposals for research will look at the involvement of partners, effects of CenteringPregnancy on biochemical parameters of stress and well-being, and the effect of CenteringPregnancy on care providers. *The positive results seen thus far are encouraging and provide strong support to continue the implementation of CenteringPregnancy in the Netherlands.*

References (Titles translated from the Dutch indicated by brackets)

Aalhuizen, I., & Rijnders, M. (2015a). [CenteringPregnancy in a hospital can be done!] Tijdschrift voor Verloskunde. *Dutch Journal of Midwifery, 6,* 12–13.

Aalhuizen, I., & Rijnders, M. (2015b). [What does CenteringPregnancy offer in case of a fourth pregnancy?] Tijdschrift voor Verloskunde, *Dutch Journal of Midwifery, 2,* 14–15.

Kraan van der, A., Rijnders, M., Groessen, K., & Aalhuizen, I. (2015). [Centering-Pregnancy: Experiences of students and lecturers]. Tijdschrift voor Verloskunde. *Dutch Journal of Midwifery, 3,* 16–17.

Kweekel, L., Gerrits, T., Rijnders, M., & Brown, P. (2016). The role of trust in CenteringPregnancy: Building interpersonal trust relationship in group-based prenatal care in the Netherlands. *Birth.* doi:10.1111/birt.12260

Mohangoo, A. D., Buitendijk, S. E., Hukkelhoven, C. W., Ravelli, A. C., Rijninks-van Driel, G. C., Tamminga, P., & Nijhuis, J. G. (2008). [Higher perinatal mortality in the Netherlands than in other European countries: the Peristat-II study]. *Ned Tijdschr Geneeskd, 152*(50), 2718–2727.

Rijnders, M., & Aalhuizen, I. (2016). [Integrated CenteringPregnancy; Facilitate together] Tijdschrift voor Verloskunde. *Dutch Journal of Midwifery, 1,* 45.

Rijnders, M., Kraan van der, A., Aalhuizen, I., Nalonya Laan van der, N., Groessen, K., Goudsmit, M., & Lijster de, K. (2015). [CenteringPregnancy: An exciting way to provide care!] Tijdschrift voor Verloskunde. *Dutch Journal of Midwifery, 1,* 33–34.

van der Velden, J. (2009). *A good beginning: Safe care around pregnancy and birth: Advice of the steering group pregnancy and birth.* Retrieved from www.rijksoverheid .nl/enzwangerschap-en/x-cz-2978049b.pdf

Acknowledgments: Inger Aalhuizen, Katja van Groessen, Annemiek van der Kraan, Nalonya van der Laan KNOV (Royal Dutch Organization of Midwives), TNO Child Health
Note: All references of TNO are based on the actual name of the organization the Netherlands Organization for Applied Scientific Research.

Field Notes: CenteringPregnancy-Based Group Antenatal Care in Achham District, Nepal

Sheela Maru, MD, MPH

Instructor in Obstetrics and Gynecology, Boston University School of Medicine

Women's Health Advisor, Possible and Health Care Systems Design Group

Research Fellow, Division of Women's Health, Brigham and Women's Hospital

Globally, 800 women die from preventable causes related to childbirth every day, and 99% of these deaths occur in low-resource countries. Increasing institutional birth rates is a central strategy in reducing maternal mortality. Nepal is a paradigmatic case of the challenges in increasing institutional birth rates and reducing maternal mortality. Maternal mortality in Nepal is 281 per 100,000, and only 35% of births take place in a health facility (Central Bureau of Statistics—National Planning Commission Secretariat, Government of Nepal, 2012). Nepal is South Asia's most impoverished country. This Centering initiative is located in Achham District in Nepal's Far-Western Development Region, an economically, geographically, and politically isolated rural area, 14 hours from the nearest major referral hospital. Most people have average monthly incomes of under US$30 (Ministry of Health and Population, New ERA, ICF International Inc., 2012). The initiative was started by Possible, a nonprofit health care organization that independently manages the government-owned, district hospital and community health care in 14 surrounding village clusters via a public–private partnership model with the Ministry of Health. Possible employs 170 full-time staff, 80% of whom are local.

Our research here has shown that almost all women recognize institutional delivery is safer and prefer it to a home birth (Maru et al., 2016). Poverty, rugged terrain, and lack of infrastructure inhibit transportation to a skilled birth facility. In this patriarchal society, women need male family member support to access a skilled birth facility, but obtaining support can be difficult due to male migration for labor or contradicting beliefs among in-laws. ANC should help women plan to obtain support and manage logistics for timely and safe arrival at a skilled birth facility. However, less than 50% of women in rural Nepal complete the four recommended ANC visits.

To address underutilization of institutional birth, we found inspiration in the CenteringPregnancy model. Group care for dispersed rural populations held the potential for creating social support and detailed birth planning with counseling, and sharing of context-specific advice from peers. Additionally, Group ANC could also strengthen the relationship between women and their providers—skilled birth attendants based in village-level skilled birthing facilities. We hypothesized that this novel intervention that we called "Group ANC" would lead to increased institutional birth by addressing the drivers of underutilization and drawing on the strength within communities of women to change health-seeking behaviors.

Preparation

Because CenteringPregnancy was not designed for our setting, a significant amount of adaptation was necessary. Nepali government ANC protocols based on the World Health Organization's (WHO) Focused Antenatal Care (FANC) are for four visits. We designed a six-visit model that met WHO and Nepali standards that incorporated essential elements of CenteringPregnancy. We also integrated community-based women's participatory action groups, where groups are guided through a process of planning, action, observation, and reflection about local issues by community women trained as facilitators. Women's groups have been effective in several rural developing-country contexts, including Nepal (Prost et al., 2013). Due to the dispersed population and difficult topography of the region, we planned to deliver Group ANC in village-level clinics, more proximate to where women lived than the hospital. We integrated group ANC within a broader program to strengthen village skilled-birthing facilities by enhancing provider counseling skills and using the gestational-age matched groups of CenteringPregnancy to enable mobile ultrasound and antenatal lab testing beyond HIV screening. We obtained approval for the intervention from the district health officer and the mid-level practitioners who run the village-level clinics. The district health officer was initially favorable to the idea, while there was a mixed response from the clinic administrators.

Pilot

The first 6 months of running the nascent program were considered a pilot phase. Regular observations by supervising community health nurses and other supervisors highlighted several challenges: substandard clinical care documentation, poor time management, highly variable facilitation quality, and incomplete implementation of the participatory action portion of the model.

We then worked to further modify the program by addressing each of these concerns. To improve documentation, we created a simpler paper registry. For improved time management, we asked women to discuss the importance of arriving on time, adjusted some start-times, and streamlined our facilitator guides. Time management also improved with experience of the facilitators. To improve facilitation quality, we increased feedback to facilitators and timed feedback to immediately follow each group. The community health nurses used a form on their mobile phones that included components covered and Likert scales rating group dynamics and facilitation and shared their observations immediately after the session. Despite detailed planning and on-site consultation from another Nepali group experienced in participatory learning and action groups, we struggled to fully implement this portion of the model. No group was able to get to the "action" part of the cycle. After much brainstorming, the team decided to narrow the focus of problem solving to specifically creating birth plans for each participant.

Our most contentious and difficult adaptation came from a conflict with a specific government policy. The national Safe Motherhood Program provides a financial incentive to women who complete four ANC visits, but only if those visits are completed during specific months of gestation. The government tracks this and rewards the clinics with the highest rates. Problematically, these windows are often defined and calculated inconsistently, making it difficult to predict when a woman would be considered eligible for the incentive. To achieve fidelity to the CenteringPregnancy model, groups were composed of women who would deliver in the same month; to maximize incentive eligibility the visits were scheduled on different days each month. The government nurse–midwives felt the scheduling was too "chaotic" and preferred fixed dates (Focus group, December 23, 2015). Government officials were not receptive to more flexible eligibility policies despite multiple attempts at compromise. We agreed to modify the program to have a fixed monthly "ANC Day" that women attend according to their gestational age so they meet the government eligibility windows. This adaptation loosens Centering Pregnancy's requirement for stable groups but maintains some gestational-age focus by separating groups into a second trimester (fourth to sixth month) and a third trimester (eighth to ninth) group each month.

Expansion and Evaluation

The adapted CenteringPregnancy-based Group ANC model, with monthly group visits by gestational age, is now being offered in six village development clusters (VDCs). Group ANC is acceptable to women, as demonstrated by median ANC attendance of eight (interquartile range: 3–12), survey data identifying group ANC as more enjoyable than individual care, and focus group data that group ANC participation generates a sense of empowerment and self-respect that women value. One nurse-midwife observed this powerful transformation:

> *Initially, when they come in, they have their faces covered, they [are] shy from introducing themselves. . . . In the beginning, they are unable to even say their names . . . . Then, gradually, as they come in for the sessions, they feel more comfortable introducing themselves. By the fourth visit, all women are able to introduce themselves, to speak up.*

Feasibility of the intervention has greatly improved due to the simplicity of the new scheduling system, which also increased compatibility with government protocols and organizational workflow. We identified core components of our CenteringPregnancy-based Group ANC as leading to a supportive, empowering atmosphere with high-quality counseling and basic diagnostics. Quality of facilitation, rated from 0 (like a class) to 5 (peer group discussion), is improving, from a median of 2 to median of 4 on a scale of 1 to 5 since April 2015. Content coverage is excellent, with 100% of content discussed at least once. Data regarding exam coverage are not yet available. Staff identified that a new community health worker (CHW) home-visit program complements Group ANC by deepening CHW–client relationship, reinforcing the importance of ANC attendance, and providing additional time for follow-up of issues like high-risk conditions and complex social situations

Long-Term Evaluation

Our overall evaluation will employ a mixed methods analysis of the intervention using quantitative data, longitudinal cohort focus groups, key informant interviews, and process metrics to validate the Group ANC model, investigate its mechanisms of impact, and assess the implementation process. To evaluate our primary outcomes, Institutional Birth Rate, and ANC completion, we are conducting a prospective nonrandomized controlled trial in the six VDCs receiving Group ANC and eight VDCs receiving individual ANC. Both areas also have the same CHW home-visit program. Outcomes are measured using a household census of the catchment area in 2014 to 2015, repeated in 2016, to provide data for all women giving birth in the catchment area. We also followed a cohort of 140 women (60 in the intervention and 80 in the control group) throughout their pregnancy to assess change in knowledge, practices, and satisfaction, especially regarding maternal and neonatal danger signs, available health services, and planning for an institutional birth.

Lessons Learned

As others have found, implementing CenteringPregnancy-based Group ANC is challenging due to the degree of practice change required, from adjusting staffing and scheduling systems to facilitating an empowering learning experience rather than didactically imparting medical knowledge. In rural Nepal, these challenges were compounded by working within a public health care system where strict policy and incentives around ANC scheduling are not compatible with a stable gestational age group model. The necessity of adaptation in this environment is clear, but few roadmaps exist. Our evaluation will give us some insight into whether this adapted CenteringPregnancy-based Group ANC model will be effective in our setting. Many questions may be left unanswered: How might variations on scheduling stable groups differently affect outcomes? How does our CHW home-visit program contribute to women's knowledge and practices, and how does that interact with Group care? How valuable are birth-planning activities with and without participatory learning and action cycles? How is facilitation of groups affected by joint care delivery between nurse-midwives and CHWs?

For our team at Possible and for our government partners, group care has opened the door to true collaborative care delivery, decentralization of specialized services, improved efficiency of provider time, and greatly increased participation of women in their care. These benefits have pushed us to start to design group care for mothers and their newborn children through 1 year of life. With CenteringParenting as a model, we are starting to create a new model of Group Dyad Care for mothers and infants, hand in hand with our government partners, to fit our context in rural Nepal.

References

Central Bureau of Statistics – National Planning Commission Secretariat, Government of Nepal. (2012). *Nepal National Living Standards Survey 2010-2011*. Kathmandu: Central Bureau of Statistics.

Maru, S., Rajeev, S., Pokhrel, R., Poudyal, A., Mehta, P., Bista, D., Borgatta, L., & Maru, D. (2016). Determinants of institutional birth among women in rural Nepal: A mixed-methods cross-sectional study. *BMC Pregnancy and Childbirth , 16*(1), 252. doi:10.1186/s12884-016-1022-9

Ministry of Health and Population, New ERA, ICF International Inc. (2012). *Nepal Demographic and Health Survey 2011*. Kathmandu.

Prost , A., Colbourn, T., Seward, N., Azad, K., Arri, C., Copas, A., . . . Costello, A. (2013). Women's groups practising participatory learning and action to improve maternal and newborn health in low-resource settings: A systematic review and meta-analysis. *Lancet*, 381, 1736–1746.

Acknowledgments: Community Health and Impact teams, especially Isha Nirola, David Citrin, Alex Harsha, Poshan Thapa, Bishal Belbase, Jasmine Lama, and Duncan Maru. Nepal Ministry of Health collaborators, especially Sabita KC, Mukesh Adhikari, and Sharad Baral.

Field Notes: Malawi and Tanzania

Crystal L. Patil, PhD, and Kathleen F. Norr, PhD
University of Illinois at Chicago, College of Nursing

*Since we started Focused Antenatal Care . . . we saw that it is impossible to talk
with every mother. You have 100 pregnant mothers, how are you going to finish?
So we decided to talk in a group to cover all things in focused antenatal care.
According to the program, we are supposed to do this individually. The one who
decided this is the one in the office, not the one in the practice area.
Practice—it is impossible! Focused care is very difficult.
—Midwife in-charge, rural ANC clinic Tanzania*

Malawi and Tanzania have high rates of poverty, maternal and infant
mortality, and fertility (Malawi Demographic and Health Survey, 2010;
Tanzania, National Bureau of Statistics and ORC Macro, 2010). A national
health system provides free or low-fee services to all, but acute health
workers shortages and underfunded health systems mean quality of care
is low. Both use the FANC, designed to provide fewer but more intense
woman-centered visits, but this model has failed to improve care.

This initiative to improve quality of ANC in these two African countries began when we formed a team of two social scientists and three
doctorally prepared midwives, one each from Malawi, Tanzania, and the
United States. Our team's observations confirmed prior observations in
both countries that what actually occurs in ANC is a very brief visit with
an associated health promotion lecture. Disrespectful interactions with
health workers and long wait times were not uncommon. After learning about CenteringPregnancy, our team recognized the potential that
continuity of care, building of trusting relationships, and opportunity
to offer respectful care could have in the congested and stressful health
care environments in sub-Saharan Africa. Our team's long-term goal is to
test the efficacy of a CenteringPregnancy-based group ANC to improve
quality of care and perinatal outcomes model in sub-Saharan Africa.

Preparation

Our first step was to describe CenteringPregnancy to midwives and women
at ANC clinics in Malawi and Tanzania to get their initial thoughts on
this model of care. After listening to a description of CenteringPregnancy,

a pregnant woman from Tanzania said, "I think women will like this. Because many fail or are afraid to ask the nurse questions because they are there alone." Providers also noted CenteringPregnancy's potential but voiced a few concerns, including whether women would actually talk and that asking women to do their own self-care measures would be interpreted as them not doing their job. Overall, both women and providers introduced to the idea of group ANC felt that group care had a lot of potential. All wanted to see how it worked in practice.

Based on these positive responses and potential challenges or barriers, we conducted a small feasibility and acceptability study. We consulted with Sharon Rising at CHI and training workshops to be sure that we understood the model. In 2013, we trained 12 health care workers and organized two trial sessions to be conducted at a rural hospital and small clinic in Malawi. This work established that group ANC was feasible and acceptable to provider and women (Patil et al., 2013).

In developing a CenteringPregnancy-based group ANC model for two different contexts in the Africa region, we emphasized maintaining fidelity to the original innovation's core components while making appropriate adaptations to enhance acceptability, sustainability, and eventual scale-up. Key adaptations were a substantial reduction in the number of ANC visits and incorporation of region-specific health promotion content, especially malaria, HIV, and prevention of mother-to-child transmission (PMTCT). To promote sustainability and to accommodate low literacy levels, we moved away from written materials and reading-based activities and replaced these with activities that respect strong oral traditions of the region as well as commonly used group activities, such as role-playing. We worked with each clinic to develop a process for recruiting women, scheduling groups and continuity of facilitators, reserve dedicated space, and assign responsibility for maintaining each task. We retained CenteringPregnancy's basic session structure and modeled our training and supporting materials after CenteringPregnancy to reinforce fidelity and build needed skills.

Pilot

In the next step, we tested the adapted model in a small pilot with random assignment of 180 women to group or individual care, with outcome evaluation using surveys at baseline, late pregnancy, and postdelivery. Process evaluation used structured observations and focus groups. We selected one very large ANC clinic in urban Dar es Salaam, Tanzania, and a rural hospital and one of its smaller satellite clinics in Malawi, and each site selected administrators, midwives, and co-facilitators for training.

The pilot began with a 2-day training workshop in each country conducted by Sharon Rising, developer of CenteringPregnancy and chief executive officer of the CHI, and our team's experienced trainer, Carrie Klima. Although the language of education in both countries is English, we found that training in the primary spoken language would be best, so our Malawi and Tanzania team members each provided concurrent translation. At training, administrators and future facilitators learned the core components of CenteringPregnancy-based group ANC both cognitively and experientially. Interactive learning, using facilitative leadership, is a core component related to outcomes (Novick et al., 2013); but health workers are more comfortable with a didactic teaching modality. Therefore, our training focused on building facilitative leadership skills through practice and corrective feedback. The Facilitator's Guide also provided pretested activities for the topics. The last activity gave administrators and health workers time to make implementation plans specific to their clinic.

Expansion and Evaluation

Based on the pilot's very positive results, we began preparing for expansion of this innovative CenteringPregnancy-based group ANC model. At late pregnancy, women in group care had significantly higher ANC care satisfaction, HIV transmission and PMTCT knowledge, and pregnancy-related empowerment scores and less mental distress as measured by the WHO's Self-Reporting Questionnaire integrating depressive, anxiety, and somatic symptoms. At the postbirth interview, women in group care had significantly more ANC visits, postpartum checkups, and exclusive breastfeeding. There were no differences in adverse birth outcomes, but the pilot was not powered to be able to detect these.

Equally important, qualitative focus groups with pregnant women and providers experiencing group ANC documented their overwhelming perception that group ANC greatly improves quality of care. Health workers expressed this by describing what women talked about and changes they have seen. One midwife said,

Here they are able to be open, to talk about the real problems that they have. If there's a breakdown in care they know what to do . . . They are really learning, especially about communicating with their husband. At the last session, some brought their husbands . . . [The] husbands were saying was that women have really learned . . . Now they can be more open to ask for what they need.

In reflecting on how the model affected the job, a midwife said,

This has brought good to my profession, taught me how to make a woman talk about things they have been brought up not to talk about—how to probe, be a good listener, be patient, and not always rush [so I can] find out more about the problem.

In addition to expressing overwhelming support for group ANC, health workers and women both suggested that we expand the program to include well-baby/well-woman visits so that groups can stay together. We are looking into ways to adapt the CenteringParenting program to continue along the continuum of care.

After this pilot, we made the difficult decision that, in order to move forward with this initiative, we needed to pursue a randomized controlled trial (RCT) in only one country. The logistics of implementation in two languages was challenging. We realized that the usual funding mechanisms were not likely to provide sufficient funding to conduct an RCT in two sites. We decided to begin our expansion in Tanzania, primarily because the medical officer in charge of the municipality invited our team to help him introduce this CenteringPregnancy-based group ANC model throughout the municipality. We have begun the critically important work of networking with the ANC systems leaders and stakeholders. Representatives in the Ministry of Health are supportive and would like to see the model tested for efficacy. We have enlisted the support of the professional organizations in Tanzania, such as the Tanzanian Midwives Association. Moreover, our Tanzania principal investigator has begun integrating modules for group care into their midwifery curriculums.

The major barrier to expansion is obtaining funding for an RCT adequately powered to explore impacts of CenteringPregnancy on perinatal outcomes/adverse events. Because these events are rare, even when rates are relatively high, a large sample is required. We are preparing proposals for research funding to support an RCT, and our Tanzanian collaborators are seeking program funds.

Lessons Learned

In our adaptation, we substantially reduced the number of visits from the CenteringPregnancy model in the United States to enhance feasibility and sustainability in these low-resource settings. However, new evidence regarding potential negative impacts of a four-visit FANC model highlights the need for further evidence to determine the optimal number of ANC visits in low-resource settings. An additional consideration is that many women are coming for their first ANC visit closer to the recommended 8 to 12 weeks gestation. A four-visit schedule means a long delay between visits for these women, and often the midwife informally advises them to return earlier, so that they in fact have a total of more than four visits. Thus, it is likely that policy changes regarding the number of ANC visits will be forthcoming soon, and at that time we can revisit the number of sessions for group ANC.

Contrary to advice we received during session development, women in group ANC readily discussed sensitive topics like sexuality, limiting family size, HIV transmission, and the gendered power of husbands over wives. Women welcomed the opportunity to discuss these issues in a safe setting. We documented dramatic changes in knowledge about HIV and its transmission process—topics no longer discussed at a typical ANC visit. Given that HIV prevalence, unintended pregnancy, and gender-based violence are still high in both countries, the benefits of including these sensitive topics are many.

As such, we see the CenteringPregnancy-based group model not just as setting for impact on a single pregnancy but as the beginning of changes that can impact a woman and her family's future health.

Improvements in quality of ANC can provide an exemplar that inspires quality improvement across the continuum of care for childbearing women and their families and the health care system as a whole. Even with severe health worker shortages, we saw that a CenteringPregnancy-based model of group ANC is a low-technology innovation with the power to reframe the antenatal health care experience in settings in these two countries. A model that makes more effective use of health workers' time, reduces crowding, and changes the structure of relationships between health workers and women addresses several important aspects of ANC quality in the African region and elsewhere. A key strength of this model lies in its impact on the social dimensions of the health care experience, increasing trust in the health care system and motivating women to make important knowledge gains and behavioral changes, affecting not only the current pregnancy but also future pregnancies, health care utilization, and overall health for women and their families. Overall, we feel confident in saying the CenteringPregnancy is ideally suited to contexts of Malawi and Tanzania and likely elsewhere in sub-Saharan Africa. As it will take several decades to produce a suffi-cient health care workforce, the CenteringPregnancy model focuses on patient–provider relationships, respect for experience, and viewing the woman as a whole person and not just a pregnancy, all of which help the model overcome so many of the structural obstacles inherent to low-resource health care settings. In closing, we want to share the song women in Malawi wrote, which they sang and danced to at the close of each session, capturing the essence of group care.

Centering has brought unity, built relationships and taught us a lot.

When walking in a centering group, we belong!

We show our pride in centering group.

When dancing in a centering group, we belong!

—*Malawi group*

References

National Bureau of Statistics [Tanzania] & ICF Macro. (2011). *Tanzania Demographic and Health Survey 2010*. Dar es Salaam, Tanzania: Author.

National Statistical Office ICF Macro. (2011). *Malawi Demographic and Health Survey 2010*. Zomba, Malawi, and Calverton, MD: Author.

Novick, G., Reid, A. E., Lewis, J., Kershaw, T. S., Ickovics, J. R., & Rising, S. S. (2013). Group prenatal care: Model fidelity and outcomes. *American Journal of Obstetrics & Gynecology, 209*(2), 112.e1–112.e6. Retrieved from http://linking hub.elsevier.com/retrieve/pii/S0002937813003001

Patil, C. L., Abrams, E. T., Klima, C., Kaponda, C. P., Leshabari, S. C., Vonderheid, S. C., . . . Norr, K. F. (2013). CenteringPregnancy-Africa: A pilot of group antenatal care to address millennium development goals. *Midwifery, 29*(10), 1190–1198. doi:10.1016/j.midw.2013.05.008

Acknowledgments: This research was funded by the National Institutes of Health through the National Institute for Nursing Research (Grant NR014413). We especially acknowledge the hard work and support of Sebalda C. Leshabari, Lugano Mafwenga, C. P. N. Kaponda, and Willy Sangu. The members of the ministries of health, health facility administrators, midwives, and health workers as well as the women who participated all provided invaluable feedback throughout the adaptation process and piloting of the program.

Index